Techniques in Histopathology and Cytopathology

Techniques in Histopathology and Cytopathology

A Guide for Medical Laboratory Technology Students

Sadhana Vishwakarma
MSc PhD (Chemistry)
Professor
Department of Engineering Chemistry
Technocrats Institute of Technology
Bhopal, Madhya Pradesh, India

Formerly
Head, Department of Medical Laboratory Technology
Gramin Polytechnic
Nanded, Maharashtra, India

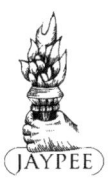

The Health Sciences Publisher

New Delhi | London | Panama

Jaypee Brothers Medical Publishers (P) Ltd

Headquarters
Jaypee Brothers Medical Publishers (P) Ltd
4838/24, Ansari Road, Daryaganj
New Delhi 110 002, India
Phone: +91-11-43574357
Fax: +91-11-43574314
Email: jaypee@jaypeebrothers.com

Overseas Offices

J.P. Medical Ltd
83 Victoria Street, London
SW1H 0HW (UK)
Phone: +44 20 3170 8910
Fax: +44 (0)20 3008 6180
Email: info@jpmedpub.com

Jaypee Brothers Medical Publishers (P) Ltd
17/1-B Babar Road, Block-B, Shaymali
Mohammadpur, Dhaka-1207
Bangladesh
Mobile: +08801912003485
Email: jaypeedhaka@gmail.com

Jaypee-Highlights Medical Publishers Inc
City of Knowledge, Bld. 235, 2nd Floor, Clayton
Panama City, Panama
Phone: +1 507-301-0496
Fax: +1 507-301-0499
Email: cservice@jphmedical.com

Jaypee Brothers Medical Publishers (P) Ltd
Bhotahity, Kathmandu
Nepal
Phone: +977-9741283608
Email: kathmandu@jaypeebrothers.com

Website: www.jaypeebrothers.com
Website: www.jaypeedigital.com

© 2017, Jaypee Brothers Medical Publishers

The views and opinions expressed in this book are solely those of the original contributor(s)/author(s) and do not necessarily represent those of editor(s) of the book.

All rights reserved. No part of this publication may be reproduced, stored or transmitted in any form or by any means, electronic, mechanical, photocopying, recording or otherwise, without the prior permission in writing of the publishers.

All brand names and product names used in this book are trade names, service marks, trademarks or registered trademarks of their respective owners. The publisher is not associated with any product or vendor mentioned in this book.

Medical knowledge and practice change constantly. This book is designed to provide accurate, authoritative information about the subject matter in question. However, readers are advised to check the most current information available on procedures included and check information from the manufacturer of each product to be administered, to verify the recommended dose, formula, method and duration of administration, adverse effects and contraindications. It is the responsibility of the practitioner to take all appropriate safety precautions. Neither the publisher nor the author(s)/editor(s) assume any liability for any injury and/ or damage to persons or property arising from or related to use of material in this book.

This book is sold on the understanding that the publisher is not engaged in providing professional medical services. If such advice or services are required, the services of a competent medical professional should be sought.

Every effort has been made where necessary to contact holders of copyright to obtain permission to reproduce copyright material. If any have been inadvertently overlooked, the publisher will be pleased to make the necessary arrangements at the first opportunity.

Inquiries for bulk sales may be solicited at: jaypee@jaypeebrothers.com

Techniques in Histopathology and Cytopathology

First Edition: **2017**

ISBN 978-93-5270-109-4

Printed at Sanat Printers

Dedicated to

*My Father and Mother
Late Shri Chhotelal Sharma
and
Shrimati Tara Sharma*

Preface

The decision of writing this book is based on my experience as a classroom teacher and unavailability of the textbook related to histopathological and cytopathological techniques for medical laboratory technology (MLT) students. This book is therefore written primarily for students and trainees of medical laboratory technology.

This book covers the full range of basic histological and cytological techniques used in medical laboratories and pathology departments. It provides a thorough grounding in all aspects of histological technology, from basic methods of section preparation and staining to advanced diagnostic techniques like cytology.

Each chapter is comprehensively divided into basic theory, procedure, difficulties encountered, and important subjective and objective questions. Recent developments in this field like immunochemistry, automation, microarray, etc. are also incorporated to the extent required.

This book provides text in simple language with diagrammatic explanation of procedure, and diagrams and figures that are neat and simple so that students can reproduce them in the examinations without any difficulty. It also provides, sufficient material to the students from examination point of view. It is a suitable resource for both the beginners in histological and cytological area and for the fully qualified laboratory technicians.

This book is written in such a manner that it covers all the topics of histological and cytological techniques included in PGMLT, BMLT, DMLT, and CMLT of different boards and universities.

Students or teachers are ultimately the right judge of whether I have done justice to this book. Since this is the first edition, the possibility of errors and omissions is difficult to rule out. Suggestions for further improvement of the book are most welcomed and will be gratefully acknowledged.

Sadhana Vishwakarma

Acknowledgments

Many people have contributed in different ways and to acknowledge their individual advice and assistance is impossible. However, I owe special thanks to Dr PM Patil, Professor and Reader, Nanded Education Society's Science College, Nanded, Maharashtra, India, for his advice and valuable suggestions. My thanks are also to the colleagues I worked with during the lifetime of this book. My thanks to Dr JG Pakwanne, Mr OS Darak, and Mr C Khan, who assisted in the preparation of manuscript. With deep gratitude, I acknowledge Dr VS Power, Principal, Gramin Polytechnic, Vishnupuri, Nanded, Maharashtra, India, for his continuous, interest and support.

I express my deep appreciation to my husband Chandrakant for his moral support, encouragement and time to time help, my in-laws Shri Tulsiramji Vishwakarma and Shrimati Kesar Vishwakarma, who elevated my ambition, and my children Sanskruti and Aditya, who endured gracefully past painful days I devoted to writing this book. I owe my special thanks to Shri PS Kokas for his advice and moral support.

My thanks are due to Shri Jitendar P Vij (Group Chairman) and Mr Ankit Vij (Group President) of M/S Jaypee Brothers Medical Publishers (P) Ltd, New Delhi, India, especially for Shri Prasun Bhattacharya for taking great efforts in bringing out this book in a nice and attractive manner.

Contents

Chapter 1   **Cell and Tissues**   1

Cell   1
Cell Division   2
Cell Metabolism   5
Tissues   6
Liquid Connective Tissue   11

Chapter 2   **Microscopy**   17

History of Optical Microscope   17
Basic Terminology in Microscopy   17
Parts of Microscope   18
Care of Microscope   20
Types of Microscopy   21
Bright Field Microscopy   21
Dark Field Microscopy   22
Phase Contrast Microscopy   24
Fluorescence Microscopy   24
Electron Microscopy   25
Types of Electron Microscope   26
Confocal Scanning Optical Microscopy   28
Deconvolution Microscopy and Image Reconstruction   29
Polarization Light Microscopy   29

Chapter 3   **Introduction and Importance of Histopathology**   32

Importance of Histopathology   32
Decomposition and Putrefaction   32
Various Steps of Histological Techniques   33
Specimen Collection   33
Logging of Specimen   34
Tissue Marking and Orientation   36
Methods of Examination of Tissues   37
Special Instructions on Specimen Collection and Handling   37
Duties and Responsibilities   38

Chapter 4 Tissue Fixation 40

Functions of fixatives 40
Properties of Fixatives 40
Types of Fixatives 41
Properties and Action of Some Important Fixatives 42
Fixation of Specific Substances 48
Artefacts 47
Preservation and Storage of Tissues 48
Points to be Remember During Fixation of Tissues 48
Special Fixatives for Special Tissue Samples 48

Chapter 5 Decalcification 51

Properties of Decalcifying Agents 51
Technique of Decalcification 51
Tests for Completion of Decalcification 52
Decalcifying Agents 53
Treatment after Decalcification 54
Surface Decalcification 54
Factors Affecting the Rate of Decalcification 55
Tips for Proper Decalcification 55

Chapter 6 Tissue Processing 57

Principle of Tissue Processing 57
Selection and Labeling of Tissues 57
Completion of Fixation before Processing 57
Post-fixation Procedures 57
Dehydration 58
Clearing 59
Impregnation and Infiltration 61
Automatic Tissue Processing 64
Manual Tissue Processing 66
Paraffin Wax Embedding 70
Storage of Paraffin Blocks 71
Celloidin and Low Viscosity Nitrocellulose Embedding 72
Gelatin Embedding 72
Plastic Embedding 73
Resin Embedding 73
Double Embedding 74
Re-embedding 74

Chapter 7 Microtomy and Section Cutting 77

Microtomes 77
Microtome Knives 79
Section Cutting 83
Attaching the Sections to Slides 89

Chapter 8   Frozen Sections and Cryostat   93

Principle of Frozen Sections   93
Theory of Freezing   93
Cryoprotectants   94
Cryogen selection   94
Freezing Microtome   95
Methods of Cutting Frozen Sections   95

Chapter 9   Staining   100

Principle of Staining   100
Types of Dyes and Stains   101
Classification of Dyes or Stains   102
Types of Staining Processes   103
Staining Procedures   106
Hematoxylin Stains   107
Counter Stains   109
Standard Hematoxylin and Eosin Staining Method for Paraffin Sections   110
Special Staining Methods   110
Staining of Frozen Sections   123
Precautions Taken during Staining   125
Causes of Poor Staining   125

Chapter 10   Mounting of Sections   129

Characteristics of Mountant   129
Types of Mountant   129
Restaining   133
Labeling and Storage of Slides   133
Coverslips   133
Ringing Media   133

Chapter 11   Cytopathology   135

Types of Exfoliation   135
General Cytological Changes in Cells during Malignancy   135
Cytology of Normal Genital Tract   136
Methods of Specimen Collection and Submission   137
Gynecological Sample Collection   138
Non-gynecological sample collection   140
Fine Needle Aspiration Cytology   142
Preservation of cytological specimens   144
Preparation of Smears   145
Fixation and Fixatives   146
Cytological Staining Techniques   148
Special Stains   150
Mounting of Smear of Cell Samples   154

Chapter 12 Museum Techniques   156

Functions of Pathology Museum   156
Safety in the Museum   159

Chapter 13 Safety in Histopathology Laboratory   160

Staff Training   160
Basic Organization and Common Sense   160
Infectious Hazards   160
Radiations Hazard   161
Equipment Hazards   162
Practical Safety in Routine Use   162

Chapter 14 Advances in Histopathology and Cytopathology   165

Microwave Irradiation of Primary Tissue Fixation   165
Ultrasonic Decalcification   165
Microwave-stimulated Tissue Processing   166
Ultrasound-stimulated Tissue Processing   167
Automatic Knife Sharpners   168
Ultramicrotomy   168
Automatic Staining Method   169
Endoscopy   169
Colposcopy   170
Autoradiography   171
Immunohistochemistry   172
Tissue Microarrays   173

Chapter 15 Solution and Reagents   176

Important Definitions   176
Preparation of Standard Solutions   176

Bibliography   *179*

Glossary   *181*

Index   *187*

CHAPTER 1

Cell and Tissues

CELL

It is the basic functional unit of all living systems. It can be described as a mass of protoplasm enclosed within a membrane (plasma/cell membrane). The cells are of different types performing specialized functions, but they have the same common characteristics. The cell is made up of water, protein, carbohydrates, lipids, and inorganic salts.

Structure of a Cell

The various structures present within the protoplasm are nucleus, cytoplasm, and cell membrane (Fig. 1.1).

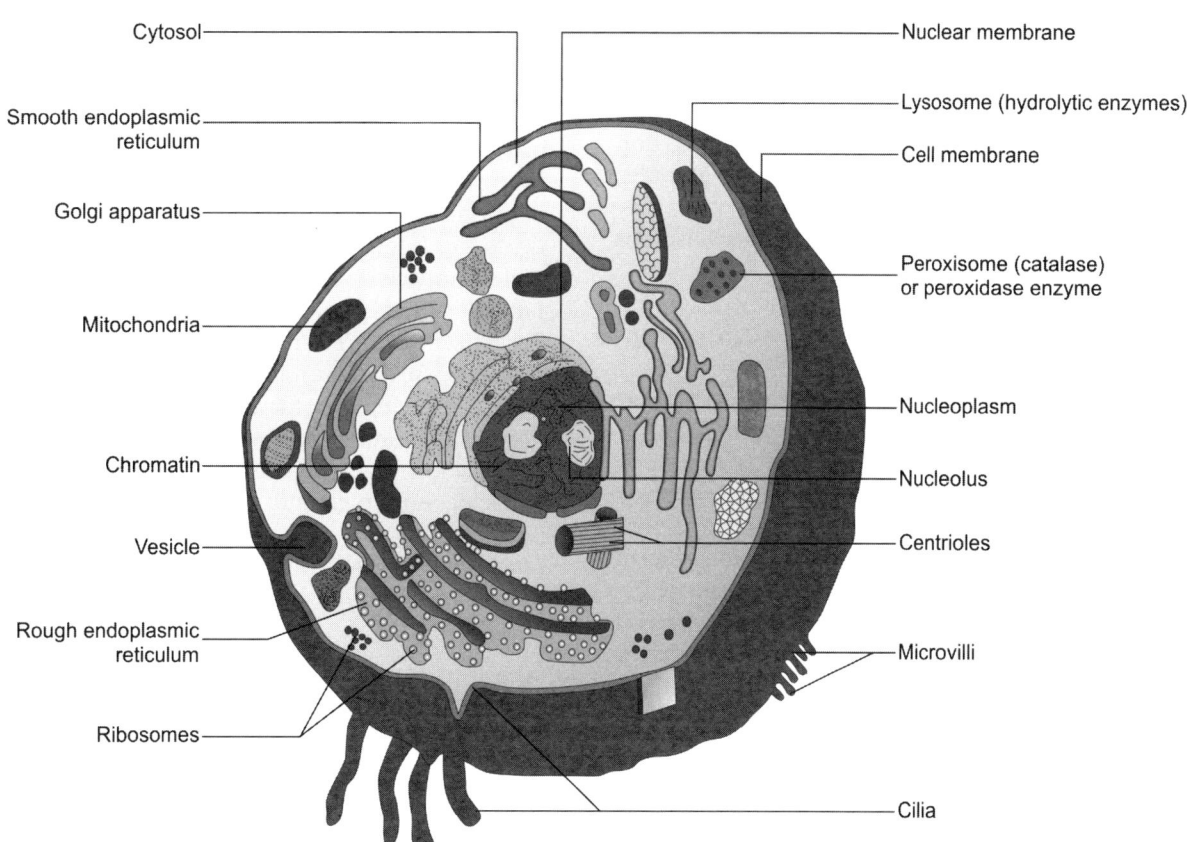

Fig. 1.1: Structure of a cell

Nucleus

It is a somewhat rounded structure present at the center of the cell. It contains genetic materials of the cells. It is bounded by two membranes called as nuclear membrane. The outer membrane contains large number of minute pores called as nuclear pores which are open to the cytoplasm. The nucleus contains a colloidal solution of proteins called nucleoplasm. It contains nucleic acid, DNA and RNA. DNA plays important role in the cell division and transmission of hereditary characters. RNA plays important role in the synthesis of various proteins. RNA is mostly concentrated in a small spherical body present within the nucleus and is called as nucleolus. Aggregations of granules are scattered throughout the nucleus and are called as chromatin granules. Chromosomes appear during cell division and are small thread like structure.

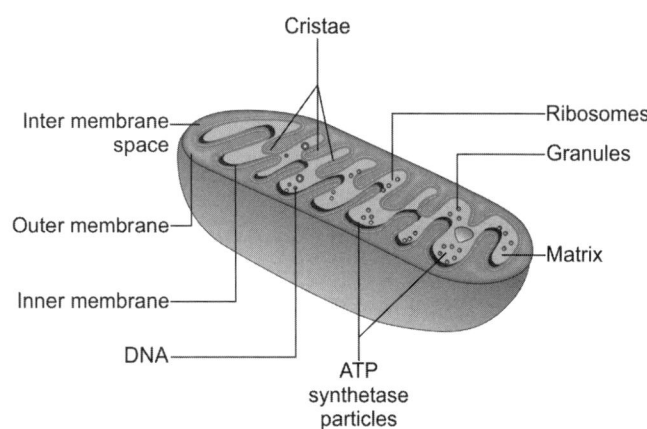

Fig. 1.2: Structure of mitochondrion

Cytoplasm

It is a watery and homogenous solution of proteins, sugars and various salts. It contains other organelles like endoplasmic reticulum. Golgi apparatus, mitochondria, centrosome, lysosome, and cytoplasmic inclusions.

- **Endoplasmic/Cytoplasmic reticulum:** Cytoplasm contains a network of fine branching tubules known as endoplasmic reticulum (ER). There are two types of ER namely smooth and rough ER. Smooth ER are not coated with ribosomes and are also called as agranular ER, they are responsible for the synthesis of lipids and similar substances. Rough ER are coated with granules of ribosomes and are also called as granular ER, they are associated with protein synthesis. Free ribosomes are also present in the cytoplasm.
- **Golgi apparatus:** These are a series of flattened sacs with bulbous parallel ends. Secretory products are concentrated in this area.
- **Mitochondria:** These are small filamentous or granular bodies may be distributed evenly throughout the cytoplasm or accumulated in selected sites according to cell types. They are bounded by double membranes. The inner most membrane is reflected to run across the inside of the mitochondria at several points to form shelves called cristae. Mitochondria are called as the power house of the cell and are concerned with cell respiration and enzymatic activity. They supply energy in the form of ATP (Fig. 1.2).
- **Lysosome:** This is a spherical organelle bounded by a single membrane and contain a large number of hydrolytic enzymes such as acid phosphatases. These enzymes break down complex molecules into small molecules. Rupture of the lysosome membrane causes release of these enzymes which digest the cell (autolysis). Lysosome play important role in the intracellular digestion of foreign matter within the cell (phagocytosis).
- **Centrosomes:** The centrosomes or centrioles present in all the cells and are visible during cell division. They are short, cylindrical bodies whose walls are composed of microtubules arranged longitudinally. During mitosis the two centrioles move to the opposite poles of the cell and support the formation of the spindle along which chromosomes arranged themselves after cell division.
- **Cytoplasmic inclusions:** These are non-protoplasmic, nonliving substances found within the cytoplasm. They usually consist of stored nutrients, materials produced by the cell, or ingested particles. Following are some of important inclusions:

Glycogen: It found in the cytoplasm of liver cells and skeletal muscles.

Lipid: It stored in lipid cells as fat globule.

Secretion granules: They are products of cellular synthesis and they are found in the cytoplasm of specialized cells having secretory functions.

Pigments: It may be exogenous or endogenous in nature. Endogenous pigments are melanin, hemosiderin, etc. and exogenous pigments are foreign particles like coal dust, etc.

Mucin: It appears as minute granules mainly in mucin producing cells.

CELL DIVISION

Both mitosis and meiosis are types of cell divisions. Mitosis occurs in both reproductive cells and body or somatic cells while meiosis occurs in germ cells or reproductive cells. The former is called as mutiplication, division or replica division as the two daughter cells produced resemble the parent cells. Mitosis occurs in order to favor growth and differentiation of an organism. Meiosis called as reduction division as it results in reduction of total number of chromosomes in the daughter cells, in order to maintain a constant chromosome number thereby race is maintained.

■ Mitosis

Mitosis is the visible part of cell division (Fig. 1.3). By the time mitosis begins all the 'heavy lifting' in the form of DNA replication and production of elements necessary for division has already been done. At the start of mitosis, the duplicated DNA exists as chromatin joined at its centromere, but has not yet been packaged in its chromosomal form.
- **Interphase:** It occurs just before mitosis begin. DNA is replicated along with organelles and other cellular components and the cell prepares for division.
- **Prophase:** The centriole divides, and the chromatin starts to condense. The centrioles are pushed to the poles of the cell by microtubules, i.e. 'spindles'. The star like configuration, the asta that surrounds the centrioles is also made up of microtubules and actin strands.
- **Prometaphase:** The chromatin condenses into chromosomes. The nuclear membrane disappears, and the chromosomes attach themselves to the spindles.
- **Metaphase:** The chromosomes align along the equator.
- **Anaphase:** The chromosomes divide at their centromere, and start to move along the spindles to their respective poles.
- **Telophase:** The nuclear membranes reform round the chromosomes, the chromosomes unwind to form chromatin.
- **Cytokinesis:** The actual splitting of the daughter cells into two separate cells is called cytokinesis.

■ Meiosis

Meiosis only occurs in germ cells, and produces ova in females and sperm in males. In the process of meiosis, the genetic material is reshuffled, and the chromosomes are reduced to their haploid number. During fertilization when the ovum and sperm unite, the diploid number is restored. There are two phases of meiosis viz: meiosis I and meiosis II (Fig. 1.4).

Meiosis I: Meiosis I separates homologous chromosomes, producing two haploid cells (23 chromosomes, N in humans), so meiosis I is referred to as a reductional division. A regular diploid human cell contains 46 chromosomes and is considered 2N because it contains 23 pairs of homologous chromosomes. However, after meiosis I, although the cell contains 46 chromatids it is only considered as being N, with 23 chromosomes.
- **Prophase I:** During prophase I, DNA is exchanged between homologous chromosomes in a process called homologous recombination. This often results in chromosomal crossover. The new combinations of DNA created during crossover are a significant source

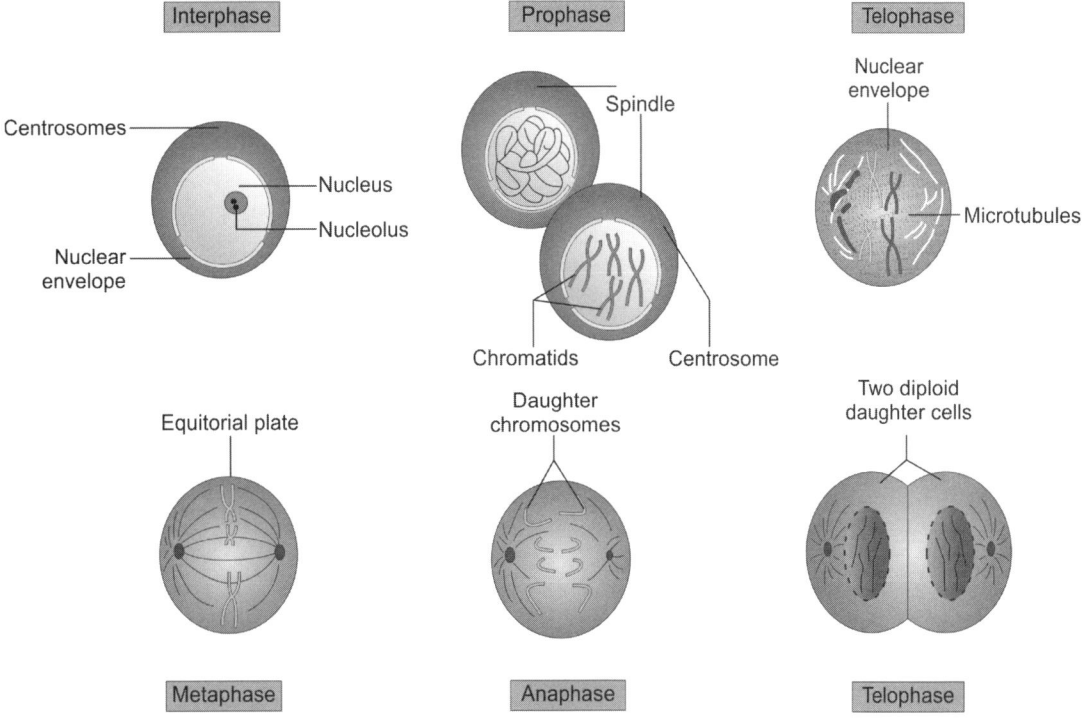

Fig. 1.3: Various stages of mitosis

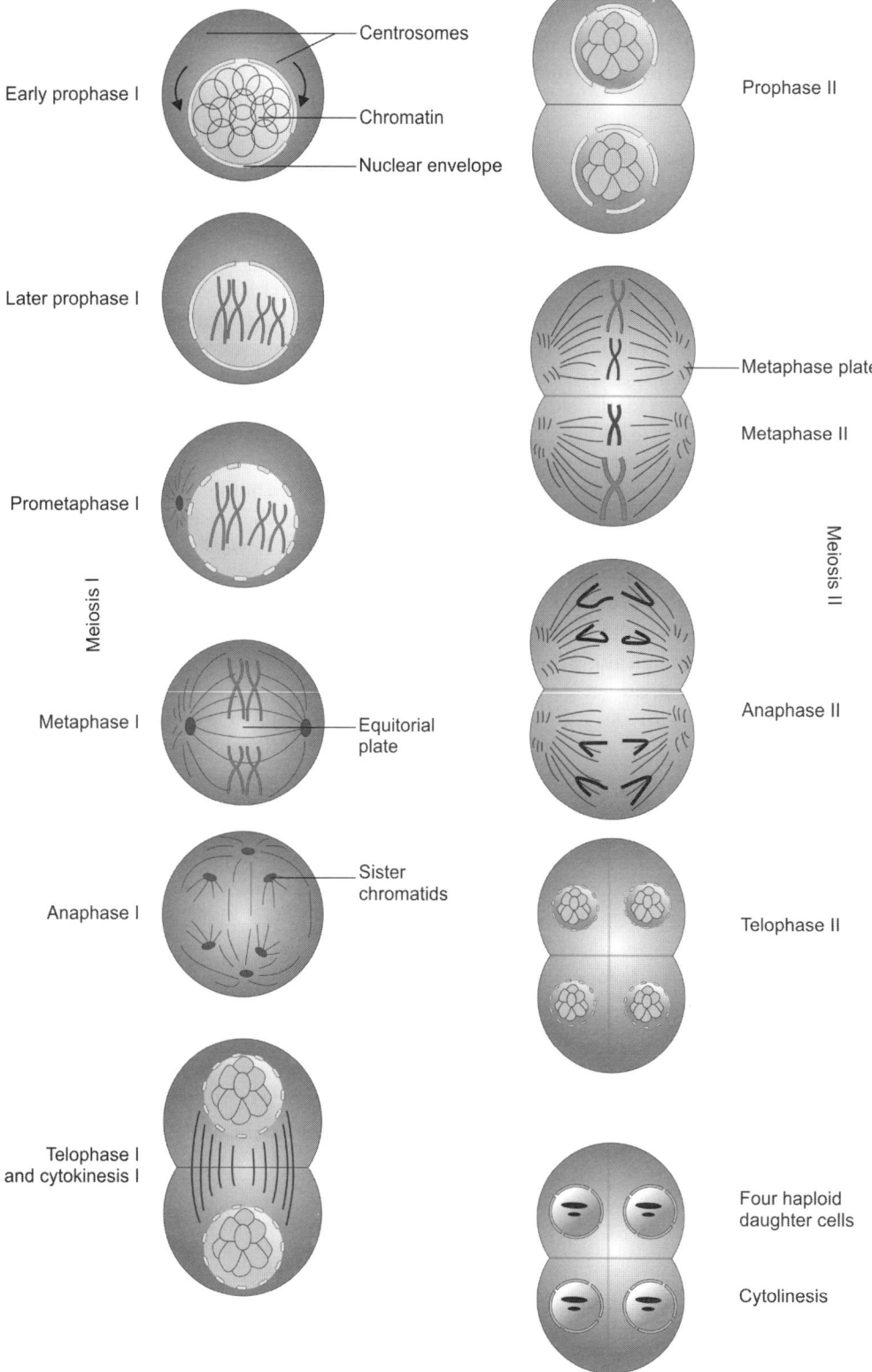

Fig. 1.4: Various stages of meiosis

of genetic variation, and may result in beneficial new combinations of alleles. The paired and replicated chromosomes are called bivalents or tetrads, which have two chromosomes and four chromatids, with one chromosome coming from each parent. At this stage, non-sister chromatids may crossover at points called chiasmata (plural; singular chiasma).
- **Metaphase I:** Homologous pairs move together along the metaphase plate. As kinetochore microtubules from both centrioles attach to their respective kinetochores, the homologous chromosomes align along an equatorial plane that bisects the spindle, due to continuous counterbalancing forces exerted on the bivalents by the microtubules.
- **Anaphase I:** Kinetochore microtubules shorten, severing the recombination nodules and pulling homologous chromosomes apart. Since each chromosome has only one functional unit of a pair of kinetochores, whole chromosomes are pulled toward opposite poles, forming two haploid sets. Each chromosome still contains a pair of sister chromatids. Nonkinetochore microtubules lengthen, pushing the centrioles farther apart. The cell elongates in preparation for division down the center.
- **Telophase I:** The last meiotic division effectively ends when the chromosomes arrive at the poles. Each daughter cell now has half the number of chromosomes but each chromosome consists of a pair of chromatids. The microtubules that make up the spindle network disappear, and a new nuclear membrane surrounds each haploid set. The chromosomes uncoil back into chromatin. Cytokinesis, the pinching of the cell membrane in animal cells or the formation of the cell wall in plant cells, occurs, completing the creation of two daughter cells. Sister chromatids remain attached during telophase I.
- **Interphase II:** Cells may enter a period of rest known as interkinesis or interphase II. No DNA replication occurs during this stage.

Meiosis II: Meiosis II is the second part of the meiotic process. Much of the process is similar to mitosis. The end result is production of four haploid cells (23 chromosomes, 1N in humans) from the two haploid cells (23 chromosomes, 1N each of the chromosomes consisting of two sister chromatids) produced in meiosis I. The four main steps of meiosis II are: Prophase II, metaphase II, anaphase II, and telophase II.
- **Prophase II**: It takes an inversely proportional time compared to telophase I. In this prophase, we see the disappearance of the nucleoli and the nuclear envelope again, as well as the shortening and thickening of the chromatids. Centrioles move to the polar regions and arrange spindle fibers for the second meiotic division.
- **Metaphase II:** In metaphase II, the centromeres contain two kinetochores that attach to spindle fibers from the centrosomes (centrioles) at each pole. The new equatorial metaphase plate is rotated by 90 degrees when compared to meiosis I, perpendicular to the previous plate.
- **Anaphase II:** In anaphase II the centromeres are cleaved, allowing microtubules attached to the kinetochores to pull the sister chromatids apart. The sister chromatids by convention are now called sister chromosomes as they move toward opposing poles.
- **Telophase II:** Telophase II is similar to telophase I, and is marked by uncoiling and lengthening of the chromosomes and the disappearance of the spindle. Nuclear envelopes reform and cleavage or cell wall formation eventually produces a total of four daughter cells, each with a haploid set of chromosomes. Meiosis is now complete and ends up with four new daughter cells.

Significance

Meiosis facilitates stable sexual reproduction. Without the halving of ploidy, or chromosome count, fertilization would result in zygotes that have twice the number of chromosomes as the zygotes from the previous generation. Successive generations would have an exponential increase in chromosome count. In organisms that are normally diploid, polyploidy, the state of having three or more sets of chromosomes, results in extreme developmental abnormalities or lethality. Polyploidy is poorly tolerated in most animal species. Plants, however, regularly produce fertile, viable polyploids. Polyploidy has been implicated as an important mechanism in plant speciation.

Most importantly, recombination and independent assortment of homologous chromosomes allow for a greater diversity of genotypes in the population. This produces genetic variation in gametes that promote genetic and phenotypic variation in a population of offspring.

CELL METABOLISM

Cell metabolism is the process by which living cells process nutrient molecules and maintain a living state. Cell metabolism involves extremely complex sequences of controlled chemical reactions called metabolic pathways.

Anabolism: Anabolism is a constructive metabolic process whereby energy is consumed to synthesize or combine simpler substances, such as amino acids, into more complex organic compounds, such as enzymes and nucleic acids.

Catabolism: Catabolism is a type of metabolic process occurring in living cells by which complex molecules are broken down to produce energy. On balance, catabolic reactions are normally exothermic.

Carbohydrate catabolism: Carbohydrate catabolism is the breakdown of carbohydrates into smaller units. The empirical formula for carbohydrates, like that of theirs monomer counterparts, is $C_x(H_{2Y}O_Y)$. Carbohydrates literally undergo combustion to retrieve the large amounts of energy in their bonds.

Fat catabolism: Fat catabolism, also known as lipid catabolism, is the process of lipids or phospholipids being broken down by lipases. The opposite of fat catabolism is fat anabolism, involving the storage of energy, and the building of membranes.

Protein catabolism: Protein catabolism is the breakdown of proteins into amino acids and simple derivative compounds, for transport into the cell through the plasma membrane and ultimately for the polymerization into new proteins via the use of ribonucleic acids (RNA) and ribosomes.

TISSUES

Tissue is a group of cells having similar origin and structure, which performs specific functions. A group of different tissues results in the formation of **organ** of the body like stomach, lungs, esophagus, etc. Various organs may join together to perform a vital function of the body and are called **system** like respiratory system, digestive system, etc.

Tissues are classified according to the size, shape and functions of the cells. There are four main types of tissues each of which has subdivision. They are:
- Epithelial tissues
- Connective tissues
- Muscular tissues
- Nervous tissues.

■ Epithelial Tissues

Epithelial tissues form the covering of the body and lining of cavities and tubes. It is also found in glands. The cells of epithelial tissues are very closely packed and the intercellular (matrix) substance is very less.

The cells are resting on the basement membrane which is made up of an inert connective tissue. These cells are classified on the basis of their structure and functions such as protection, absorption, excretion, sensory, conduction of materials and regeneration. Epithelial tissues are further subdivided into
1. Simple epithelium
2. Stratified epithelium.

Simple Epithelium

Simple epithelium consists of a single layer of similar cells. Depending upon the shape and size of the cells they are further divided into four types. It is usually found on absorptive or secretory surfaces where single layer increases these processes. The types are named according to the shape of the cells, which differ according to their functions. The more active the tissue, the taller are the cells.
- Squamous epithelium
- Cuboidal epithelium
- Columnar epithelium
- Ciliated epithelium.

Squamous Epithelium

It consists of flat and plate like cells. The cells fit closely together like flat stones forming a thin and very smooth membrane. Each cell has a polygonal shape and is filled with cytoplasm with a flattened nucleus (Fig. 1.5). Complete layer of squamous epithelium rest on a basement membrane. Diffusion takes place freely through this thin, smooth and inactive lining. It is present lining the following organs- heart, blood vessels, lymph vessels, alveoli of the lungs, Bowman's capsule, membranous labyrinth of internal ear, etc.

Functions: Diffusion of the substances and protection of organs.

Cuboidal Epithelium

The cuboidal epithelium consists of cube shaped cells fitting closely together lying on a basement membrane (Fig. 1.6). These cells are present in the form of a single layer in the internal lining of uriniferous tubules in the kidney,

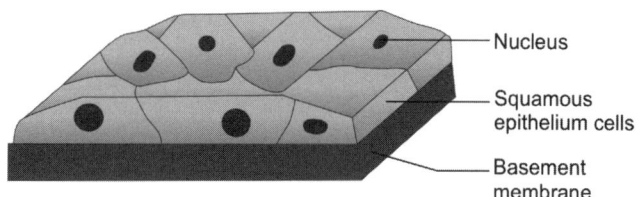

Fig. 1.5: Squamous epithelium

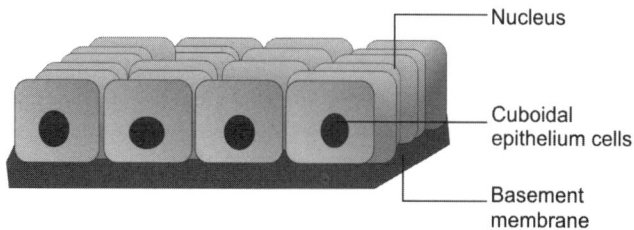

Fig. 1.6: Cuboidal epithelium

ducts of the internal ear and some glands. *Function:* They perform the function of protection, secretion, absorption and excretion.

Columnar Epithelium

As the name indicates, columnar epithelium consists of single layer of elongated, rectangular cells resting on a basement membrane. Cells have prominent nucleus. They are found lining the following organs: Stomach, small intestine, large intestine, rectum, gallbladder, alveoli and secretary glands. They perform the functions of absorption of digested products, and secretion of mucus (Fig. 1.7).

Ciliated Epithelium

As the name indicates it consists of columnar cells having many hairlike processes called cilia at their free edges. The cilia consist of microtubules inside the plasma membrane that extends from the free border of the columnar cells. By the wave like movement of the cilia, these epithelium helps in propelling the contents of the tube, which they line, in one direction only. Example in oviduct, cilia helps to push the egg towards the uterus, while in nasal passage, they prevent the entry of dust, foreign particles and mucus into respiratory tubes and lungs. Ciliated epithelium is found lining the organs like nasal lining, trachea, bronchial tubules, oviducts and uterus (Fig. 1.8).

Stratified Epithelium

Stratified epithelium consists of several layers of cells of various shapes. The superficial layers grow up from below. Basement membranes are usually absent. The main function of stratified epithelium is to protect underlying structures from mechanical wear and tear. There are two main types of stratified epithelium namely stratified squamous epithelium and transitional epithelium.

Stratified Squamous Epithelium

It consists of several layers of cells of different shapes. In the deepest layer the cells are columnar and as they grow towards the surface, they become flattened and are then shed (Fig. 1.9).

Non-keratinized stratified epithelium: It is mostly found on the moist surfaces like buccal cavity, pharynx, esophagus, anal canal, lower portion of urethra, and vagina, conjunctiva of the eyes etc. where they protect the organs from drying, wear and tear.

Keratinized stratified epithelium: The dry surfaces are mostly found to be covered with keratinized stratified epithelium like skin, hair, nails, etc. They protect the surface from wear and tear. This epithelium consists of dead cells containing keratin (protein). This forms a tough, relatively waterproof protective layer that prevents drying of the underlying live cells.

Transitional Epithelium

It is a compound epithelium in which basement membrane is absent. It is composed of several layers of pear shaped cells which are comparatively thinner and have more elasticity. Its outermost layer is composed of pear-shaped cells and innermost layer is composed of cuboidal cells. They

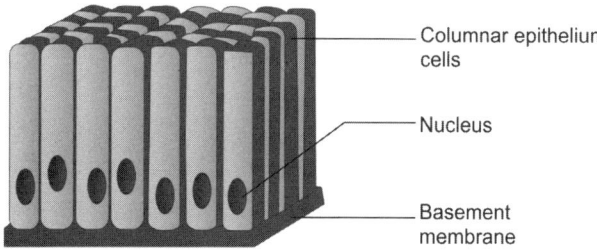

Fig. 1.7: Columnar epithelium

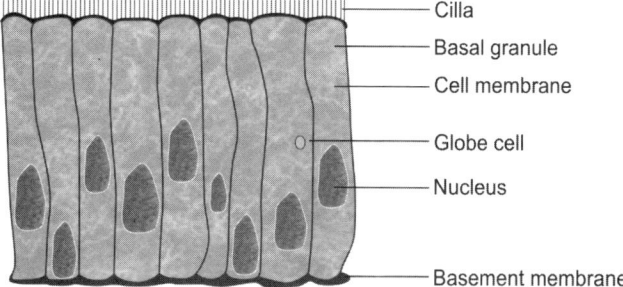

Fig. 1.8: Ciliated epithelium

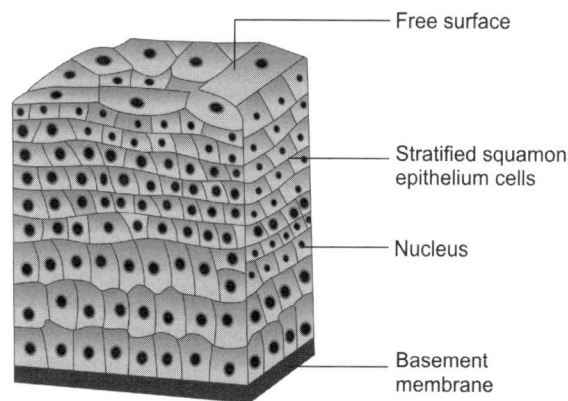

Fig. 1.9: Stratified squamous epithelium

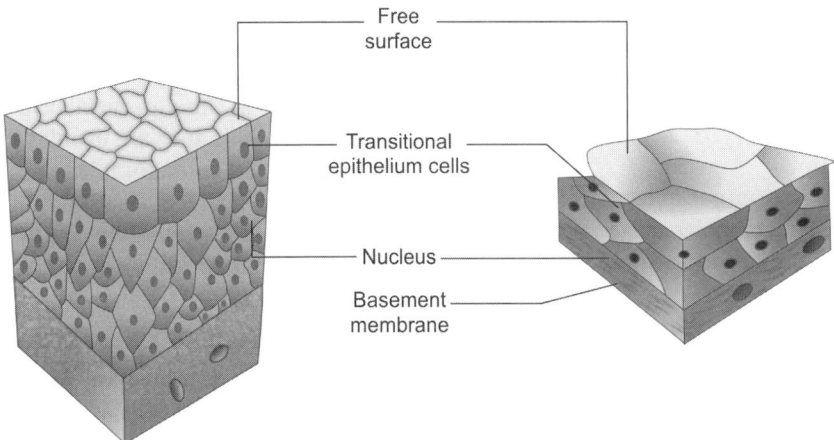

Fig. 1.10: Transitional epithelium unstretched and stretched

are found lining the pelvis of the kidney, urinary bladder, ureters and upper part of the urethra. It allows stretching of these organs when they are filled (Fig. 1.10).

Connective Tissues

These are extensively spread throughout the body. They are found connecting the various parts of the body and provide them suitable support. The cells forming the connective tissues are more widely separated from each other than those forming the epithelium. An intracellular substance, i.e. matrix is present in large amounts. Depending upon the structure and functions connective tissues are classified into following categories.
- Connective tissue proper
- Supporting connective tissues
- Fluid connective tissues.

Connective tissue proper: It consists of a large amount of intercellular materials. It is further classified into loose connective tissue and dense connective tissue.

Loose connective tissue: It is a mass of widely scattered cells whose matrix is a loose weave of fibers. Many of the fibers are strong protein fibers called collagen. Loose connective tissue is found beneath the skin and between organs. It is a binding and packing material whose main purpose is to provide support and hold other tissues and organs in place. Three types of loose connective tissue are recognized. These include areolar, adipose, and reticular types.

Areolar connective tissue: It is loose connective tissue that consists of a mesh-work of collagen, elastic tissue, and reticular fibers with many connective tissue cells in between the mesh-work of fibers. The different types of cells embedded within the areolar tissue are fibroblasts, plasma cells, adipocytes, mast cells, and macrophages. The fibers and cells are embedded in a semifluid ground matrix. Areolar tissue binds skin to the muscles beneath. The key functions of areolar tissue are support, strength and elasticity (Fig. 1.11).

Adipose tissue: It is a loose fibrous connective tissue packed with many cells (called "adipocytes") that are specialized for storage of triglycerides, i.e. "fats". Each adipocyte cell is filled with a single large droplet of fat. As this occupies most of the volume of the cell, its cytoplasm, nucleus, and other components are pushed towards the edges of the cell which is bounded by the plasma membrane. Adipose tissue acts as an insulating layer, helping to reduce heat loss through the skin. It also has a protective function, providing mechanical protection ("padding") and support around some of the major organs, e.g. kidneys. Adipose tissue is also a means of energy storage. Food that is excess to requirements is converted into fat and stored within adipose tissue in the body (Fig. 1.12).

Reticular connective tissue: Reticular connective tissue is named for the reticular fibers which are the main structural part of the tissue. These fibers are present in many types of connective tissue and are particularly heavily concentrated in reticular connective tissue. The cells that make

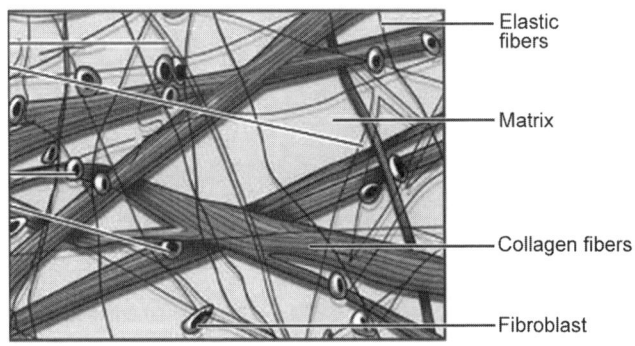

Fig. 1.11: Areolar connective tissue

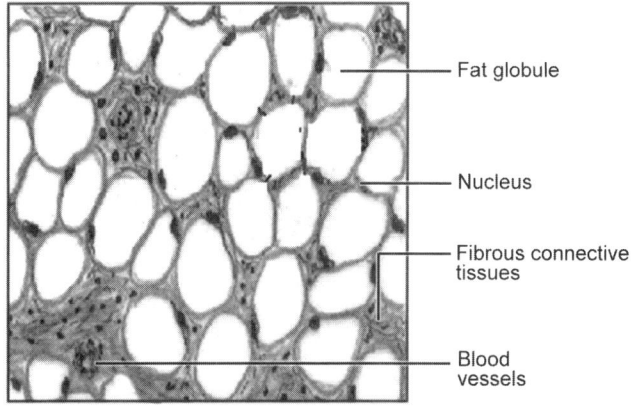

Fig. 1.12: Adipose connective tissue

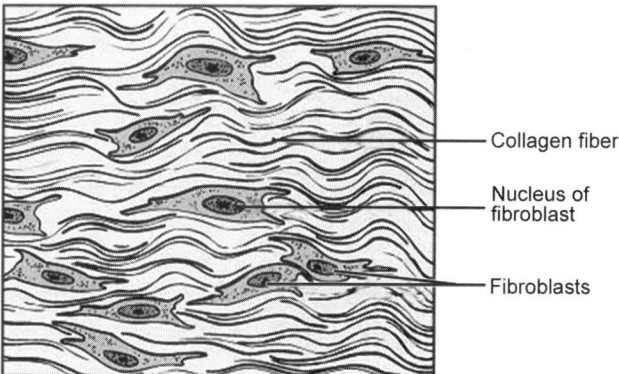

Fig. 1.14: Dense regular connective tissue

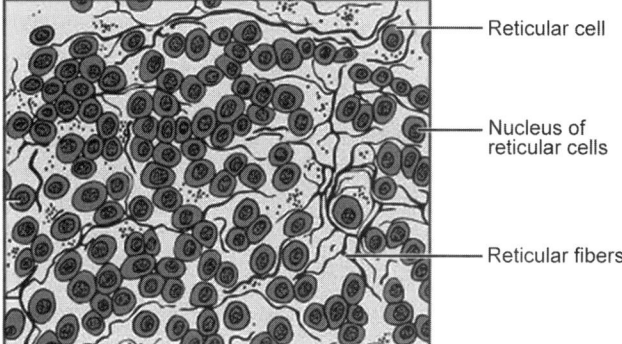

Fig. 1.13: Reticular connective tissue

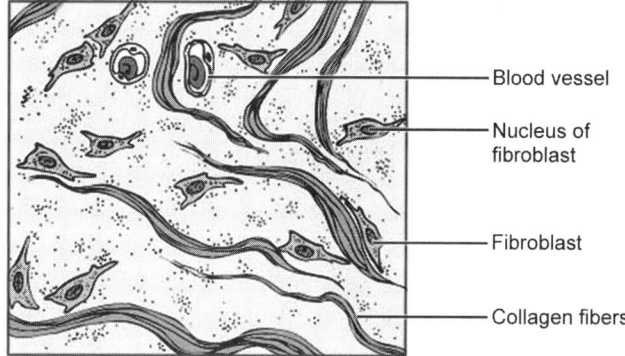

Fig. 1.15: Dense irregular connective tissue

the reticular fibers are fibroblasts called reticular cells. Reticular connective tissue forms a scaffolding for other cells in several organs, such as lymph nodes, liver, spleen and bone marrow (Fig. 1.13).

Dense connective tissue: They are also called dense fibrous tissue and has fibers as its main matrix element. Dense connective tissue is mainly composed of collagen fibers. Crowded between the collagen fibers are rows of fibroblasts, fibre forming cells, that manufacture the fibers. In addition, these body tissues also contain ground substance - the material that fills in the gaps between fibroblasts and holds the fibers themselves. Ground substance contains fluids and cell adhesion proteins, which essentially act as the glue that keeps the connective tissue attached to the extracellular matrix. Dense connective tissue forms strong, rope like structures such as tendons and ligaments. Tendons attach skeletal muscles to bones; ligaments connect bones to bones at joints. Ligaments are more stretchy and contain more elastic fibers than tendons. Dense connective tissue also makes up the lower layers of the skin (dermis), where it is arranged in sheets.

There are three different types of dense connective tissue: Dense regular connective tissue, dense irregular connective tissue, and elastic connective tissue.

Dense regular connective tissue (White fibrous): In this type of tissue, the collagen fibers are densely packed, and arranged in parallel. This type of tissue is found in ligaments and tendons. These are powerfully resistant to axially loaded tension forces, but allow some stretch (Fig. 1.14).

Dense irregular connective: Tissue has an irregular, somewhat disorderly, dense weave of thick collagen fibers, with bundles of fibers oriented in all directions. With its high tensile strength, dense irregular connective tissue effectively binds various tissues together to form organs and passively translates mechanical forces in all directions without tearing. It is found in several locations: The dermis of the skin, the walls of large tubular organs, such as the alimentary canal, in glandular tissue, and in organ capsules (Fig. 1.15).

Elastic connective tissue: They are thicker and do not exists as bundles. They form ligaments which join the bone with another tissue. They also form the pinna or lobe of the ear,

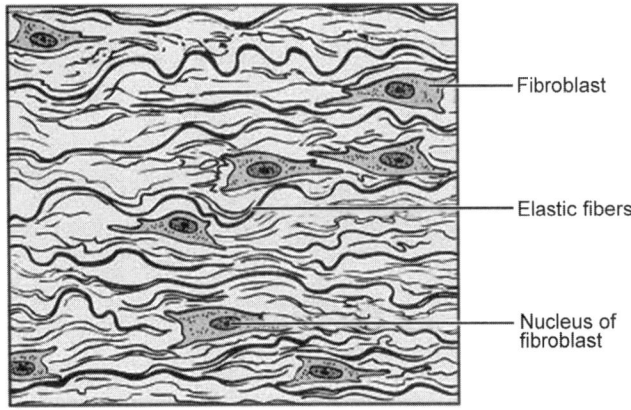

Fig. 1.16: Elastic connective tissue

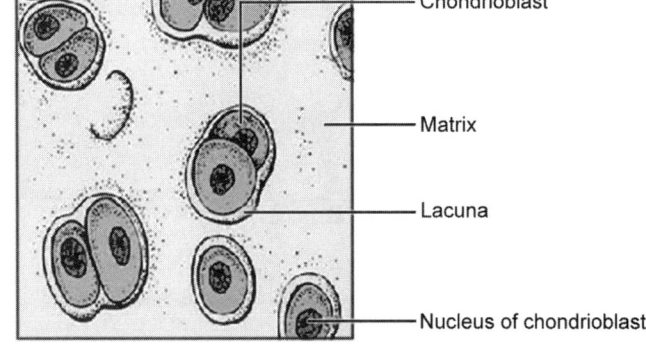

Fig. 1.17: Hyaline cartilage

the epiglottis and part of the tunica media of blood vessel walls (Fig. 1.16).

Supporting connective tissues: These tissues are responsible for the formation of the skeleton of the body. They are further classified into cartilage and bone.

■ Cartilage

It is a supporting tissue. The cells are nearly rounded in shape and the intercellular spaces are filled with a substance called as matrix. The matrix is tough, gelatinous and elastic in nature formed of chondrin and hence is also called as chondrion. A cartilage consists of cells called chondroblasts which are packed in the matrix. The entire tissue is covered by a tough and fibrous membrane called as perichondrium. Cartilages are of following types hyaline cartilage, fibrocartilage, and elastic cartilage.

Hyaline cartilage: It is composed of collagen fibers which are packed in a translucent and elastic matrix. It has semi transparent and glossy matrix. It is found in the hyoid apparatus (at the base of tip tongue), larynx, trachea, sternum and the end of limb bones. It is also present at the tip of nose (Fig. 1.17).

Fibro cartilage: It has a compact matrix with large amounts of white fibers. It is present in the movable parts of the body which require extra strength like knee joints, joints between scapular and humerus bone of upper arm, intervertebral discs and pubic region (Fig. 1.18).

Elastic cartilage: It contains a network of branching and rejoining collagenous fibers which are yellowish in color. It is present at the tip of the nose, eustachian tube, and pinna. It is highly elastic in nature (Fig. 1.19).

Bone: It is hardest of all the cartilages because its matrix contains fine granular calcium carbonate. It is present in scapula, and spongy ends of the bones (Fig. 1.20).

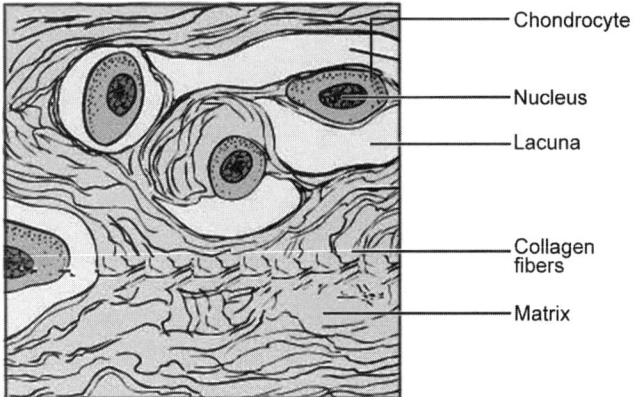

Fig. 1.18: Fibrocartilage connective tissue

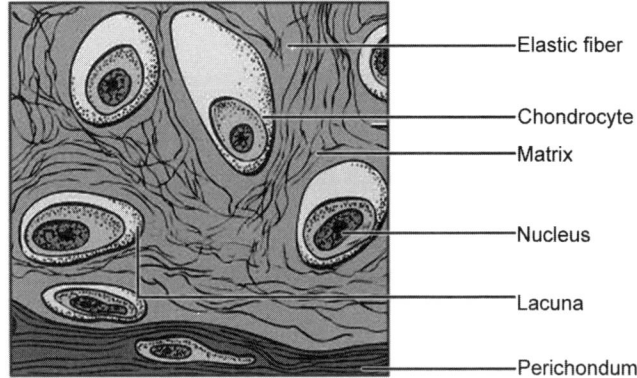

Fig. 1.19: Elastic cartilage connective tissue

It is also called as osseous tissue. It is the hardest tissue in the body after tooth enamel. It contains a specialized fibrous tissue, which is hardened by deposits of mineral salts mainly calcium phosphate, calcium carbonate, calcium fluoride, and magnesium phosphate.

The long bones of the body, such as those of legs and arms, (femur and humerus) are hollow in the central part

Cell and Tissues

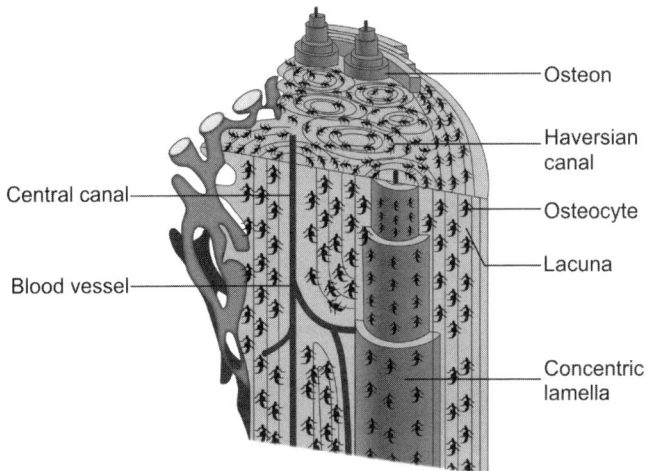

Fig. 1.20: Cross-section of bone

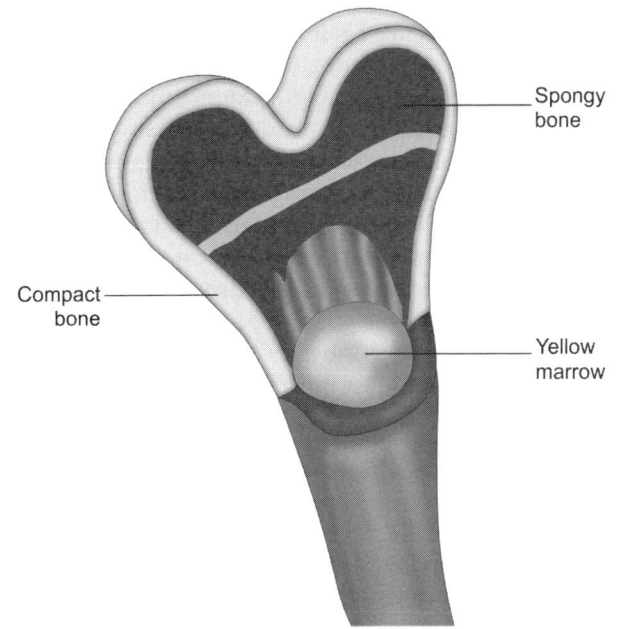

Fig. 1.21: Compact and spongy bone

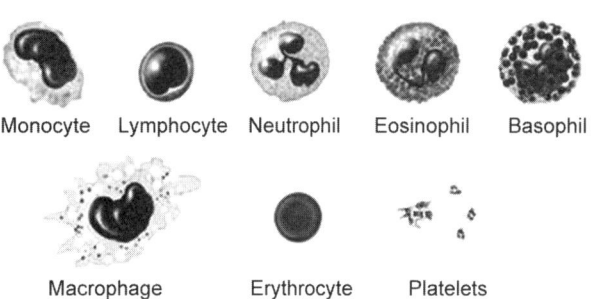

Fig. 1.22: Types of blood cells

central canal called as **Haversian canal** which contain artery and a vein for blood supply and a nerve. This canal is surrounded by several concentric rows of **lamellae.** Between the lamella there are spaces called **lacunae** containing lymph and bone cells called **osteocytes**. All the lacunae are connected to each other through narrow spaces called **canaliculi** which permit the flow of food materials and waste matter. The lymph carrying nourishment flows through the canaliculi. In the spaces between the Haversian system there are **interstitial lamellae** (Fig. 1.20).

Spongy bone: It is also called as cancellous bone. The Haversian canals are much larger and there are fewer lamellae as compared to compact bone. Red bone marrow is always present with cancellous tissue.

LIQUID CONNECTIVE TISSUE

These are those connective tissues which circulate throughout the body and transport various metabolites. Basically, they are of two types: Blood and Lymph.

Blood: It is a constantly circulating fluid providing the body with nutrition, oxygen, and waste removal. Blood is mostly liquid, with numerous cells and proteins suspended in it, making blood "thicker" than pure water. The average person has about 5 liters (more than a gallon) of blood. A liquid called plasma makes up about half of the content of blood. Plasma contains proteins that help blood to clot, transport substances through the blood, and perform other functions. Blood is composed of blood cells: Erythrocytes, i.e. red blood cells, leukocytes, i.e. white blood cells and thrombocytes, i.e. platelets (Fig. 1.22).

Erythrocytes: They are non-nucleated biconcave discs, containing hemoglobin. They are responsible for transportation of oxygen, carbon dioxide and minerals.

Leukocytes: They are part of the body's immune system; they destroy and remove old or aberrant cells and cellular debris, as well as attack infectious agents and foreign

which is filled with soft pulp like fatty tissue called bone marrow. All the bone consists of four parts periosteum, endosteum, matrix and bone marrow. Periosteum is the outermost thick and tough part made of fibrous connective tissue and a layer of bone cells called osteoblasts (bone forming cells). The endosteum the is innermost layer that lines the cavity of the bone. Matrix lies in between periosteum and endosteum and forms the major part of the bone. There are two types of bone tissues namely compact bone and spongy bone (Fig. 1.21).

Compact bone: It consists of a large number of units called **Haversian systems.** The Haversian system consists of a

substances. There are several different types of white blood cells, these are granulocytes and agranulocytes.

Granulocytes (polymorphonuclear leukocytes): Leukocytes characterized by the differential staining of the granules in their cytoplasm. There are three types of granulocytes: neutrophils, basophils, and eosinophils which are named according to their staining properties.
- **Neutrophils:** The are most abundant white blood cells. They are "C" shaped with segmented nucleus. They play a crucial role in fighting infection.
- **Basophils:** They are least numbered white blood cells. They have coarse granules with a single, deeply stained nucleus. They are responsible for the production and secretion of antibodies.
- **Eosinophils:** These are characterized by large coarse granules having two or more lobed nucleus. They are found in increasing number in chronic bronchitis, asthma and in certain allergies.

Agranulocytes (mononuclear leukocytes): Leukocytes characterized by the apparent absence of granules in their cytoplasm. The cells include lymphocytes, monocytes, and macrophages.
- **Lymphocytes:** These are non-granular cells with a very large nucleus. They show some amoeboid movement, but are not actively phagocytes. They are concerned with the production of antibodies.
- **Monocytes:** They are the largest of the white blood cells and have a horse-shoe shaped nucleus. They are most powerfully phagocytic and act, mostly as scavengers.
- **Microphages:** A type of white blood cell that ingests foreign materials. Macrophages are key players in the immune response to foreign invaders of the body, such as infectious microorganisms.

Thrombocytes also called platelets, are responsible for blood clotting. They change fibrinogen into fibrin. This fibrin creates a mesh onto which red blood cells collect and clot, which then stops more blood from leaving the body and also helps to prevent bacteria from entering the body.

Lymph

The fluid "lymph" can be described as a tissue in its own right in the same way as the fluid "blood" can be described as "blood tissue". Lymph is a clear fluid that is similar to plasma, but contains less protein. It flows through lymphatic vessels throughout the body and includes chemicals and cells whose composition vary according to location within the body. Despite being a fluid, lymph is classified as a connective tissue. The major functions of lymph is draining interstitial fluid, transporting dietary lipids is vitamin K, and protecting the body against invasion/infection as it contains leukocytes (particularly lymphocytes and macrophages) (Fig. 1.23).

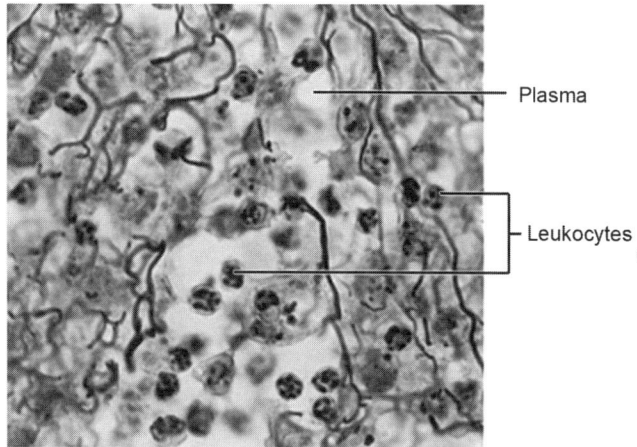

Fig. 1.23: Lymph

Muscular Tissues

It is a type of connective tissue, which help in the movement of body parts by articulating bones with each other. It is contractile and is therefore able to produce movements. The cells, which form this tissue are different from the normal cells as they are shorten or contract. The cells are like long fibers of variable lengths. Each fiber is made of very fine fibers called myofibrils which are arranged in the form of bundles. The muscle fibers may or may not be covered by a layer of connective tissue called **sarcolemma.** The cytoplasm of the muscular cells is termed as **sarcoplasm.** There are three types of muscle fibers:
- Smooth or involuntary muscle
- Striated muscle fibers
- Cardiac muscle.

Smooth Muscle

It is also called as involuntary, plain or visceral muscle. It is not under control of the will. The muscle cells are long and spindle-shaped with a nucleus present in the center of the spindle. The cells of these muscles are uninucleate and each nucleus is surrounded by sarcoplasm. These cells generally occur in the form of sheets made of loosely packed fibers of connective tissue (Fig. 1.24). The myofibrils in the sarcoplasm are also present longitudinally and the sarcolemma is absent. In its place the muscle fibers are covered by the plasma membrane. These muscles are present in the lower part of the esophagus, stomach intestine, lungs, walls of blood vessels, urinary bladder and eyes.

Striated Muscle Fibers

The striated muscles are also sometimes called as skeletal muscles, because they are attached to bones where they extend from one bone to the other and help in their

Cell and Tissues

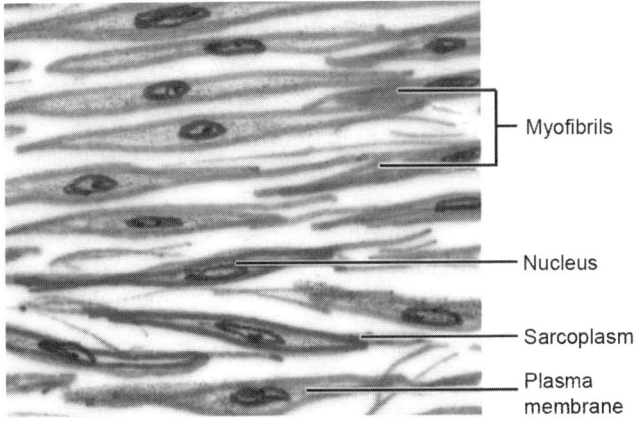

Fig. 1.24: Smooth muscle

muscle a characteristic striped or banded appearance. These muscle fibers are present in those movable parts of the body which are under the will of a person, such as tongue, body wall, muscles of arms and legs and the walls of pharynx and esophagus.

Cardiac Muscle

These are found only in the heart where they are capable of constant rhythmic contractions. They are also unique in having the characteristics of both striped and unstriped muscle fibers. The muscle cells are arranged in the form of cylindrical units which are without sarcolemma. The fibers have few branches. All the fibers united and branched in such a way that a network of muscle fibers is formed. The myofibrils have regions of different densities so that their cytoplasm presents an irregular striated appearance. The transverse band-like appearance is also proved by the cell membranes of the adjacent cell walls (Fig. 1.26).

■ Nervous Tissues

The nervous tissue carries out the special function of carrying messages of stimuli within the body. The properties of **'irritability'** and **'conductivity'** are specially developed in the nervous tissue. The nervous tissue is made of nerve cells called **neurons.** The neurons are supported by a special type of connective tissue called **neuroglia.**

movements by their contractions. It works under the control of will hence are called as voluntary muscle. The cells are about 10 to 40 mm in length and are roughly cylindrical in shape (Fig. 1.25).

The sarcolemma is a fine sheath which surrounds each muscle fiber and several nuclei are situated under it. These muscle fibers are present in the form of bundles of muscle fibers or muscle fibrillation. They appear striated because their fibers have regions of different densities, which occur at very precise regular intervals so as to give the whole

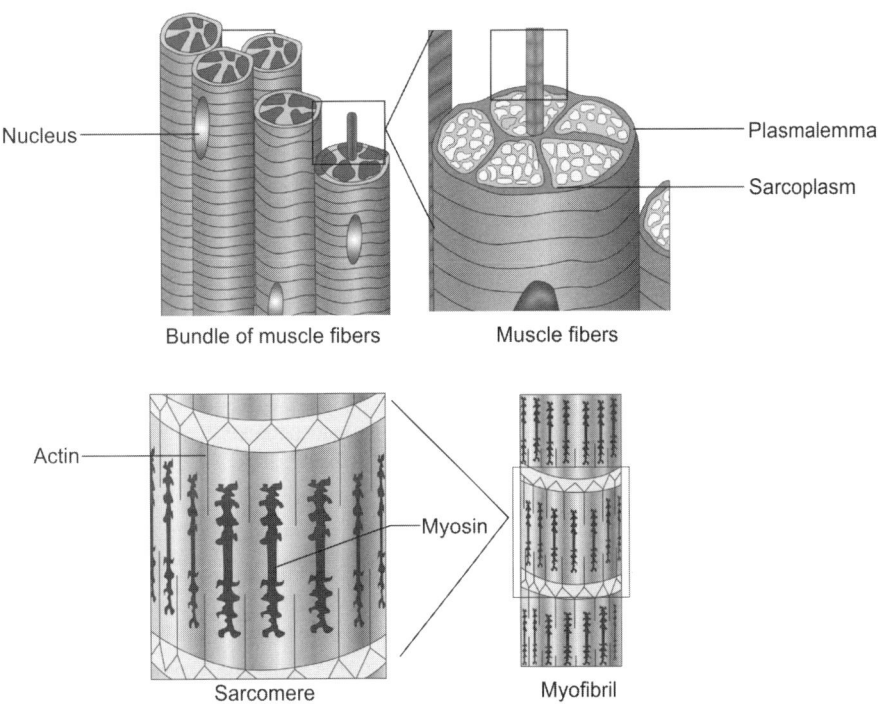

Fig. 1.25: Striated muscle fibers

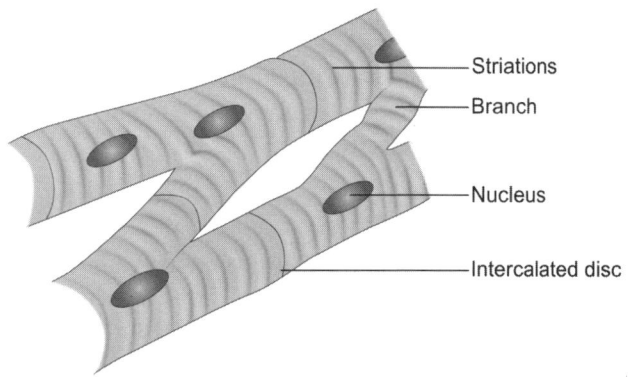

Fig. 1.26: Cardiac muscle

- **Nerve cells:** The nerve cells or neurons considerably vary in size and shape. They form gray matter of the nervous system and are found at the periphery of the brain, in the center of the spinal cord, in groups called ganglia outside the brain and spinal cord and as single cells in walls of organs.
- **Axons and dendrites:** These are the processes of nerve cells and form the white matter of the nervous system. They are found deep in the brain and at the periphery of the spinal cord and called as nerves or nerve fibers outside the brain and spinal cord.
- **Axon:** It consists of **axolemma**, a membrane of axon and contains **axoplasm** and **myelin,** which is a sheath of fatty material surrounding most of the axons and given them white appearance. The myelin sheath is absent at intervals along the length of the axon and near its branching end. These intervals are called **"Nodes of Ranvier"** and they contribute to rapid transmission of nerve impulse along **myelinated fibers**. The axons of the neurons which do not possess myelin sheath together form **non-myelinated fibers.** The axons of all peripheral nerves are surrounded by a very fine delicate membrane called as **neurilemma**. It consists of a series of **'Schwann Cells'** which surround the axon and myelin sheath.
- **Dendrites:** These are the processes on nerve cells which carry impulses towards nerve cells. These are shorter as compared to axon and each neurons has many dendrites (Fig. 1.27).

Types of Neurons

- **Sensory or afferent neurons:** These neurons transmit impulses from the periphery of the body to the spinal cord and then to the brain where they are interpreted and sensed e.g. sense of taste, sight, touch, etc.
- **Motor or efferent neurons:** These neurons convey impulses from the brain and spinal cord to other parts of body stimulating glandular secretion or causing muscle contraction.
- **Inter calculated neurons:** These are found between sensory and motor neurons and form links in the pathways of nerves.

Synapse

In the transmission of nerve impulse, whether sensory or motor more than one neuron is always involved. The point at which the nerve impulse passes from one to another is called synapse. Various chemicals known as transmitters are secreted in the synapse and they are involved in the transmission of information across the synapse.

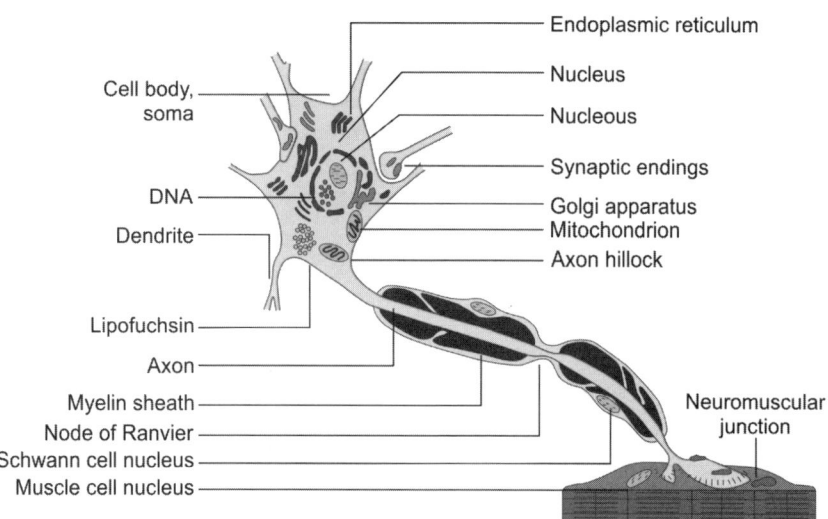

Fig. 1.27: A nerve cell

EXERCISE

1. Define cell. Describe the structure of a cell in detail.
2. Draw well labeled diagram of a cell.
3. What is cell division? Describe various types of cell division.
4. What is meiosis? Describe the various steps involved in the process of meiosis.
5. What is mitosis? Describe phases of mitosis.
6. Differentiate between meiosis and mitosis.
7. What is the importance of meiosis and mitosis?
8. Define metabolism. What are anabolism and catabolism?
9. What are tissues? Classify tissues with examples.
10. Describe various epithelial tissues with their functions.
11. Discuss various simple epithelial tissues with respect to their structure, location and functions.
12. Describe different stratified epithelium.
13. What are connective tissues? Give classification with description of each.
14. What is cartilage? Write about different cartilages present in our body.
15. What is bone? Describe TC of a bone with the help of well labeled diagram.
16. Define muscular tissues. Describe types of muscular tissues.
17. Describe the structure of nervous tissue or neuron with the help of diagram.
18. Give an account of different types of neurons.
19. Write short notes on following:
    i. Cytoplasmic inclusions
    ii. Ciliated epithelium
    iii. Stratified epithelium
    iv. Bone
    v. Cardiac muscle
    vi. Nervous tissues

OBJECTIVE QUESTIONS

1. Which of the following is not an animal tissue?
   a. Connective tissue   b. Xylem
   c. Epithelial   d. Nervous

2. Tissues are made of _____.
   a. Groups of cells that perform a different set of functions
   b. Collections of cells that perform similar or related functions
   c. Subcellular structures that aid in the performance of the cell's role
   d. None

3. Which of these is not a function of epithelial tissue ?
   a. Covering surfaces
   b. Secretion
   c. Support of the body
   d. Lining internal exchange areas

4. Layered epithelial tissue is referred to as which of these?
   a. Squamous   b. Stratified
   c. Voluntary   d. Pseudostratified

5. Which of these cell types covers the nasal lining?
   a. Stratified epithelium
   b. Cartilage
   c. Blood
   d. Cuboidal epithelium

6. Protection of the body from infectious organisms is accomplished by which of these tissues?
   a. Bone   b. Muscle
   c. Nerve   d. Blood

7. The tissue that link a bone to another bone in a skeletal system is _____ tissues.
   a. Epithelial   b. Connective
   c. Muscular   d. Nervous

8. Tissues that line the tubules in the kidney are made up of _____.
   a. Adipose
   b. Squamous epithelium
   c. Cuboidal epithelium
   d. Stratified epithelium

9. _____ tissues are the storage of fat.
   a. Adipose
   b. Squamous epithelium
   c. Cuboidal epithelium
   d. Stratified epithelium

10. Glands are composed of ___ tissues.
    a. Epithelium   b. Connective
    c. Muscle   d. Nervous

11. Hard part of the body is made of ____ tissue.
    a. Blood   b. Bone
    c. Muscle   d. Nerves

12. Bone acts as a reservoir for which of these elements?
    a. Carbon   b. Hydrogen
    c. Calcium   d. Nitrogen

13. The major function of bone is _____.
    a. Covering body surface
    b. Support
    c. Movement
    d. Integration of stimulus

14. Formation of blood takes place in _____.
    a. Matrix   b. Bone marrow
    c. Liver   d. Adipose tissues

15. The blood cell that transport oxygen within the body are the ___.
    a. Macrophages   b. Erythrocytes
    c. Platelets   d. Leukocytes

16. _____ is the liquid part of the blood.
    a. Plasma   b. Adipose
    c. Cartilage   d. Platelets

17. _____ tissues helps in the contraction of heart.
    a. Cardiac   b. Skeletal
    c. Smooth   d. Bone

18. During birth uterus is contracted with the help of the _____ tissue.
    a. Cardiac   b. Skeletal
    c. Smooth   d. Transitional epithelium

19. The junction between nerve cells are known as ____.
    a. Gap junction b. Synapses
    c. Tight junction d. Villi

20. The function unit of the nerves system is ____.
    a. Neuron   b. Axon
    c. Dendrite   d. Nephron

ANSWERS

1-b, 2-a, 3-b, 4-b, 5-d, 6-d, 7-c, 8-c, 9-a, 10-a, 11-b, 12-c, 13-b, 14-b, 15-b, 16-a, 17-a, 18-d, 19-b, 20-a.

CHAPTER 2

Microscopy

HISTORY OF OPTICAL MICROSCOPE

The first powerful magnifier was probably made by Anthony Leeuwenhoek (1632-1723) while working with magnifying glasses in a dry goods store. He used the magnifying glass to count the threads in woven cloth. He became so interested that he learned how to make lenses. By grinding and polishing, he was able to make small lenses with great curvatures. These rounder lenses produced greater magnification, and his microscopes were able to magnify up to 270X. Because it had only one lens, Leeuwenhoek's microscope is now referred to as a single-lens microscope. Its convex glass lens was attached to a metal holder and was focused using screws. With such microscope, he discovered microorganisms – bacteria, yeast, blood cells and many tiny animals swimming about in a drop of water, thereby founding the science of microbiology and providing the basis for the development of the germ theory of disease. From his great contributions, many discoveries and research papers, Anthony Leeuwenhoek has since been called the "**Father of Microscopy**".

Microscope is an instrument for producing a magnified image of a small object. There are many types of microscopes, ranging from simple, single-lens instruments (magnifying glasses) to compound microscopes and high-powered electron microscopes.

BASIC TERMINOLOGY IN MICROSCOPY

- **Scale of microorganisms**
  Micrometer (μm) = 10^{-6} meters <= bacteria cell (0.1 μm ~ viruses); nanometer (nm) = 10^{-9} meters ~ an amino acid; angstrom (Å) = 10^{-10} meters ~ an atom.
- **Resolution:** Resolution is defined as the ability to distinguish two very small and closely-spaced objects as separate entities. Resolution is best when the distance separating the two tiny objects is small. Resolution is determined by certain physical parameters that include the wavelength of light, and the light-gathering power of the objective and condenser lenses. A simple mathematical equation defines the smallest distance (d_{min}) separating the two very small objects:

  d_{min} = 1.22 × **wavelength** / **N.A.** $_{objective}$ + **N.A.** $_{condenser}$

  This is the theoretical resolving power of a light microscope. In practice, specimen quality usually limits d_{min} to something greater than its theoretical lower limit.
- **Numerical aperture (NA)** is a mathematical calculation of the light-gathering capabilities of a lens. The N.A. of each objective lens is inscribed in the metal tube, and ranges from 0.25-1.4. The higher the NA, the better the light-gathering properties of the lens, and the better the resolution. Higher NA values also mean shorter working distances (you have to get the lens closer to the object). NA values above 1.0 also indicate that the lens is used with some immersion fluid, such as immersion oil. From the equation above, you should be aware that the NA of the condenser is as important as the NA of the objective lens in determining resolution. It is for this reason that closure of the condenser diaphragm results in a loss of resolution.
- **Wavelength:** Viewing things through a microscope usually means passing something (e.g. light) through a specimen (an object). The shorter the wavelength, the higher the resolution. Blue light, for example, has a shorter wavelength than red light (blue light is also more energetic than red light). Thus, a light microscope that was limited to employing blue light can theoretically achieve a higher resolution than an otherwise similar light microscope that employs only red light (or all wavelengths of visible light).
- **Electron:** Light is not the only thing that has a wavelength. All objects have an associated wavelength, and the larger the object, the shorter the wavelength.

Electrons, though small objects, are much larger than photons (photons are the "objects" of light). Electrons thus have much smaller wavelengths than light (especially visible light), so consequently, a microscope that employs electrons rather than light has a much higher theoretically (and actually) achievable resolution.

- **Refract:** Another thing that can influence the resolution (in addition to wavelength and numerical aperture) is refraction. The occurrence of refraction causes objects to appear fuzzy (i.e. lowers resolution). To achieve high resolutions under high magnification, refraction must be minimized. To do this, one employs immersion oil between objects and lenses.
- **Illumination:** An essential factor in producing a good image with the light microscope is obtaining adequate levels of light in the specimen, or object plane. The best way to illuminate the specimen involves the use of yet another lens system, known as a condenser. The front element of the condenser is usually a large, flattened lens that sits directly beneath the specimen. Its placement on a movable rack provides the means to focus the light beam coming past the object and maximize the intensity and control the uniformity of illumination. Two apertures in the illumination system allow to regulate the diameter of the illumination beam by closing or opening iris diaphragms. One of these diaphragms, housed within the bright field condenser and known as the condenser diaphragm, allows to increase contrast, but at the cost of worsening resolution. The second of these diaphragms, known as the field aperture diaphragm, does not affect resolution as dramatically and is regularly adjusted for optimal illumination.

PARTS OF MICROSCOPE

▪ Specimen Control

- **Stage clips**: These are the basic stage slide holders. Supplied in pairs, they are adequate for general slide manipulation up to a maximum of 400X (if properly adjusted, which can be tricky). In the hands of a skilled operator a good pair can serve very well in this magnification range.
- **Stage:** This is the platform or "stage" that supports the specimen (which are typically mounted on glass slides).
- **Micromanipulator:** It is a device that allows to move the specimen in controlled, small increments along the x and y axes (useful for scanning a slide).

▪ Illumination

- **Aperture iris diaphragm:** This device is a part of the substage condenser. It serves to control the angle of the cone of light emerging from the top of the condenser. When adjusted so that the back lens of the objective, as viewed through the eyepiece tube, is just filled with light, the full numerical aperture (NA) of the objective is being utilized. Under these conditions the objective provides maximum resolution, but some glare may be present, which reduces image contrast. If the aperture iris is adjusted to fill about 75% of the objective's back lens this is reduced and contrast is improved, without significant lose of image detail. Closing the iris further will increase contrast, but some image detail will be lost. A further problem will be the introduction of details ("artifacts") that are not actually present in the specimen. Therefore, it is very import that the iris not be used to control light intensity (Fig. 2.1).
- **Condenser:** It is a vital part of the illumination system, and is designed to collect, control and concentrate light from the lamp onto the specimen. As with objectives, the optical elements can introduce a variety of aberrations which are corrected to varying degrees, depending on the type of condenser one is using. Condensers (as well as filters and objectives) are available to provide specialized, contrast enhancing illumination such as darkfield, polarization, differential interference contrast, and phase contrast (Fig. 2.2).
- **Filter holder (Carrier):** A swing-out circular carrier, or C-shaped frame, attached to the underside of the condenser body. Filters for reducing light intensity (neutral density), providing near monochromatic light (color specific, e.g. "daylight"), polarized light or introducing other special lighting characteristics are placed here. The diameter of hold ers ranges between 30 and 32 mm. However, with today's digital color imaging, colored filters are not used that often.

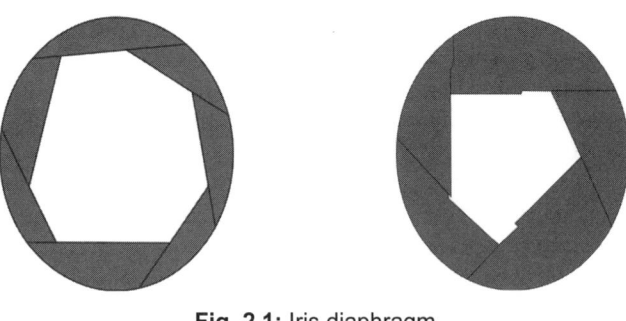

Fig. 2.1: Iris diaphragm

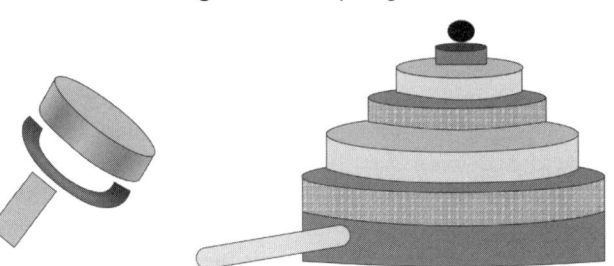

Fig. 2.2: Mirror and condenser

Lenses Systems

- **Magnification and imaging:** Most microscopes in current use are known as compound microscopes, where a magnified image of an object is produced by the objective lens, and this image is magnified by a second lens system (the ocular or eyepiece) for viewing. Thus, final magnification of the microscope is dependent on the magnifying power of the objective times the magnifying power of the ocular. Objective magnification powers range from 4X to 100X. Ocular magnification ranges are typically 8X–12X though 10X oculars are most common. As a result, a standard microscope will provide a final magnification range of ~40X up to ~1000X (Fig. 2.3).
- **Eyepiece (Ocular):** The optics in this component magnify the "virtual image" formed by the objective. In addition, as the virtual image cannot be seen directly by the eye (but can be projected onto a sheet of paper), the eyepiece converts it to a "real image", which the eye can see. The top element is an achromatic doublet, and it provides a large, flat, well corrected field of view. In addition the higher eye point makes viewing more pleasurable (Fig. 2.3).
- **Objective:** This, together with the condenser, is the microscope. Objective lenses are very tiny and as a result great care is needed to form and assemble such lens systems. Objectives were generally shorter, typically having an adjustment distance of 37 mm (measured from the shoulder of the attached objective to the plane of focus in the specimen). A revolving nosepiece permits rapid changeover between objectives.
- **Immersion oil (Index of refraction):** Immersion oil possesses an index of refraction (that is, the speed with which light passes through a substance) that is identical to that of glass, with both different from that of air. When light passes from a glass slide into the air, the light bends; this bending causes a scattering of the light exiting a specimen so consequently there is a reduction in resolution (i.e. there is an increase in fuzziness). Because immersion oil possesses the same index of refraction as glass, light passing out of a specimen and slide will pass through the oil without bending and then will go directly into the immersed lens (Fig. 2.3).

Focus

- **Coarse adjustment knob:** As the name suggests, this control (typically a pair, one on each side) moves either the body tube, or the stage/sub-stage, up or down in a quick manner. This is accomplished by means of a rack and pinion assembly. The pinion is a toothed wheel (the knobs are attached to either end of the axial) that rides along a diagonally grooved bar or "rack", attached to the stage or body tube. A good coarse focus control will provide smooth, backlash free movement, often adequate for initial focusing at magnifications as high as 400X.
- **Fine focus knob:** This control allows for precise focusing of the specimen. It is absolutely essential that this control works smoothly, with zero rebound effect (e.g. set the focus and leave for five minutes, the image should remain razor sharp). Therefore, this control should be checked carefully under viewing conditions, before investing in a microscope.

Support and Alignment

- **Body tube:** This part supports the eyepiece and objectives. It is critical that the tube be constructed so that these optics share a common axis.
- **Condenser focus knob:** This control is used to precisely adjust the vertical height of the condenser.
- **Draw tube:** At one time, "all good instruments" had a body tube equipped with an inner sliding draw tube. This tube enabled us to adjust the mechanical tube length when certain accessories were screwed on between the eyepiece and objective, or when using objectives designed for longer mechanical tube lengths.
- **Eyepiece tube:** A fixed tube into which the eyepiece is inserted. For mainstream, "professional" scopes, the inside diameter is either 23 mm or 30 mm.
- **Foot (Base):** It rests on the bench top and supports the stage and body of the microscope, and in many cases also houses the lamp. A well designed base will ensure that the image does not dance about during focusing, or while manipulating the specimen. There are a vast number of different base designs.

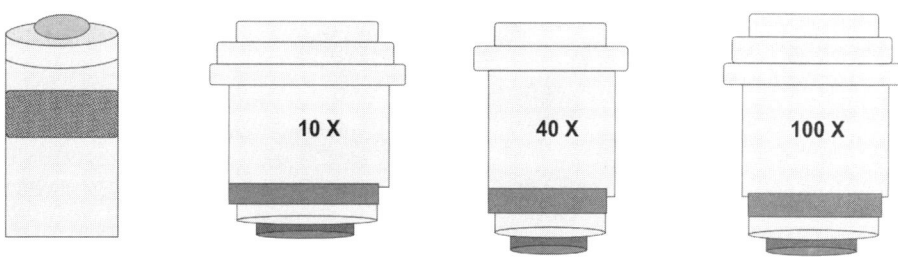

Fig. 2.3: Eyepiece and objectives 10X, 40X and oil immersion 100X

- **Limb (Arm):** The arm is attached to the foot and supports the body tube. This arm is very strong and can better support additional equipment, such as video cameras.
- **Nose-piece (Objective Changer):** A rotating device to which objectives are attached. It should move smoothly, and most importantly, should have a distinct click or feel when an objective is properly "seated". Most older nose-piece can accommodate four objectives. Figure 2.4 shows various parts of a microscope.

CARE OF MICROSCOPE

- Microscope should be properly carried, handled, used and stored when not in use.
- Microscope must be covered when not in use. This should be done even if they are stored in a cabinet.
- Never store a microscope with the eyepiece removed or uncovered, since dust will collect in the body tube and be very difficult to clean. Keep the body tube sealed at all times.
- When finished using a microscope with an electric illuminator, turn the illuminator off and let it cool for several minutes before moving the scope to put it away. This cooling off period will extend the life of the bulb.
- If oil immersion is used, the high power objective lens and the lens of the condenser should be thoroughly cleaned before microscope storage.
- Always make sure the stage and lenses are clean before putting away the microscope.
- Never store microscopes in chemical storage areas where corrosive fumes might etch lenses or destroy metal parts.
- Lenses should be treated with care. Never use a hard instrument (such as a dissecting needle, etc.) or abrasive to clean a lens.
- Never use a paper towel, or any material other than good quality lens tissue or a cotton swab (must be 100% natural cotton) to clean an optical surface. Organic solvents may separate or damage the lens elements or coatings.
- Most microscopes require periodic cleaning, lubricating and minor adjustment of their mechanical parts.
- Never over-tighten or use force when doing any repair/maintenance of your microscope.
- Sliding surfaces on the microscope can be cleaned and lubricated. This should be done on an annual basis.
- Focus smoothly, do not try to speed through the focusing process or force anything.

■ Cleaning of Microscope Slides and Coverslips

Reagent: Acid alcohol (1% HCl in 70% alcohol) add 10 mL concentrated HCl in 1000 mL of 70% ethyl alcohol. Clean the used slides and coverslips in acid alcohol. Rinse in water and then place in 95% alcohol. Finally, take out

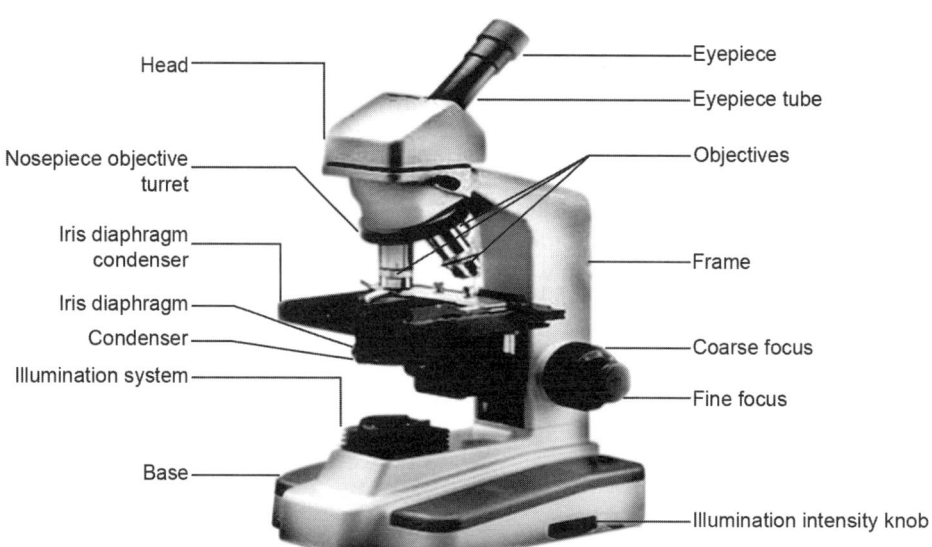

Fig. 2.4: Various parts of microscope

from the alcohol, polish, and dry each with a lintless cloth (e.g. surgical gauze). Cleaned slides and coverslips should be stored in clean, covered boxes or in dishes with lids. For routine work, dip new slides and coverslips in 95% alcohol and polish. Slides and coverslips to be used in fluorescence microscopy must be thoroughly cleaned with acid alcohol.

TYPES OF MICROSCOPY

The science of investigating small objects using microscope is called microscopy. Different types of microscopy are:
- Bright field microscopy
- Dark field microscopy
- Phase contrast microscopy
- Fluorescence microscopy
- Electron microscopy
- Confocal scanning optical microscopy
- Deconvolution microscopy and image reconstruction
- Polarization light microscopy.

BRIGHT FIELD MICROSCOPY

Use of a compound microscope, such that the image observe is the product of light that has passed through the specimen. It is called bright field because the background is brighter than the specimen. Because bright field microscopy relies solely on refraction, most specimens are difficult to see without staining.

■ Compound Microscopes

Compound microscopes are two lens systems. The object lens is positioned close to the object to be viewed. It forms an upside-down and magnified image called a real image because the light rays actually pass through the place where the image lies. The ocular lens, or eyepiece, acts as a magnifying glass for this real image. The eyepiece makes the light rays spread more, so that they appear to come from a large inverted image beyond the object lens. Because light rays do not actually pass through this location, the image is called a virtual image (Fig. 2.5).

■ Using a Bright Field Microscope

The various steps of using a bright field microscope are as follows:
- **Mount the specimen on the stage**: Adjust the slide manually on the slide holder or by using mechanical stage. The slide may or may not have coverslip. High magnification objective lenses cannot be focused through a thick glass slide hence must be brought close to the specimen.

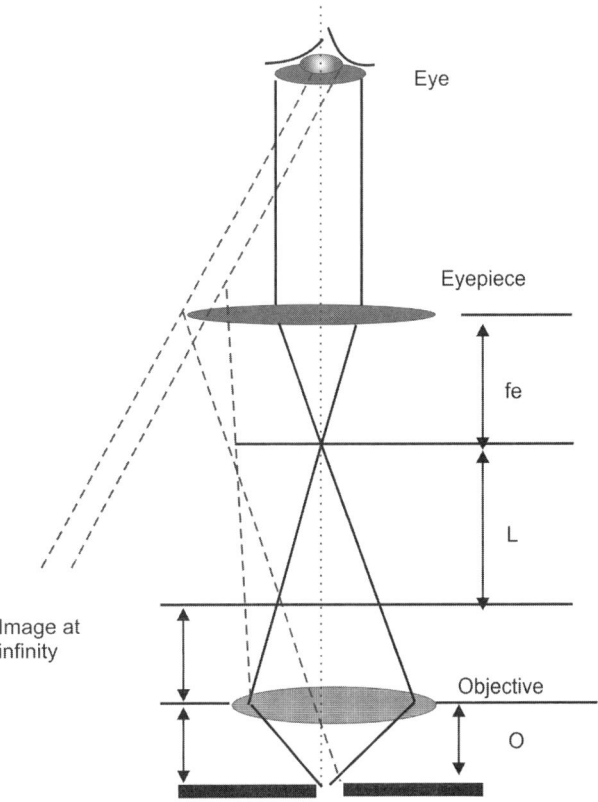

Fig. 2.5: Bright field microscopy

- **Optimize the lighting:** Some microscope is provided with a built-in-illuminator and simple microscope requires an external light source. The light must aimed toward the middle of the condenser. Adjust illumination so that the field is bright without hurting the eyes.
- **Adjust the condenser:** If the condenser is focusable, position it with the lens as close to the opening in the stage as you can get it. If the condenser has selectable options, set it to bright field. Start with the aperture diaphragm stopped down (high contrast). The light that comes up through the specimen change brightness as we move the aperture diaphragm lever.
- **Think about what we are looking for:** It is harder to find something when we have no expectations as to its appearance. How big is it? Will it be moving? Is it pigmented or stained, and if so what is its color?
- **Focus, locate, and center the specimen:** Start with the lowest magnification objective lens. It is rather easy to find and focus on sections of tissues, especially if they are fixed and stained, as with most prepared slides. However, it can be very difficult to locate living, minute specimens such as bacteria or unpigmented protists. A suspension of yeast cells makes a good practice specimen for finding difficult objects.
  - Start with the specimen out of focus so that the stage and objective must be brought closer together. The

first surface to come into focus, as we bring the stage and objective together, is the top of the cover slip. With smears, a cover slip is frequently not used, so the first thing we see is the smear itself.
- If we are having trouble, focus on the edge of the cover slip or an air bubble, or something that we can readily recognize. The top edge of the cover slip comes into focus first, then the bottom, which should be in the same plane as your specimen.
- Once the specimen is found, adjust contrast and intensity of illumination, and move the slide around until you have a good area for viewing.

- **Adjust eyepiece:** With a single ocular, there is nothing to do with the eyepiece except to keep it clean. With a binocular microscope (preferred) we need to adjust the eyepiece separation. One or both of the eyepieces may be a telescoping eyepiece, that is, we can focus it. Since very few people have eyes that are perfectly matched, most of us need to focus one eyepiece to match the other image. Look with the appropriate eye into the fixed eyepiece and focus with the microscope focus knob. Next, look into the adjustable eyepiece (with the other eye, of course), and adjust the eyepiece, not the microscope.
- **Select an objective lens for viewing:** The lowest power lens is usually 3.5X or 4X, and is used primarily for initially finding specimens. The most frequently used objective lens is the 10X lens, which gives a final magnification of 100X with a 10X ocular lens. For very small protists and for details in prepared slides such as cell organelles or mitotic figures, a higher magnification is needed. Typical high magnification lenses are 40X and 97X or 100X. The latter two magnifications are used exclusively with oil in order to improve resolution. We can move up in magnification step by steps. Each time we go to a higher power objective, re-focus and re-center the specimen. Higher magnification lenses must be physically closer to the specimen itself, which poses the risk of jamming the objective into the specimen.
- **Adjust illumination for the selected objective lens:** The apparent field of an eyepiece is constant regardless of magnification used. So, it follows that when we raise magnification the area of illuminated specimen become smaller, and less light reaches the eye, and the image darkens. With a low power objective, we may have to cut down on illumination intensity. With a high power we need all the light we can get, especially with less expensive microscopes.

■ When to Use Bright Field Microscopy

Bright field microscopy is best suited to viewing stained or naturally pigmented specimens such as stained prepared slides of tissue sections or living photosynthetic organisms. It is useless for living specimens of bacteria, and inferior for non-photosynthetic protists or metazoans, or unstained cell suspensions or tissue sections. Here is a not-so-complete list of specimens that might be observed using bright field microscopy, and appropriate magnifications.

- Prepared slides: Stained - bacteria (1000X), thick tissue sections (100X, 400X), thin sections with condensed chromosomes or specially stained organelles (1000X), large protists or metazoans (100X).
- Smears: Stained - blood (400X, 1000X), negative stained bacteria (400X, 1000X).
- Living preparations (wet mounts, unstained): Pond water (40X, 100X, 400X), living protists or metazoans (40X, 100X, 400X occasionally), algae and other microscopic plant material (40X, 100X, 400X). Smaller specimens will be difficult to observe without distortion, especially if they have no pigmentation.

■ Limitations

Limitations of standard bright field microscopy lie in three areas:
- The technique can only image dark or strongly refracting objects effectively.
- Diffraction limits resolution to approximately 0.2 micrometer.
- Out of focus light from points outside the focal plane reduces image clarity.

Live cells, in particular generally lack sufficient contrast to be studied successfully, internal structures of the cell are colorless and transparent. The most common way to increase contrast is to stain the different structures with selective dyes, but this involves killing and fixing the sample. Staining may also introduce artifacts, apparent structural details that are caused by the processing of the specimen and are thus not a legitimate feature of the specimen.

These limitations have all been overcome to some extent by specific microscopy techniques which can non-invasively increase the contrast of the image. In general, these techniques make use of the differences in the refractive index of cell structures.

DARK FIELD MICROSCOPY

In dark field microscopy there is an opaque disk in the condenser which blocks all light passing in a straight line from the condenser, through the specimen, into the objective lens. As a consequence, only scattered and reflected light is observed and the background is dark. This is one way of observing microorganisms without staining and therefore is useful for observing bacteria which are not easily stained. It necessarily gives a different image from that seen when employing brightfield microscopy and staining. Dark field microscopy is somewhat archaic since today more sophisticated methods are available for visualize stain-resistant bacteria.

■ Transmitted Dark Field Illumination

Transmitted dark field illumination can be used to increase the visibility of specimen lacking sufficient contrast for satisfactory observation and imaging by ordinary bright field microscopy techniques.

■ Reflected Dark Field Illumination

A dark field illumination with reflected light enables visualization of grain boundaries, surface defects, and other features that are difficult or impossible to detect with bright field illumination. The technique relies on an opaque occluding disk, which is placed in the path of the light travelling through the vertical illuminator so that only the peripheral rays of light reach the deflecting mirror. These rays are reflected by the mirror and pass through a hollow collar surrounding the objective to illuminate the specimen at highly oblique angles.

Figure 2.6 is illustrating the light path through a dark field microscope.
- Light enters the microscope for illumination of the sample.
- A specially sized disc, the patch stop blocks some light from the light source, leaving an outer ring of illumination.
- The condenser lens focuses the light towards the sample.
- The light enters the sample. Most are directly transmitted, while some is scattered from the sample.
- The scattered light enters the objective lens, while the directly transmitted light simply misses the lens and is not collected due to a direct illumination block (see figure). Only the scattered light goes on to produce the image, while the directly transmitted light is omitted.

■ Advantages of Dark Field Microscopy

- Dark field microscopy is a very simple yet effective technique and well-suited for uses involving live and unstained biological samples, such as a smear from a tissue culture or individual water-borne single-celled organisms.
- The quality of images obtained from this technique is impressive.
- Dark field microscopy techniques are almost entirely free of artifacts, due to the nature of the process. However, the interpretation of dark field images must be done with great care as common dark features of bright field microscopy images may be invisible, and vice versa.

■ Limitations of Dark Field Microscopy

- The main limitation of dark field microscopy is the low light levels seen in the final image. This means the sample must be very strongly illuminated, which can cause damage to the sample.
- While the dark field image may first appear to be a negative of the bright field image, different effects are visible in each. In bright field microscopy, features are visible where either a shadow is cast on the surface by the incident light, or a part of the surface is less reflective, possibly by the presence of pits or scratches.
- Raised features that are too smooth to cast shadows will not appear in bright field images, but the light that reflects off the sides of the feature will be visible in the dark field images.

■ Uses of Dark Field Microscopy

Dark field microscopy is used for:
- Initial examination of suspensions of cells, such as yeast, bacteria, small protists, or cell and tissue fractions including cheek epithelial cells, chloroplasts, mitochondria, even blood cells (small diameter of pigmented cells makes it tricky to find them sometimes despite the color).
- Initial survey and observation at low powers of pond water samples, hay or soil infusions, purchased protist or metazoan cultures.
- Examination of lightly stained prepared slides. Initial location of any specimen of very small size for later viewing at higher power.
- Determination of motility in cultures.

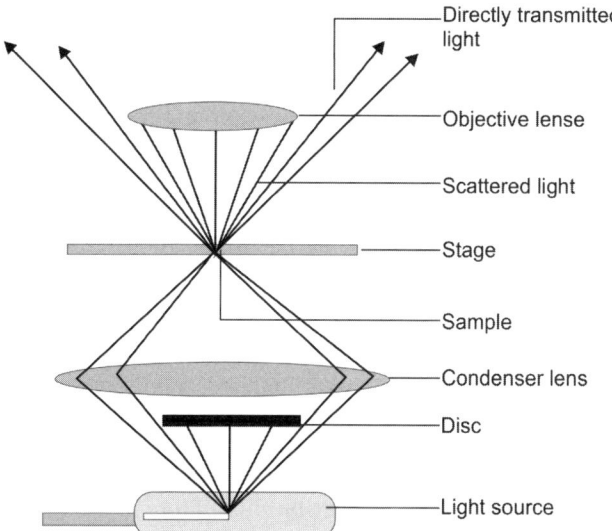

Fig. 2.6: Dark field microscopy

PHASE CONTRAST MICROSCOPY

The phase contrast microscope is widely used for examining such specimens as biological tissues. It is a type of light microscopy. A phase microscope is a device which causes the difference in refractive index between an object and its surrounding medium to be made visible in the form of an ordinary black and white image. The phase contrast microscope is able to show components in a cell or bacteria, which would be very difficult to see in an ordinary light microscope.

■ Altering the Light Waves

The phase contrast microscope uses the fact that the light passing through a transparent part of the specimen travels slower and, due to this is shifted compared to the uninfluenced light. This difference in phase is not visible to the human eye. However, the change in phase can be increased to half a wavelength by a transparent phase-plate on the microscope and thereby causing a difference in brightness. This makes the transparent object shine out in contrast to its surroundings (Fig. 2.7).

■ The Invisible Can Be Seen

The phase contrast microscope is a vital instrument in biological and medical research. When dealing with transparent and colorless components in a cell, dyeing is an alternative but at the same time stops all processes in it. The phase contrast microscope has made it possible to study living cells, and cell division is an example of a process that has been examined in detail with it.

■ Applications of Phase contrast Microscopy

- Phase contrast is an excellent method for enhancing the contrast of thin, transparent specimens without loss of resolution, and has proven to be a valuable tool in the study of dynamic events in living cells.
- The technique of phase contrast is widely applied in biological and medical research, especially throughout the fields of cytology and histology. Phase contrast enables internal cellular components, such as the membrane, nuclei, mitochondria, spindles, mitotic apparatus, chromosomes, Golgi apparatus, and cytoplasmic granules from both plant and animal cells and tissues to be readily visualized.
- In addition, phase contrast microscopy is widely employed in diagnosis of tumor cells and the growth, dynamics, and behavior of a wide variety of living cells in culture.
- Specialized long-working distance phase contrast optical systems have been developed for inverted microscopes employed for tissue culture investigations.
- Other areas in the biological arena that benefit from phase contrast observation are hematology, virology, bacteriology, parasitology, paleontology, and marine biology.
- Industrial and chemical applications for phase contrast include mineralogy, crystallography, and polymer morphology investigations. Colorless microcrystals, powders, particulate solids, and crystalline polymers, having a refractive index that differs only slightly from that of the surrounding immersion liquid, are often easily observed using phase contrast microscopy.
- Incident light phase contrast microscopy is useful for examination of surfaces, including integrated circuits, crystal dislocations, defects, and lithography.

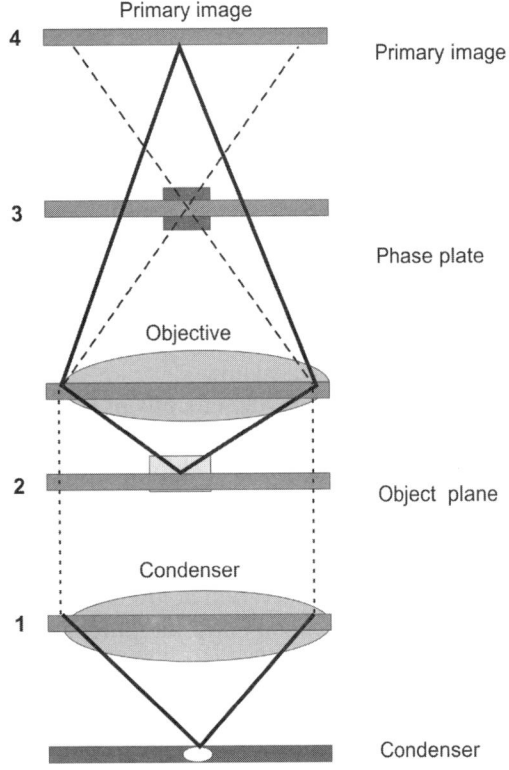

Fig. 2.7: Phase contrast microscopy

FLUORESCENCE MICROSCOPY

When certain compounds are illuminated with high energy light, they then emit light of, lower frequency. This effect is known as fluorescence. Often specimens show their own characteristic autofluorescence image, based on their chemical makeup. Fluorescence has the advantage of providing a very high signal-to-noise ratio, which enables us to distinguish spatial distributions of rare molecules.

This method is of critical importance in the modern life sciences, as it can be extremely sensitive, allowing the

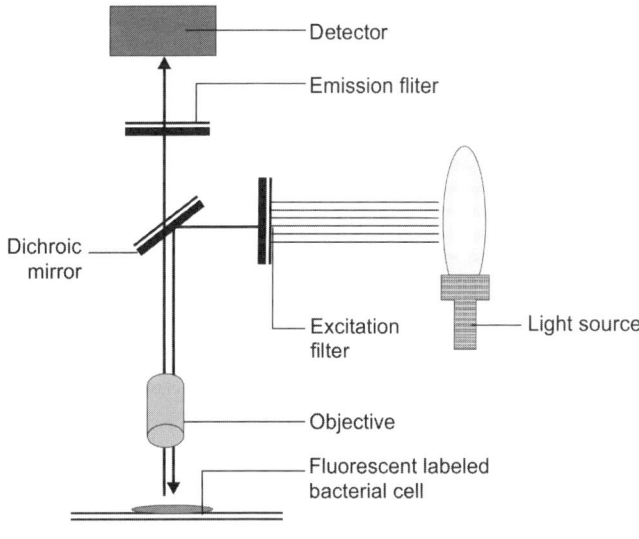

Fig. 2.8: Illustration showing components of fluorescence microscope

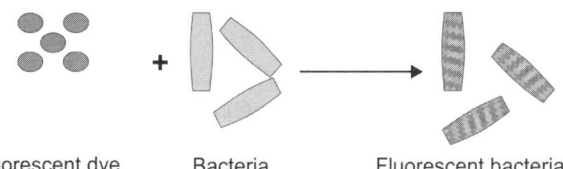

Fig. 2.9: Fluorochroming

light (of a different color than the absorbed light). The illumination light is separated from the much weaker emitted fluorescence through the use of an emission filter. Typical components of a fluorescence microscope are the light source (xenon lamp or mercury-vapor lamp), the excitation filter, the Dichroic mirror (or dichromatic beamsplitter), and the emission filter (Fig. 2.8). The filters and the dichroic are chosen to match the spectral excitation and emission characteristics of the fluorophore used to label the specimen. In this manner, a single fluorophore (color) is imaged at a time. Multi-color images of several fluorophores must be composed by combining several single-color images.

Immunofluorescence or Fluorescent Antibody Technique

Antibodies are natural defense molecules that are produced by humans and many animals in reaction to a foreign substance or antigen. Fluorescent antibodies (FA) to a particular antigen are obtained as follows: An animal is injected with a specific antigen, such as a bacterium, the animal then begins to produce specific antibodies against that antigen. After a sufficient time, the antibodies are removed from the serum of the animal. Then a fluorochrome is chemically combined with the antibodies (Fig. 2.10). These fluorescent antibodies are then added to a microscope slide containing an unknown bacterium. If this unknown bacterium is the same bacterium that was injected into the animal, the fluorescent antibodies bind to antigens on the surface of the bacterium, causing it to fluorescent. This technique can detect bacteria or other pathogenic microorganisms, even within cells, tissues or other clinical specimens. FA can be used to identify a microbe in minutes. Immunofluorescence is especially useful in the diagnosis of syphilis or rabies.

ELECTRON MICROSCOPY

A microscope employing electrons instead of light to image specimens. Electron microscopy (EM), is capable of much better resolution than light microscopes because the wavelength of electrons is much smaller than that of the photons of visible light.

The electron microscope is a type of microscope that uses electrons to create an image of the target. It has much higher magnification or resolving power than a normal light microscope, up to two million times, allowing it to see smaller objects and details.

The basic steps involved in all EMs regardless of type:
- A stream of electrons is formed (by the electron source) and accelerated toward the specimen using a positive electrical potential.

detection of single molecules. To utilize fluorescence, we need to label the specimen (a cell, a tissue, or a gel) with a suitable molecule (a fluorochrome) whose distribution will become evident after illumination (Fig. 2.9). Many different fluorescent dyes/fluorochromes can be used to stain different structures or chemical compounds. One particularly powerful method is the combination of antibodies coupled to a fluorochrome as in immunostaining. Examples of commonly used fluorochromes are fluorescein, rhodamine, green fluorescent protein (GFE) or DyLight 488. The antibodies can be made tailored specifically for a chemical compound. For example, one strategy, often in use is the artificial production of proteins, based on the genetic code (DNA). These proteins can then be used to immunize rabbits, which then form antibodies which bind to the protein. The antibodies are then coupled chemically to a fluorochrome and then used to trace the proteins in the cells under study. The fluorescence microscope is ideally suited for the detection of particular fluorochromes in cells and tissues.

The specimen is illuminated with light of a specific wavelength (or wavelengths) which is absorbed by the fluorophores, causing them to emit longer wavelengths of

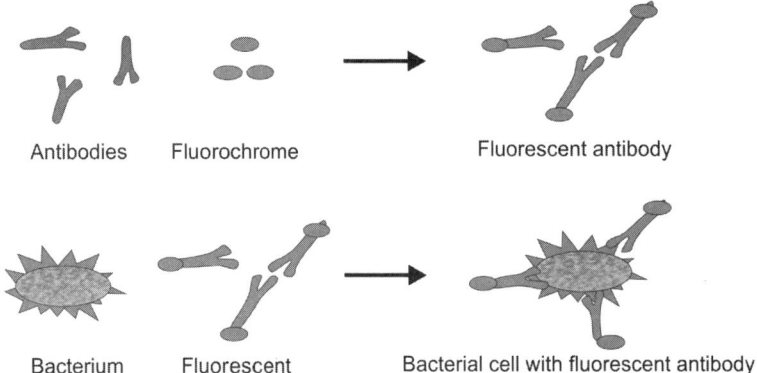

Fig. 2.10: Fluorescent antibody (FA) technique

- This stream is confined and focused using metal apertures and magnetic lenses (condenser) into a thin, focused, monochromatic beam.
- This beam is focused onto the sample using a magnetic lens.
- Interactions occur inside the irradiated sample, affecting the electron beam.
- These interactions and effects are detected and transformed into an image, which contains information such as structure and composition.

TYPES OF ELECTRON MICROSCOPE

Transmission Electron Microscope

The original form of electron microscopy, i.e. transmission electron microscopy (TEM) involves a high voltage electron beam emitted by a cathode and formed by magnetic lenses. The electron beam that has been partially transmitted through the very thin (and so semitransparent for electrons) specimen carries information about the inner structure of the specimen. The spatial variation in this information (the "image") is then magnified by a series of magnetic lenses until it is recorded by hitting a fluorescent screen, photographic plate, or light sensitive sensor such as a CCD (charge-coupled device) camera (Fig. 2.11). The image detected by the CCD may be displayed in real time on a monitor or computer. The conventional electron microscopy is now a days called TEM (transmission electron microscopy). The ray of electrons is produced by a pin-shaped cathode heated up by the current. The electrons are collected by the anode. The accelerating voltage is between 50 and 150 KV. The higher it is, the shorter is the electron waves and the higher is the power of resolution. But this factor is hardly ever limiting. The power of resolution of electron microscopy is usually restrained by the quality of the lens-systems and especially by the technique with which the preparation has been achieved. Modern gadgets have powers of resolution that range from 0.5–10 nm. The useful magnification is therefore more than 1,000,000X.

Scanning Electron Microscope

Unlike the TEM, where electrons are detected by beam transmission, the scanning electron microscope (SEM) produces images by detecting secondary electrons which are emitted from the surface due to excitation by the primary electron beam. In the SEM, the electron beam is rastered across the sample, with detectors building up an image by mapping the detected signals with beam position (Fig. 2.12). Generally, the TEM resolution is about an order of magnitude better than the SEM resolution, however, because the SEM image relies on surface processes rather than transmission it is able to image bulk samples and has a much greater depth of view, and so can produce images that are a good representation of the 3D structure of the sample. The path of the electron beam within the SEM differs from

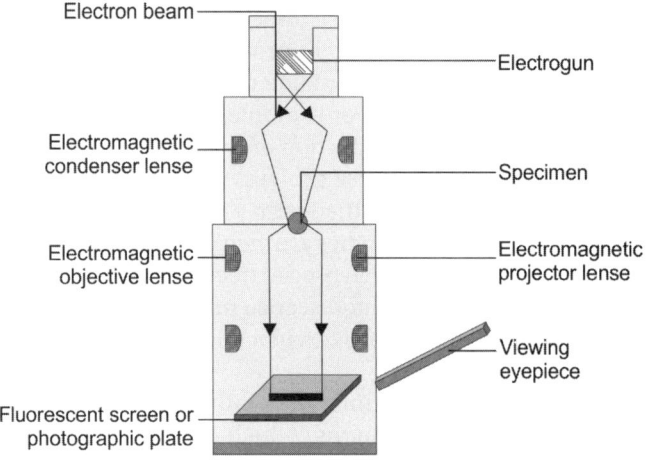

Fig. 2.11: Transmission electron microscope

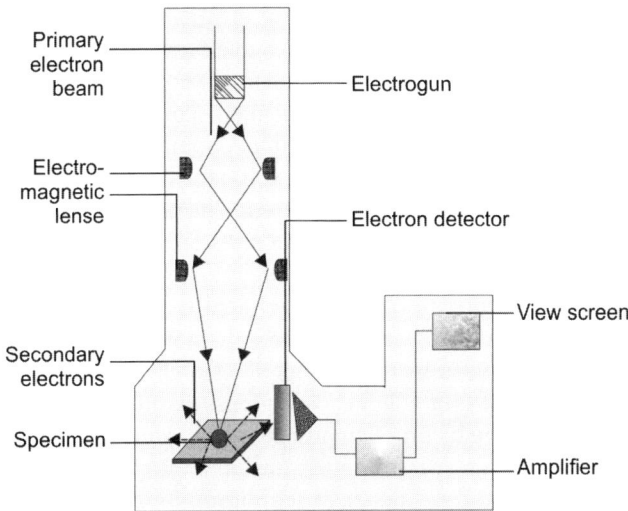

Fig. 2.12: Scanning electron microscope

that of the TEM. The technology used is based on television techniques. The method is suitable for the depiction of preparations with conductive surfaces. Biological objects have thus to be made conductive by coating with a thin layer of heavy metal (usually gold is taken). The power of resolution is normally smaller than in transmission electron microscopes, but the depth of focus is several orders of magnitude greater.

The surface of the object is scanned with the electron beam point by point whereby secondary electrons are set free. The intensity of this secondary radiation is dependent on the angle of inclination of the object's surface. The secondary electrons are collected by a detector that sits at an angle at the side above the object. The signal is then enhanced electronically. The magnification can be chosen smoothly and the image appears a little later on a viewing screen.

Reflection Electron Microscope

In addition, there is a reflection electron microscope (REM). Like TEM, this technique involves electron beams incident on a surface, but instead of using the transmission (TEM) or secondary electrons (SEM), the reflected beam is detected. This technique is typically coupled with reflection high energy electron diffraction and reflection high-energy loss spectrum (RHELS).

Sample Preparation

Materials to be viewed under an electron microscope may require processing to produce a suitable sample. The technique required varies depending on the specimen and the analysis required:

- **Cryofixation:** Freezing a specimen so rapidly, with liquid nitrogen or even liquid helium temperatures, that the water forms vitreous (non-crystalline) ice. This preserves the specimen in a snapshot of its solution state. An entire field called cryoelectron microscopy has branched from this technique. With the development of cryoelectron microscopy (CEMOVIS), it is now possible to observe virtually any biological specimen close to its native state.
- **Fixation:** Preserving the sample to make it more realistic. Glutaraldehyde—for hardening—and osmium tetroxide—which stains lipids black—are used.
- **Dehydration:** Replacing water with organic solvents such as ethanol or acetone.
- **Embedding:** Infiltration of the tissue with a resin such as araldite or epoxy for sectioning.
- **Sectioning:** Produces thin slices of specimen, semi-transparent to electrons. These can be cut on an ultra-microtome with a diamond knife to produce very thin slices. Glass knives are also used because they can be made in the lab and are much cheaper.
- **Staining:** Uses heavy metals such as lead, uranium or tungsten to block electrons to give contrast between different structures, since many (especially biological) materials are nearly "transparent" to electrons (weak phase objects).
- **Freeze-fracture or Freeze-etch:** A preparation method particularly useful for examining lipid membranes and their incorporated proteins in "face on" view. The fresh tissue or cell suspension is frozen rapidly (cryofixed), then fractured by simply breaking or by using a microtome while maintaining at liquid nitrogen temperature. The cold fractured surface (sometimes "etched" by increasing the temperature to about −100°C for several minutes to let some ice sublime) is then shadowed with platinum or gold at an average angle of 45° in a high vacuum evaporator. A second coat of carbon, evaporated normal to the average surface plane is often performed to improve stability of the replica coating. The specimen is returned to room temperature and pressure, then the extremely fragile "pre-shadowed" metal replica of the fracture surface is released from the underlying biological material by careful chemical digestion with acids, hypochlorite solution or SDS detergent. The still-floating replica is thoroughly washed from residual chemicals, carefully fished up on EM grids, dried then viewed in the TEM.
- **Ion beam milling:** Thins samples until they are transparent to electrons by firing ions (typically argon) at the surface from an angle and sputtering material from the surface. A subclass of this is focused ion beam milling, where gallium ions are used to produce an electron transparent membrane in a specific region of the

sample, for example, through a device within a microprocessor. Ion beam milling may also be used for cross-section polishing prior to SEM analysis of materials that are difficult to prepare using mechanical polishing.
- **Conductive coating:** Thin-film deposition, or sputtering of carbon, gold, gold/palladium, platinum or other conductive material to avoid charging of non-conductive specimens in a scanning electron microscope.

Disadvantages

- Electron microscopes are expensive to buy and maintain.
- As they are sensitive to vibration and external magnetic fields, suitable facilities are required to house microscopes aimed at achieving high resolutions.
- The samples have to be viewed in a vacuum, as the molecules that make up air would scatter the electrons.
- The samples have to be prepared in many ways to give proper detail, which may result in artifacts purely the result of treatment. This gives the problem of distinguishing artifacts from material, particularly in biological samples.

CONFOCAL SCANNING OPTICAL MICROSCOPY

In the incident light fluorescence microscope, a light beam passes through a chromatic beam splitter and then the objective lens to illuminate a specimen. This light beam is used to excite electrons in fluorochrome molecules present in the object. As some of those excited electrons return to their ground state, the emission of light is detectable through the oculars of the microscope, or with a camera or video printer. The image is generated continuously, across the entire field of view. A primary problem with the fluorescence images generated in this way is that out-of-focus fluorescence appears as 'flare' in the object, and reduces the signal substantially. In addition, human eyes are not sufficiently sensitive photodetectors for the lowest levels of fluorescence, and most video-based imaging systems are only slightly better than our eyes. Under conditions where there is sufficient signal to easily observe fluorochrome distribution patterns, the excitation light can be of sufficient intensity to photooxidize (i.e. burn) our specimen. Much information can be lost with just a few seconds of exposure to the excitation lamp. It is an expensive piece of instrumentation that illuminates the object with a small beam of light in a point-by-point (i.e. serial) fashion, eliminates most of the photo-oxidation problems, permitting the observation of objects for extended periods at very high resolution with little loss of signal. The placement of a small aperture in the beam path generates a small depth of field, and effectively eliminates out of focus information in image formation.

The confocal scanning optical microscope is designed to illuminate an object in a serial fashion, point by point, where a small beam of light (from a LASER) is scanned across the object rapidly in an X-Y raster pattern. The raster pattern can be created in several ways, but in one of the more popular instruments, it occurs as a consequence of the simultaneous rotation and vibration of a polygonal mirror. The vibration is caused by the activity of a servogalvanometer, while the rotation is caused by the activity of a small electric motor. Thus, a bright spot of light scans across an object from top to bottom, line by line. The image is also generated point-by-point. Image formation is translated into intensities at each spot in the X-Y raster by a photomultiplier tube. The intensity information is digitized and stored in a computer. A complex image processing software package permits visualization and manipulation of the images. Resolution is limited by spot size for the LASER and approaches 0.12–0.15 μm for an ideal specimen and with the best available objective lenses.

The confocal scanning optical microscopes include a pinhole diaphragm at a very special place in the optical path, near to the site of the photomultiplier tube. This pinhole is situated in a plane where the light from the in-focus part of the image converges to a point. Light from object planes above or below that of the focused image do not converge on the spot in the optical path occupied by the pinhole. Because of this design, out of focus image information is darkened to the extent that it is not detectable (Fig. 2.13). The consequence is that all out of focus information is removed from the image and the confocal image is basically an 'optical section' of what could be a relatively thick object. The 'thickness' of the optical section may approach the limit of resolution, but in practice, the resolution in the Z-direction is somewhat greater, approximately 0.4–0.8 μm. The value of optical sectioning is best realized with fluorescence microscopy, where out-of-focus information alters, distorts, or even degrades the image. Because the confocal images are stored in a computer, it is possible to stack them up and generate three-dimensional reconstructions. The image processing programs also enable us to rotate these images and observe three-dimensional aspects of cellular structure. It may be clear to you that the computer responsible for these image manipulations must be fast and powerful. The biggest problem is one of image storage, where single images can routinely occupy >1,000,000 bytes of space. In rather short periods of use, it is easy to accumulate sufficient numbers of images to fill the largest of hard discs.

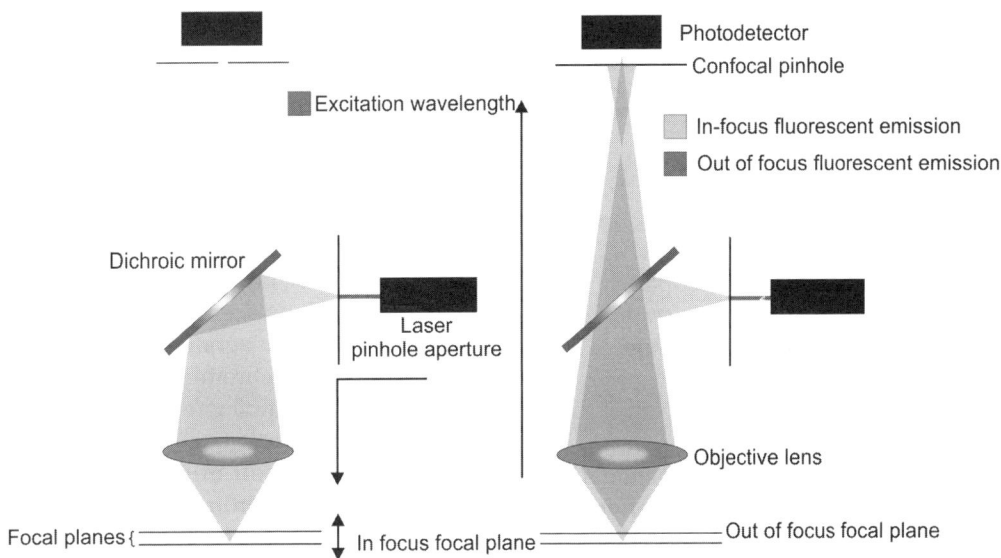

Fig. 2.13: Simplified schematic representation of a confocal microscope

DECONVOLUTION MICROSCOPY AND IMAGE RECONSTRUCTION

An alternative approach for eliminating flare from fluorescent image stacks is to perform intensive, interactive image analysis and processing, from objects that have been illuminated and photographed at multiple, adjacent focal planes. The images are obtained with a high-performance CCD camera, operating at very high magnification, using standard incident light fluorescence microscopy. The excitation source is a mercury arc lamp, and filters placed in rotating filter wheels control bandwidth for excitation and emission. The lamp is stabilized and the beam is randomized for uniform illumination of the specimen. Unlike confocal scanning instruments, the whole field of view is illuminated simultaneously with this microscope. It is possible to perform rapid sequential imaging (4 colors) from multiple fluorochromes with this microscope. At very high magnification, fluorescence from any spot in a cell acts as a point source. By knowing the image spread functions above and below the plane of focus, it is possible to determine points of origin for fluorescence, and spreading beams of light from that point source, above and below the plane of focus. An iterative algorithm, which is essentially a linear combination is performed by a computer on the adjacent pixels within a single image plane, and in successive image planes through the thickness of the object. Spreading light beams are subtracted from the reconstructed image stack, and that light is added back to the source, thereby reducing noise and increasing signal, respectively.

POLARIZATION LIGHT MICROSCOPY

■ Birefringence

When light passes through an object, it interacts with some or all of the atoms and molecules present in that object. In these interactions, sometimes light of a particular wavelength (i.e. color) is absorbed by the atoms or molecules, while sometimes light is scattered. The interaction of light with a translucent object often results in a slight reduction in the velocity of the light beam. The extent of this reduction in velocity can be measured as the refractive index of the object. For certain kinds of objects, especially those with high order in particular axes of the object, such a crystalline or paracrystalline arrays, the interaction with light beam is vastly different, depending on the orientation of the object relative to the impinging light beam. As a result, the refractive indices are measurably different in different axes of the object. Such an object with multiple refractive indices is termed **birefringent**. Birefringence (multiple refractive indices) results from the alignment of atoms or molecules in particular planes of an object; these atoms or molecules interact strongly with light beams impinging on them from a particular direction, and to a far lesser extent with light beams impinging on them from a different direction. There are two kinds of birefringence, *intrinsic birefringence*, which results from the atomic or molecular order in a crystalline or paracrystalline array (i.e. calcite crystals, membranes) and *form birefringence*, which results from supramolecular associations in paracrystalline arrays (i.e. microtubules in a spindle).

EXERCISE

1. Define microscopy. Write importance of microscope.
2. Define the following terms:
    i. Resolution
    ii. Numerical aperture
    iii. Refract
    iv. Wavelength
3. Describe various parts of the microscope.
4. Draw well labeled diagram of a microscope.
5. Describe following parts of the microscope:
    i. Iris diaphragm
    ii. Condenser
    iii. Objectives
6. What is iris diaphragm? What are its functions?
7. Define condenser. Write importance of condenser.
8. Describe illumination system of microscope.
9. Write about various lens systems of microscope.
10. What is oil immersion? Write its advantages.
11. Write a note on caring of microscope.
12. Describe the procedure of clearing of microscopic slides and coverslips.
13. What is microscopy? Enlist various types of microscopy.
14. Describe bright field microscopy with respect to principle, ray diagram and working of it.
15. When is bright field microscopy used? What are its limitations?
16. Write detailed account of dark field microscopy.
17. Write limitations and applications of dark field microscopy.
18. Differentiate between bright field and dark field microscopy.
19. What is phase contrast microscopy? Write its principle and describe ray diagram and applications.
20. Describe fluorescence microscopy with respect to its principle and diagram.
21. What is fluorochroming? Explain it.
22. What is immunofluorescence or fluorescent antibody (FA) technique?
23. Define electron microscopy. Write basic steps involved in electron microscopy.
24. Describe various types of electron microscopy. Give applications of electron microscopy.
25. Write a note on transmission electron microscopy and scanning electron microscopy.
26. Draw well labeled ray diagram of TEM and SEM.
27. Describe the processing of the sample or tissue to be viewed under and electron microscope.
28. What is confocal scanning optical microscopy?
29. Write a note on deconvolution microscopy and polarization light microscopy.

OBJECTIVE QUESTIONS

1. The first powerful magnifier was probably made by _____
    a. Anthony Leeuwenhoek
    b. Robert Hooke
    c. Marvin Minsky
    d. Frits Zernike

2. One micrometer (µ1-m) is equal to _____
    a. 10^{-6} m
    b. 10^{-4} m
    c. 10^{-5} m
    d. 10^{-10} m

3. One nanometer (nm) is equal to _____
    a. 10^{-6} m
    b. 10^{-4} m
    c. 10^{-9} m
    d. 10^{-10} m

4. One angstrom (A°) is equal to _____
    a. 10^{-6} m
    b. 10^{-12} m
    c. 10^{-9} m
    d. 10^{-10} m

5. The vital part of the illumination system designed to collect, control and concentrate light from the lamp onto the specimen is _____
    a. Condenser
    b. Objective
    c. Iris diaphragm
    d. Eyepiece

6. It serves to control the angle of the cone of light emerging from the top of the condenser.
    a. Condenser
    b. Objective
    c. Iris diaphragm
    d. Eyepiece

7. The ability to distinguish two very small and closely-spaced objects as separate entities is called as
    a. Numerical aperture
    b. Refract
    c. Illumination
    d. Resolution

8. A mathematical calculation of the light-gathering capabilities of a lens is called as
    a. Numerical aperture
    b. Refract
    c. Illumination
    d. Resolution

9. The shorter the wavelength, the _____ the resolution.
   a. Higher   b. Lower
   c. Medium   d. None

10. To achieve high resolutions under high magnification, refraction must be _____.
    a. Minimized   b. Optimized
    c. Maximized   d. None

11. Immersion oil possesses an index of refraction that is identical to that of _____.
    a. Water   b. Air
    c. Glass   d. Mountant

12. Always use a _____ to clean optical surfaces of microscope
    a. Paper towel b. Plastic gauze
    c. Cotton swab d. All

13. Bright field microscopy is best suited to viewing _____.
    a. Stained specimens   b. Pigmented specimens
    c. Unstained specimens d. Colorless specimens

14. A microscope employing electrons instead of light to image specimens is called _____.
    a. Fluorescence microscopy
    b. Dark field microscopy
    c. Bright field microscopy
    d. Electron microscopy

15. When certain compounds are illuminated with high energy light, they then emit light of a different, lower frequency. This effect is known as _____.
    a. Fluorescence   b. Phosphorescence
    c. Reflection   d. Refraction

16. Object with multiple refractive indices is termed _____.
    a. Parfocal   b. Confocal
    c. Birefringent   d. All

ANSWERS

1-a, 2-a, 3-c, 4-d, 5-a, 6-c, 7-a, 8-a, 9-a, 10-a, 11-c, 12-a, 13-a, 14-d, 15-a, 16-c.

CHAPTER 3

Introduction and Importance of Histopathology

The cells are the building blocks of all living things. Group of these cells unites to perform a specific function. These groups of cells are called tissues. The microscopic study of cells in a smear is called cytology and study of tissue is called histology (from Greek histos= tissue, logos = study).

Histology: Histology is a department of anatomy that deal with the microscopic study of the anatomy of cells and tissues of plants and animals. It is performed by examining a thin slice (section) of tissue under a light microscope or electron microscope. The ability to visualize or differentially identify microscopic structures is frequently enhanced through the use of histological stains. Histology is an essential tool of biology and medicine.

Histopathology: Means the microscopic study of diseased tissues. It is one of the important tools in anatomy and pathology for the accurate diagnosis of cancer and other diseases.

Cytopathology: It is that branch of diagnostic medicine which deals with the study of individual cells and or tissue fragments spread on a slide and stained properly.

Pathologists: Pathologists are trained medical doctors who are board certified and are the personnel who perform histopathological examination and provide diagnostic informations based on their observations.

Histotechnicians: The trained scientists who perform the preparation of histological sections are histotechnicians, histology technicians, histology technologists, medical scientists, medical laboratory technicians.

IMPORTANCE OF HISTOPATHOLOGY

- It help us to study the tissue in their original conditions with the least amount of postmortem changes.
- It provides us a continuous series of sections for studying not only a part of tissue but the entire tissue microscopically.
- The study of sections gives us the interrelationship of structures among the tissues.
- It is extremely important in clinical pathology for studying the various organs under medical examinations removed from the body (Biopsy).
- It is a basic way to study and diagnose diseased conditions in the cell (Cellular pathology), diseased conditions of tissues (Histopathology) and also helps to know the chemical disturbances in the tissues (Chemical pathology).
- It has its own importance in experimental pathology. The disease is introduced in experimental laboratory animals and the disease affected tissues of the animal are removed by biopsy and then examined by histopathology.
- It has a vital role in providing a medicolegal clues in case of suspected non-routine human death. In such cases the tissues of the victim under observation are removed from the body by autopsy/necropsy. The study of such tissues helps us to know the possible cause of death.
- It is one of the most effective means in diagnosing tissue abnormalities and cancer conditions.

DECOMPOSITION AND PUTREFACTION

Decomposition refers to the process by which tissues of a dead organism break down into simpler forms of matter.

Such a breakdown of dead organisms is essential for new growth and development of living organisms because it recycles the finite matter that occupies physical space in the biome. Bodies of living organisms begin to decompose shortly after death. It is a cascade of processes that go through distinct phases. It may be categorized in two stages by the types of end products. The first stage is characterized by the formation of liquid materials; flesh or plant matter begins to decompose. The second stage is limited to the production of vapors. Besides the two stages, historically the progression of decomposition of the flesh of dead organisms has been viewed also as four phases:

1. Fresh (autolysis),
2. Bloat (putrefaction),
3. Decay (putrefaction and carnivores) and
4. Dry (diagenesis).

Decomposition begins at the moment of death and is caused by the following factors:

1. **Autolysis:** The breaking down of tissues by the body's own internal chemicals and enzymes.
2. **Putrefaction:** The breakdown of tissues by bacteria.
3. **Black putrefaction (Carnivores):** During the putrefaction stage of decomposition number of insect start growing on it which mostly belong to Calliphoridae family.
4. **Diagenesis:** The final stage of decomposition is skeletonization. During this stage, deterioration of skeletal remains take place and is the longest process of all decompositions.

All these processes release gases that are the chief source of the putrid odor of decaying animal tissue. Most decomposers are bacteria or fungi. Scavengers play an important role in decomposition. If the body is accessible to insects and other animals, they are typically the next agent of decomposition. The most important insects that are typically involved in the process include the flesh-flies (Sarcophagidae) and blowflies (Calliphoridae). The green-bottle fly seen in the summer is a blowfly. The most important animals that are typically involved in the process include larger scavengers, such as coyotes, dogs, wolves, foxes, rats, and mice. Some of these scavengers also remove and scatter the bones which they will then ingest at a later time.

VARIOUS STEPS OF HISTOLOGICAL TECHNIQUES

A specimen brought to the histology laboratory must first be logged, identified and then subjected to specimen preparation prior to tissue processing. The various steps are:
- Sample collection
- Logging of specimen
- Preparation of tissues which include fixation and decalcification
- Processing of tissues which include dehydration, clearing, and embedding
- Preparation of sections which include process of microtomy, attachment of sections to slide and removal of pigments and precipitates
- Staining and mounting procedures which include dewaxing, hydration, staining, dehydration, clearing, and mounting.

SPECIMEN COLLECTION

Two methods which are mostly used for the specimen collection is biopsy and necropsy (autopsy). Histotechnologist do not concern with the specimen collection he only process the tissues and prepare permanent slides of the specimens. The specimen is mostly collected by the surgeon or trained nurse in the hospital.

■ Biopsy

A biopsy is a procedure in which a doctor removes a small amount of tissue for examination in a laboratory. Biopsies help doctors to diagnose many diseases, especially cancer. In some cases, biopsies help to determine the severity or stage of a disease and appropriate treatment. Doctors use different biopsy techniques depending on which tissue or organ needs to be studied.

- **Needle biopsy:** For palpable lesions it is less invasive. It can be done in the doctor's office. The surgeon obtains material for microscopic analysis using a needle with a hollow center. Results are often available in 24 hours. New technologies are helping to improve the effectiveness of needle biopsy. In some cases, a technique called needle localization guide biopsy of a non-palpable lesion (mass that cannot be felt) that was detected by mammography. A long, thin, hollow needle is placed in the lesion with the help of mammography or ultrasound to see where the needle is going. Cells are extracted through the center of the needle. A collapsible hook at the end of the needle keeps the needle in place until the surgery is done. X-rays verify that the abnormal area seen on the original X-rays is the same area into which the surgeon inserts the needle. This biopsy technique has the highest risk of "false negatives," which is when the biopsy result, says normal, even though a cancer is present. The reason for this is probably that the needle does not always pick up the cancer cells.
- **Stereotactic needle biopsy (Core biopsy):** It removes multiple pieces of a lesion. If the lesion cannot be felt, the needle is guided to the area of concern with the help of mammography or ultrasound. If a cancer is only found by MRI, then needle the biopsy may be guided by that technique. A small metal clip may be inserted

into the breast to mark the site of the biopsy. In case the biopsy proves cancerous and additional surgery is required.
- **Incisional biopsy:** It is more like a regular surgery. It involves removing a small piece of tissue for sectioning and examination. Often, incisional biopsies are done when needle biopsies are inconclusive or if the lump, mammographic change, or suspicious rash is too extensive or too big to be removed easily. There is the possibility of getting false negatives with both needle biopsy and incisional biopsy. But the advantage to each is the quick results.
- **Excisional biopsy:** It is the most involved kind of biopsy. It attempts to remove the entire suspicious lump of tissue from the breast. This is the surest way to establish the diagnosis without winding up with a false negative. Removing the entire lump also provides you some peace of mind. Both incisional and excisional biopsies can be done in an outpatient center or hospital, using local anesthesia.
- **Skin biopsy:** A sample of skin tissue is removed with a scalpel or other tool.
- **Fine-needle aspiration:** A very thin needle is inserted into an organ. The needle is attached to a syringe. Often, the procedure is accompanied by ultrasound or computed tomography (CT) scanning to guide the needle to the correct location. The doctor pulls back on the needle's plunger to suck cells from the organ into the empty syringe. The cells are spread on a slide and sent to a laboratory for examination.
- **Open biopsy:** In this an incision required in the skin. Depending on the depth of the body part to be biopsied, the complexity of the procedure varies. For example, a biopsy of an enlarged lymph node in the neck requires only a local anesthetic and often can be done in a doctor's office. An open biopsy of a lung or other organ in the abdomen has to be done in an operating room under general anesthesia.

■ Autopsy (Necropsy)

An autopsy also known as a postmortem examination, necropsy (particularly as to animals), autopsia cadaverum, or obduction—is a medical procedure that consists of a thorough examination of a corpse to determine the cause and manner of death and to evaluate any disease or injury that may be present. It is usually performed by a specialized medical doctor called a pathologist. There are two main types of autopsies:
- **Forensic autopsy:** A forensic autopsy is used to determine the cause of death. Forensic science involves the application of the sciences to answer questions of interest to the legal system. Deaths are placed in one of five manners:
    - Natural
    - Accident
    - Homicide
    - Suicide
    - Undetermined.

  In some jurisdictions, the undetermined category may include deaths in absentia, such as deaths at sea and missing persons declared dead in a court of law; in others, such deaths are classified under "Other". Following an in-depth examination of all the evidence, a medical examiner or coroner will assign a manner of death as one of the five listed above, and detail the evidence on the mechanism of the death.
- **Clinical autopsy:** Clinical autopsies serve two major purposes. They are performed to gain more insight into pathological processes and determine what factors contributed to a patient's death. Autopsies are also performed to ensure the standard of care at hospitals. Autopsies can yield insight into how patient deaths can be prevented in the future. Clinical autopsies can only be carried out with the consent of the family of the deceased person.

LOGGING OF SPECIMEN

The routine histology laboratories receive specimens in the form of biopsies or whole organs. The strict attention must be given to the problem of the specimen identifications. Tragedy may result if the specimen is interchanged in the laboratory.

In most hospitals, the operating room personnel, following biopsy, place small specimens in fixative solutions. This protects the specimen from drying. The large surgical specimen may arrive unfixed in the laboratory, but they must be put in the plastic bags or wrapped in saline soaked towels and should be kept in the refrigerator until examined by the pathologist. This slows down the hydrolysis and prevent the specimen from drying. The laboratory must maintain a log book where in each specimen is entered when first received in the laboratory (Table 3.1). From the log book the specimen receives an identification number (Fig. 3.1). After logging the specimen are first examined by the junior pathologist. The morphological description of the fixed tissue is given by the pathologist. This becomes the permanent record of the patient. After gross examination of the tissue, a portion of the tissue is trimmed by the pathologist and given to the histotechnician for laboratory processing.

After receiving the block the technician copies the identification number with a soft lead pencil on a tag that is

Table 3.1: Laboratory book maintained by technicians

Sl. No	Identification	Weight	Size	Shape	Color	Visible abnormality	Invisible abnormality	Sketch of special tissue

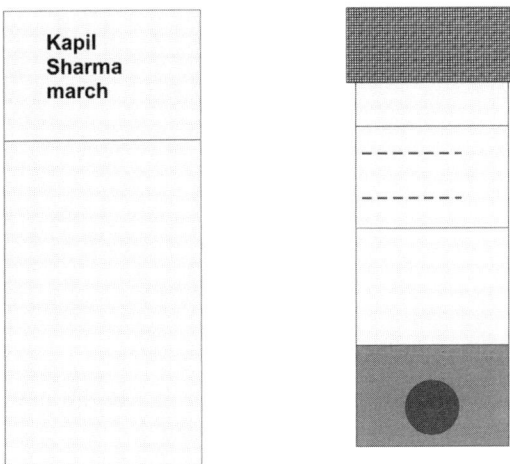

Fig. 3.1: Labeling of slide and container

always kept attached to the specimen. The technician also enters the identification number of the specimen into the laboratory register. In addition, he will draw a sketch of the specimen on a separate column in the logbook. This will help in tracking the specimen. Figure 3.2 shows the various steps of logging of specimen.

■ Labeling of Specimens

In order to ensure proper patient and specimen identification specimens sent for histopathology and cytopathology examination shall be labeled with patient's name and other identification marks like passport number, etc. The specimens with improper identification of the patient should be rendered unsatisfactory for evaluation and should be rejected without further processing.

■ Labeling of Glass Slide

Frosted-end glass slide should be used in case of making a permanent record (Fig. 3.1).

- Write the name of the patient, which should be identical to that given in the request form, in block letter on the frosted end of the glass slide.
- Write unique identification number clearly like passport number, etc.
- Skip the captions like Name:, ID:, etc. due to the limitation of the space.
- Use HB pencils.
- Always write the data in the preferred standardized format for easy checking in the laboratory.
- Do not write the name of the clinic, laboratory number, the marital status other unnecessary information.
- Cover the surface of the slice with a piece of card paper while inscribing on the frosted surface.

■ Labeling of Liquid Based Preparations (Specimen Containers)

Specimen containers should be labeled with patient's name and one or other unique identification. Serial number obtained from the request forms is not acceptable. Legible printing or pre-printed labels with two identifications are acceptable (Fig. 3.1).

■ Tissue Sampling and Identification

Tissue blocks for processing should be as thin as is consistent with the purpose for which they are required, usually 1–2 mm thick for urgent specimens and rapid processing, 3–5 mm for routine tissue processed overnight. Specimens should not be tightly packed into processing cassettes or containers but should have sufficient free space to facilitate fluid exchange. Small specimens and tissue fragments are processed in fine mesh containers, wrapped in lens tissue, sandwiched between sponge biopsy pads or more safely, double embedded in agar-paraffin wax.

Specimens are generally identified by a numbering system that is not bleached by subsequent treatment with chemicals or solvents.

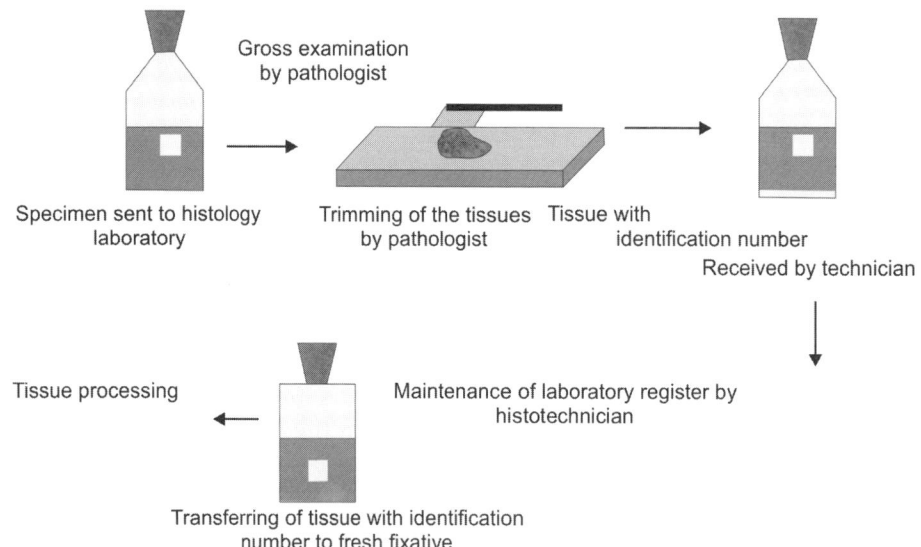

Fig. 3.2: Logging of specimen

Examples:
- A numbered card, label generated by computer-printer or hand written in soft pencil or waterproof ink.
- Color coded plastic cassettes, machine or manually labeled.

TISSUE MARKING AND ORIENTATION

Marking facilitates identification and correct orientation of particular tissue pieces or surfaces during embedding and subsequent microscopic examination. Tissue blocks are simply marked by cutting a notch on the reverse side of the block face to be sectioned, or by trimming the block to a particular shape. However, dye marking is preferred for certain surgical specimens, small tissue pieces, and for serial sectioning orientation.

Tissue Marking Substances

Criteria for the selection of a suitable tissue marker are:
- The marking substance must be relatively insoluble in fixative, processing reagents and embedding medium.
- It must survive fixation and processing and do not result in unacceptable contamination of the reagents and other tissues processed simultaneously.
- It must remain on the surface of the specimen and do not penetrate tissue.
- It should not react unfavorably with histological stains and must be clearly identifiable both macroscopically and microscopically.
- For some purposes it may be important that the marker is either radiolucent or radio-opaque.

Tissue markers are applied to the surface of the specimen using disposable swabs and allowed to dry.

India ink provides good black macro and microscopic marking is resistant to processing, but takes 15–30 minutes to dry, and may spread beyond the marked area. Silver and gold inks are not recommended as they are solvent soluble.

Silver nitrate (stick) provides a brown-black mark resistant to processing. Aqueous alcoholic silver nitrate solutions behave like India ink and are not recommended.

Artists' grade pigments are radio-opaque, processing resistant and provide good macro and microscopic contrast. Prepared by finely grinding pigment (50% w/v) to a thin paste in acetone, and store in tightly stoppered containers. These markers dry in 15–30 minutes.

Particulate pigments: 8% pigment w/v in 24% gelatin solution, dry in less than 5 minutes, or in about 10 seconds on chilled specimens. Paprika, turmeric, henna, India ink, and Bismarck brown are all inexpensive, strongly colored processing-resistant pigments with distinctive microscopic particle morphology.

Alcian blue: 1% aqueous solution, is a rapid and reliable stain for marking resection margins of fixed breast and other biopsies. The specimen is dipped into the stain for a few seconds then blotted dry. Sufficient dye remains to mark resection margins.

Eosin, erythrosin and rose Bengal: 1–2% aqueous, are used to stain small translucent specimens. Tissues are stained for 5 minutes, rinsed in water then processed. Although some dye is lost in the dehydration alcohols, sufficient remains to render the tissues visible. Alternatively dye is incorporated in the 95% ethanol dehydrant, and tissues stained during the routine dehydration step.

Tissue marking dyes is available commercially and have been favorably evaluated.

METHODS OF EXAMINATION OF TISSUES

Numerous techniques can be used to prepare tissue for microscopical examinations some are as follows.

Fresh Specimens

Fresh specimens may be examined as teased and squash preparations, smear preparation, impression smear preparation or frozen sections.

- **Teased preparation:** These are prepared by carefully dissecting the tissue to be examined with mounted needles. The specimen is immersed in an isotonic solution in a petridish or watch glass and is teased with a needle. Selected pieces are then transferred carefully to a microscope slide and mounted as wet preparation. Then it is examined by bright field microscopy under reduced illumination. This method is useful for showing the structure of a cell without staining while alive, and also make possible to see the movement of mitochondria and mitotic division. But anatomical relationship get destroyed due to teasing.
- **Squash preparations:** The cellular canteen's of smallpieces of tissue can be examined by placing the tissue in the center of a microscope slide and forcibly applying a cover slip. Placing a drop of stain at the junction of cover slip and glass slide can do staining.
- **Smear preparations:** It is useful for the examination of cellular materials in histopathology. Smears are prepared by spreading the selected portion of the specimen over the surface of the slide with a platinumloop or by using a second slide. Smear can be examined unstained or stained. The disadvantage is that the preparations are not permanent.
- **Impression smear preparations:** These are prepared by bringing into contact the surface of a clean glass slide with that of a freshly cut piece of tissue. Cell get transferred to the surface of the slide and are examined microscopically by phase contrast or after applying vital stain.
- **Frozen sections:** In this the sections are cut from frozen fresh tissues using the cryostat. Fresh tissues are rapidly frozen with the help of carbon dioxide or liquid nitrogen. The method provides rapid diagnostic information when required.

Fixed Tissue

The most effective means of studying normal and diseased tissues of the body microscopically is by the examination of thin sections, previously stained to demonstrate certain structures or inclusions and mounted on a glass slide beneath a cover slip. The sections are normally prepared from fixed tissues. A number of sections methods may be used such as paraffin sections, celloidin, nitrocellulose sections, resin sections, and froze sections using freezing microtome.

SPECIAL INSTRUCTIONS ON SPECIMEN COLLECTION AND HANDLING

- Do fix tissues thoroughly in 10% neutral-buffered formalin solution for a minimum of 24 hours prior to shipping.
- Use appropriate containers for sampling. To prevent leakage it is advised to double wrap the specimen container.
- Frozen sections will be done without fixative. Advance notice is required. Contact laboratory for specific appointment.
- Multiple small specimens, such as gastrointestinal biopsies, should be mounted on a piece of filter paper and properly labeled.
- Large specimens such as colon, should be opened, the contents cleaned out and specimen should be completely immersed in formalin. Containers must be tightly secured.
- Please tick the "URGENT" box on the General Request form; otherwise, the specimen will be processed as per normal.
- For specimens where orientation is important, mark or tag the specimen, e.g. Axillary tail of mastectomy specimens, orientation of surgical margins.
- If tissues are large (greater than 1 cm in greatest dimension), please incise through the tissue at 1 cm intervals for more rapid fixation.
- It is necessary to place tissue samples from a similar anatomic location (i.e. mammary gland, skin) into individual containers if you wish to identify each sample separately.
- It is not necessary to place each separate tissue sample from a necropsy (i.e. liver, spleen, kidney, heart, brain) into individual plastic bags for tissue identification purposes.

- Do not place tissue samples in glass bottles since many of these bottles will break prior to arrival to the laboratory.
- Do not place large tissue samples into narrow-mouth bottles. Although these tissues will usually go into these type bottles, they are much more difficult to take out of these bottles after fixation.
- Do not allow drying out of tissue samples. Ship tissue samples with a enough formalin solution to avoid drying out. Once samples dry out they are very difficult to process.
- Do not crush specimens with forceps, hemostats or other instruments.
- Do not force a large specimen in a small container. Large specimens must be completely surrounded by formalin for proper fixation.

DUTIES AND RESPONSIBILITIES

Medical laboratory testing plays a crucial role in the detection, diagnosis and treatment of disease. Histotechnicians or medical technologists and pathologists assistants are involved in laboratory testing. Although their roles may overlap in some hospitals.

Medical Technologists' Main Duties

- **Examine and analyze blood, urine, cerebrospinal and other body fluids:** Medical technologists microscopically examine blood, tissue and other body substances, looking for bacteria, fungi, parasites and other microorganisms. Analyze the chemical content of fluids, match blood types for transfusions and test for drug levels in the blood to show how a patient is responding to treatment.
- **Prepare specimens for examination:** They prepare specimens for microscopic examination, using techniques to expose special cellular tissue elements or other characteristics and count cells and look for abnormal cells.
- **Report findings to physicians:** After analysis of the results, they prepare a report for the patient's physician. They must work well under time pressure and complete reports quickly.
- **Operate automated equipment:** Automation and computer technology have made the work of medical technologists less hands-on and more analytical. Technician uses automated equipment and instruments to perform numerous, simultaneous tests.
- **Develop and modify procedures:** Technician also establish and monitor programs to ensure the accuracy of tests and modify procedures in keeping with advances in medical research.
- **Participate in training:** Some medical technologists supervise other technologists and medical laboratory technicians. With additional training, medical technologists may specialize in clinical chemistry, clinical microbiology, hematology, histotechnology, immunohematology and cytotechnology.

Pathologists' Assistants Perform Some or All of these Duties

- **Prepare for and assist with autopsies:** Assistants should have patients' medical records on hand for the pathologist. They arrange for radiographic examinations, as requested. Under a pathologists' supervision, he may assist with or perform autopsies and examine specimens.
- **Collect and analyze specimens:** They dissect, examine, weigh and photograph organs and specimens and collect tissue samples for chemical analysis and record all findings.
- **Prepare bodies for release:** Once the autopsy is complete, the assistant may be asked to prepare the body for release to a funeral home.
- **Assist in training:** They may train junior resident pathologists and train and supervise morgue attendants.

Duties and Responsibilities of Histotechnicians

- Under general supervision and according to policies and procedures, performs routine and non-routine activities involved in the preparation of slides, for microscopic evaluation by pathologist(s).
- Capable of performing all of the duties/responsibilities of a histotechnician.
- Ensure proper accessioning and labeling of all tissue samples.
- Process paper work associated with accessioning and reporting.
- Ensure proper tissue processing.
- Embed processed tissue in paraffin.
- Perform microtomy of embedded tissue.
- Prepare slides for routine hematoxylin and eosin staining.
- Perform coverslipping of stained slides either manually or automated.
- Prepare solutions and reagents for special stain procedures.
- Perform limited special stain procedures, under general supervision.
- Perform filing of finished blocks and slides.
- Perform routine maintenance and cleaning of equipment and trouble shoot minor equipment failures.
- Document remedial actions such as repairs and repeated tests.

- Adhere to laboratory's quality control policies, and document all quality control activities.
- Ensure all corporate safety, quality control and quality assurance standards are met.
- Ensure compliance with all local, federal, etc. regulations.
- Maintain a clean and well-organized work area.
- Other duties, as assigned by supervisor.

EXERCISE

1. What is histopathology? Discuss its importance.
2. Define histology, histopathology, cytology and histotechnique.
3. Write in short about specimen collection and labeling of tissues.
4. Discuss methods of examination of tissues.
5. Describe the work flow in the histopathology laboratory.
6. Write duties of technologist in histopathology department.
7. Discuss duties and responsibilities of technologist in histopathology department.
8. What is the function of reception desk worker in the histopathology?
9. Describe various steps of histological techniques.
10. Define biopsy and necropsy.
11. What is a biopsy? What are various biopsy techniques?
12. Write a note on needle biopsy.
13. Describe logging of specimen in short.
14. Write about tissue marking and orientation.
15. What are various criteria for selection of a suitable tissue marker.
16. Write about different tissue markers used in histopathology laboratories.
17. Write numerous techniques used to prepare tissue for microscopical examination.
18. Write a note on collection of specimen in histology laboratory.
19. Enlist special instructions on specimen collection and handling.

OBJECTIVE QUESTIONS

1. The building blocks of all living things are _____.
   a. Cells   b. Tissues
   c. Cartilage   d. Tendons

2. _____ deals with the study of minute structure, compositions and functions of tissues.
   a. Zoology   b. Biology
   c. Histology   d. Cytology

3. Histopathology is the study of _____.
   a. Structure of tissues   b. Diseases of tissues
   c. Functions of tissues   d. Arrangement of tissues

4. Removal of tissue from the dead body is called _____.
   a. Necropsy   b. Biopsy
   c. Endoscopy   d. Colposcopy

5. Removal of tissue from the living body is called _____.
   a. Necropsy   b. Biopsy
   c. Autopsy   d. None

6. The laboratory register in which tissue identification number, name of patient, etc. are recorded is called _____.
   a. Record book   b. Note book
   c. Log book   d. None

7. India ink is used as _____ agent in histology
   a. Clearing   b. Dehydrating
   c. Embedding   d. Tissue marking

8. Biopsy technique by which multiple pieces of a lesion are removed
   a. Core biopsy   b. Needle biopsy
   c. Skin biopsy   d. Open biopsy

9. In excisional biopsy _____ is removed.
   a. Multiple pieces of a lesion
   b. A small piece of tissue
   c. Entire suspicious tissue
   d. Cells of lesion

10. A sample of skin tissue is removed with a scalpel.
    a. Core biopsy   b. Needle biopsy
    c. Skin biopsy   d. Open biopsy

ANSWERS

1-a, 2-c, 3-b, 4-a, 5-b, 6-c, 7-d, 8-a, 9-c, 10-c.

CHAPTER 4

Tissue Fixation

INTRODUCTION

Once tissues are removed from the body, they undergo a process of self-destruction or autolysis, which is initiated soon after cell death by the action of intracellular enzymes causing the breakdown of protein and eventual liquefaction of the cell. Autolysis is independent of any bacterial action, retarded by cold, greatly increased in temperature of 30°C and inhibited by heating at 50°C.

Autolysis is more severe in tissues which are rich in enzymes, such as the liver, brain and kidney and is less rapid in tissues such as elastic fibers and collagens. Autolysis causes swelling of cytoplasm and also nuclei undergo necrosis, i.e. condensation, fragmentation and lysis. It also causes desquamation of the epithelium.

Bacterial decomposition also produces changes in tissues that resembles autolysis. It is brought about by bacterial proliferation in the dead tissue. Such bacteria may normally be present in the body during life as the nonpathogenic organisms, or may be present in diseased tissues at the time of death such as in septicemia. Thus to prevent the tissue from autolysis or bacterial putrefaction, it is subjected to a process called as **fixation**.

The objective of fixation is to preserve cells and tissue in a close a lifelike state as possible and to allow them to undergo further preparative procedures without change. Fixation arrests autolysis and bacterial decomposition and stabilizes the cellular and tissue constituents so that they can withstand the subsequent stages of tissue processing. Fixation also provides preservation of tissue substances and proteins. Fixation is, therefore, the first step and the foundation in a sequence of events that culminates in the final examination of a tissue sections.

In fixation tissues are kept in certain chemical agents called as **fixatives**. Thus fixative can be defined as a substance which will preserve the shape, size, structure, relationship and chemical composition of the tissues and cells after death.

FUNCTIONS OF FIXATIVES

- It must kill the cell quickly without shrinkage, swelling or distortion.
- It must penetrate the tissue and cells rapidly and evenly.
- It must covert soluble substances of the cell into insoluble substances and make the cell transparent.
- It must inhibit bacterial degradation and autolysis.
- It must harden the tissue and make it sensitive to the subsequent treatment.
- It must make the tissue sensitive to the staining procedure.
- It should allow the tissue to be stored for a long period of time.
- It should preserve the natural color of the tissue.
- It should be simple to prepare, nontoxic, non-hazardous and economical in use.

PROPERTIES OF FIXATIVES

The chemical and physical properties of reagents which influence processing includes polarity, concentration, miscibility with water, solvents and embedding media, evaporation rate, and viscosity. Thermal conductivity, heat capacity, boiling point and the electromagnetic conductivity of reagents are particularly important in microwave-stimulated processing.

- **Polarity:** To minimize tissue distortion there should be a gradual change in polarity of the processing fluid from highly polar aqueous fixatives and solutions to the embedding medium which is usually non-polar (hydrophobic). Tissues generally shrink when transferred to a fluid of relatively lower polarity.
- **Miscibility:** Processing reagents which are miscible with water and with the embedding medium reduce the number of processing stages and are termed universal solvents. To avoid severe tissue shrinkage

from concentration and polarity effects, they are often employed in a graded series. Many transition solvents, for example xylene, are extremely water-intolerant, and are immiscible with hydrated alcohols.
- **Evaporation rate:** The evaporation rate, rather than the vapor pressure or boiling point of a solvent, is the best predictor of the rate of elimination of a substance from molten infiltrating wax. Solvents with high evaporation rates are the most readily vaporized and are less likely to contaminate the infiltration medium.
- **Viscosity:** It is the internal friction of a particular substance which affects the rate of flow through tissues and is inversely proportional to temperature. It is particularly important in the clearing and infiltration stages of processing. Substances with high molecular weight, such as some transition solvents and waxes, have high viscosities and diffuse through the tissues more slowly than, the lower molecular weight, lower viscosity dehydrant alcohols. If tissue shrinkage or swelling is to be avoided when the specimen moves from one processing step to the next, the fluid already in the tissues must diffuse outward through the tissue pores at the same rate as the fresh medium diffuses inwards. If the viscosity difference between fluids inside and outside the tissue is too great, shrinkage will result. Hence, slow and gradual processing of tissues is necessary when viscous reagents are used (for example in nitrocellulose embedding methods).
- **Temperature:** Generally, the fixation of specimens in routine histopathological work is carried out at room temperature, for electron microscopy and some histochemical procedures, the temperature for fixation is usually 0–4°C. At this low temperature autolysis is slowed down, as in the diffusion of various cellular components, allowing a more life-like appearance of the tissues. However, fixation processes are more rapid at higher temperatures. The high temperature of 60–70°C can be used for the rapid fixation of very urgent biopsy specimens, although the risk of tissue distortion is increased.
- **Rate of penetration of fixatives:** The penetration of fixatives into tissue is a relatively slow process and tissue blocks should either be small or thin, in order to obtain satisfactory fixation. Large specimens should be opened and washed or sliced thinly before placing them in fixative.
- **Changes in volume:** Generally, during fixation, there occurs change in the volume of tissues, but the reasons behind volume change are not well-known. It may be due to inhibition of respiration, changes in membrane permeability and changes in ion transport through membranes.
- **pH and buffers:** Hydrogen ion concentration varies from fixative to fixative, but in general, the pH should be kept in the physiological range, between 6–8. This can be maintained by buffer systems. Most commonly used buffer is phosphate, S-collidine, bicarbonate, Tris, veronal acetate and cacodylate. The buffer used should not react with the fixative and at the same time it should not inhibit the enzymes.
- **Osmolarity:** The addition of buffer to the fixative solution may alter the osmotic pressure exerted by the solution. Hypertonic solutions give rise to cell shrinkage whereas, isotonic fixatives result in cell swelling and poor fixation.
- **Concentration of fixatives:** Some fixatives are effective within a range of different concentrations, for example, glutaraldehyde which may be used as a 4% solution is effective as low as 0.25%, provided the pH is maintained in the physiological range. If the concentration gradient between fluids inside and outside the tissue is too high, rapid reagent diffusion occurs. This strong diffusion current may result in shrinkage and disruption of tissues. Thus, tissues are always processed through a graded series of reagents of increasing concentration, the more delicate the tissues, the closer the gradations.
- **Duration of fixation:** It is very a important factor. It determines the extent of tissue stabilization and consequently porosity and finally influences the reactivity in histological and immunohistochemical procedures. Under fixed tissues are inadequately protected against processing reagents and exhibit a range of artefacts, including those associated with secondary fixatives by the dehydrants. Prolonged exposure to primary and secondary fixatives during processing may impair tissue reactivity and it also causes shrinkage and hardening of tissues.

TYPES OF FIXATIVES

A variety of fixatives are now available, but no single substance or known combination of substances has the ability to preserve and allow the demonstration of every tissue component. It is for this reason that some fixatives have only special and limited applications and in other instances, a mixture of two or more reagents is necessary to employ special properties of each. The selection of appropriate fixative is based on considerations such as the structures and entities to be demonstrated and the effect of short term and long term storage. Each fixatives have advantages and disadvantages, some are restrictive while others are multipurpose.

Over the years, various classifications of the fixatives have been proposed, based on functions or chemical nature, number of fixatives used and action of fixatives.

Based on action fixatives are classified into two major groups:
- Coagulants
- Non coagulants

Based on chemical nature they are classified into six categories:
- **Aldehydes:** Formaldehyde and glutaraldehyde.
- **Oxidizing agents:** Metallic ions and complexes such as osmium tetroxide and chromic acid.
- **Protein denaturing agents:** Acetic acid, methyl alcohol, ethyl alcohol, etc.
- **Unknown mechanism:** Mercuric chloride, picric acid.
- **Combined reagents:** All compound fixatives.
- **Miscellaneous:** Acrolein, glyoxal, diacetyl, etc.

Based on number of fixatives used:
- **Simple fixatives:** When a single fixative is used for fixation of the tissue then they are called as simple fixative, for example, formaldehyde, glutaraldehyde, mercuric chloride, osmium tetra oxide, picric acid, acetic acid, etc.
- **Compound fixatives:** When two or more than two chemicals are used for fixation the fixatives are called as compound/complex fixatives, for example, formal saline, Zenker's solution, Bouin's solution, Corney's fixative, etc.

Based on the action of fixatives upon cell and tissue constituents they are grouped under different groups.
- **Microanatomical fixatives:** Fixatives which preserve the tissue in a manner which permits the general microscopical study of the tissue structures and allows the various layers of tissues and cells to retain their former relationship with each other are termed as microanatomical fixatives, for example, formal saline and glutaraLdehyde fixatives
- **Cytological fixatives:** Fixatives which are employed for their specific action upon a specific part of the cell structures are termed cytological fixatives, for example, Fleming's fluid and Helly's fluid. Cytological fixatives are further classified into two groups (1) Nuclear fixatives (2) Cytoplasmic fixatives.
  - *Nuclear fixatives* are used for fixation of nuclei and nuclear materials like chromosomes, DNA chromatin, etc.
  - *Cytoplasmic fixatives* are used for fixation of cytoplasmic constituents such as mitochondria, endoplasmic reticulum, etc.
- **istochemical fixatives:** They are used for preservation of the constituents to be demonstrated, its morphological relationships and specific tissue constituents, for example, vapor fixation.

PROPERTIES AND ACTION OF SOME IMPORTANT FIXATIVES

■ Simple Fixatives

1. Formaldehyde
It is a gas, which is about 40% (by weight), is soluble in water and sold commercially as formalin. It is a powerful reducing agent and is used as a simple fixative (5% formalin) as well as compound fixative.

Action: Aldehydes form cross-links between proteins, creating a gel thus retaining cellular constituents in the tissue. Soluble proteins are fixed to structural proteins and rendered insoluble giving some mechanical strength to the entire structure which enables the tissues to withstand subsequent processing. Formalin does not precipitate proteins and only slightly precipitates other cell components. Formalin neither preserve nor destroys adipose tissue and is a good fixative for complex lipids but has no effect on neutral fats. It does not have an effect on the carbohydrates, but preserve glycogen to some extent. It favors the staining of acidic components (nuclei) with basic dyes and diminishes the effect of acid dyes on basic structures (cytoplasm).

Composition of 5% formalin	
Formalin commercial	- 5 mL
Distilled water	- 95 mL

Disadvantages:
- It gives off unpleasant vapor that causes irritation to the eyes and respiratory epithelium.
- It causes shrinkage of the tissue.
- Special precautions are required during handling of formalin.
- It reacts with the metal container and may cause corrosion of the lids.
- Formaldehyde solution produces acid formalin hematin pigment which can be seen in sites containing blood.
- After prolonged storage due to the formation of white deposit of paraldehyde the strength of the solution decreases.
- Older formaldehyde solution become acidic due to the presence of formic acid, hence should be neutralized by magnesium carbonate before use.

2. Glutaraldehyde [$(CH_2)_3$CHO-CHO]

It is used as fixative for enzymes to be studied by electron microscopy. It is a clear, colorless liquid, usually supplied commercially as 25% solution in water. It is usually diluted with phosphate buffer (pH 7.3) to give a final concentration of 1.5%.

Action: It is most efficient cross linking agent for collagen that is why it gives betters preservation of structure and rapid firing action than formaldehyde.

Disadvantages: It has poor penetration power and at pH greater than 8.0 it undergoes polymerization, it is also toxic in nature. Storage for long periods at ambient temperature caused glutaraldehyde to form precipitate which decreases its concentration.

3. Mercuric chloride ($HgCl_2$)

It is a white crystalline substance, soluble in water and alcohol.

Action: It is a powerful protein precipitant and penetrates and hardens tissue fairly quickly. It shrinks but does not distort tissue and fixes both nuclear and cytoplasm well, favoring the staining of both components. It is mostly used in conjunction with other fixing agents, particularly formalin, potassium dichromate and acetic acid.

Disadvantages:
- It is very corrosive to many metals and hence metal lid should not be used in its container.
- It is extremely poisonous and must be handled and disposed with great care.
- The most important disadvantage is that it produces a brown to black granular deposit uniformly distributed throughout the tissue called mercury pigment.
- This pigment causes hindrance during the staining procedure. Hence, the removal of mercury pigment before staining is essential. It is mostly removed either during dehydration of tissue block or before staining.

4. Potassium dichromate ($K_2Cr_2O_7$)

It is an orange crystalline substance used as a 2.5–5% solution in water.

Action: Two entirely different forms of fixation can be produced depending upon the pH of the solution. At more acidic (pH below 4.6) it fixes nucleus and precipitate cytoplasm with destruction of mitochondria. At more alkaline pH (above 4.6) the cytoplasm is homogeneously fixed along with mitochondria but nucleoproteins are not preserved. It has strong fixative action on certain lipids.

Disadvantages:
- Tissues fixed in potassium dichromate should be washed in running tap water to prevent the formation of an insoluble precipitate.
- Prolonged exposure to this fixative make tissue brittle which create problem in section cutting.
- It is unsuitable for histochemical studies.

5. Osmium tetroxide (OsO_4)

It is most commonly used for metallic ion fixation. It is referred as osmic acid. It is a yellow crystal supplied in sealed tubes as solution of OS –1% in water.

Action: Like formalin it forms additive compounds with protein. Most lipids, including myelin are blackened by the reduction of osmium tetroxide. Its penetration is poor and fixation is liable to be uneven. Minute tissues, smears of cells and thin sections may be fixed by vapors, without immersion in a fluid. Osmium tetroxide is used for preservation of fine structures in electron microscopy and is effective for small (2–3 mm^3) specimens. Vapors of this fixative are used for preservation of blood and tissue smears.

Disadvantages:
- It is extremely volatile and its vapors are irritant and causes respiratory problems.
- It undergo reduction by exposure to daylight hence should be kept in dark, and chemically clean bottle.
- Exposure of acid vapors of osmium tetroxide may cause blindness.
- Poor penetration power limits its use.
- It also interferes with many staining procedures.
- Tissues fixed in this fixative often crumble if embedded in paraffin.

6. Picric acid ($C_6H_2(NO_2)_3OH$)

It is a bright yellow crystalline substance. It is sparingly soluble in water (1%) but more in alcohol and benzene. It is normally used in saturated aqueous solution that is 1%.

Action: It precipitates nucleoproteins and causes much shrinkage, but little hardening. It enhances results with cytoplasmic stains and is a useful constituent of fixatives for glycogen. It forms picrates with proteins, which are soluble in water, hence, picrates are made insoluble by treatment with alcohol.

Disadvantages: It is explosive when dry.

7. Methyl alcohol (CH_3OH) and Ethyl alcohol (C_2H_5OH)

Methanol and ethanol are the only alcohols which have a role as fixative. They are colorless, inflammable liquids which are powerful dehydrating agent and soluble in water.

Action: Methanol and ethanol, mostly alter the structure of protein by disrupting the hydrophobic bonds responsible for tertiary structure of proteins. They can preserves the secondary structure of proteins. Absolute ethanol preserves glycogen. Methacarn a 6:3:1 mixture of absolute methanol, chloroform and glacial acetic acid is used to preserve the helical structure of proteins in myofibrils and collagens.

Disadvantages:
- Absolute alcohol causes distortion of nuclear details and shrinkage of cytoplasm.
- They are highly inflammable and not easily available.
- Methanol is highly toxic in nature.

Compound Fixatives

1. Microanatomical fixatives
- **10% formal saline:** It is mostly used for fixation of material from the central nervous system and general postmortem tissue. The periods of fixation required is 24 hours or longer depending upon the size of the tissue.

Composition of 10% formal saline	
Formaldehyde (40%)	- 100 mL
Sodium chloride	- 8.5 g
Distilled water	- 900 mL

Advantages: This is excellent fixative for postmortem materials and is most widely used fixative. It causes even fixation and produces little shrinkage. It is also used for fixation of large specimens.

Disadvantages: It is a slow fixative and causes considerable shrinkage of tissue. It also causes the formation of formalin pigment in tissues containing blood.

- **10% buffered neutral formalin:** It is used for the preservation and storage of surgical, postmortem and research specimens. The period of fixation is 24 hours or more.

Advantages: Beside advantages of 10% formal saline, it prevents the formation of formalin pigment.

Composition of 10% buffered neutral formalin	
NaH_2PO_4 (anhydrous)	- 3.5 g
Na_2HPO_4 (anhydrous)	- 6.5 g
Formaldehyde (40%)	- 100 mL
Distilled water	- 900 mL

Disadvantages: It is similar to that of formal saline. Formalin pigment is a brown, granular material, extracellular, and birefringent. It is more commonly found in, but not confined to tissues obtained postmortem and is progressive in its deposition and get heavily deposited in tissues after several days. The pigment is formed by the action of acid formalin on blood and it can be avoided by the use of neutral buffered solutions.

Removal of formalin pigments: It can be removed from the sections by treatment with a saturated alcoholic solution of picric acid for 20 minutes. or longer. The general appearance and properties of the formalin pigment are similar to those of malaria pigment.

- **Heidenhain susa fixative:** This is mostly used for biopsies. The period of fixation required is from 3–12 hours.

Composition of Heidenhain Susa fixative	
Mercuric chloride	- 45 g
Sodium chloride	- 5 g
Trichloroacetic acid	- 20 g
Glacial acetic acid	- 40 mL
Formaldehyde (40%)	- 200 mL
Distilled water	- 800 mL

Advantages: It penetrates fast producing good and even fixation, with minimum shrinkage and hardening. It allows brilliant subsequent staining results with sharp nuclear details. Large blocks of fibrous tissue may be sectioned more easily after using this fixative.

Disadvantages: Prolong fixation may cause excessive shrinkage and hardening of the tissue. RBCS are poorly preserved and some cytoplasmic granules get dissolve. It is necessary to treat the tissue with iodine to remove mercury pigment.

Zenker's solution: It is an efficient microanatomical fixative and is used as much for its beneficial effect on staining. Blocks are fixed for 12–24 hours. and are then washed in running water to remove excess of potassium dichromate.

Composition of Zenker's solution	
Mercuric chloride	- 5.0 g
Potassium dichromate	- 2.5 g
Sodium sulfate	- 1.0 g
Distilled water	- 100 mL
Add 5.0 mL glacial acetic acid just before use	

Advantages: It permits excellent staining of nuclei and of connective tissue fibers and is a good routine fixative.

Disadvantages: Penetration power is poor, and prolonged exposure causes brittleness of tissue. After fixation, it requires a post-treatment to remove mercury pigment with iodine. It cannot be used for frozen sections.

- **Helly's fluid (Zenker-Formal):** This is modified Zenker's fluid in which acetic acid is omitted from

Zenker's fluid. It is particularly suitable for use with bone marrow, spleen, lymph glands, pituitary and pancreas, where accurate preservation of cytoplasm as well as nuclei is desired. The period of fixation is from 12–24 hours.

Composition of Helly's fluid
Solution A:
Mercuric chloride	- 5.0 g
Potassium dichromate	- 2.5 g
Sodium sulfate	- 1.0 g
Distilled water	- 100 mL

Solution B:
40% Formaldehyde	- 5.0 mL

Add solution A to B immediately before use

Disadvantages: They are similar to Zenker's fluid.
Removal of mercuric pigments: Fixatives containing mercuric chloride produce a black precipitate of mercury which can be removed by placing sections in 0.5% iodine solution in 70% ethanol for 5–10 min. followed by rinsing in water, decolorization in 5% sodium thiosulfate for 5 to 6 min. and rinsing in water again.

- **Bouin's solution:** This is recommended for the fixation of embryos. The period of fixation required is from 6–24 hours.

Advantages: It penetrates evenly and rapidly and causes little shrinkage. It gives brilliant staining with cytoplasmic stains, glycogen is well preserved but kidney is badly preserved. It is used as micro-anatomical and cytological fixative when demonstration of chromosomes is desirable.

Composition of Bouin's solution
Saturated aqueous picric acid	- 5 mL
Formaldehyde 40%	- 25 mL
Glacial acetic acid	- 5 mL

Disadvantages: It causes partial or complete lysis of red blood cells and collagen fibers may be swollen. It is necessary to remove excess picric acid by washing or by alcohol treatment.

2. Cytological fixatives
   a. Nuclear fixatives
   - **Fleming's fluid:** This fixative is recommended for the preservation of nuclear structures. The period of fixation is from 24–48 hours.

Composition of Fleming's fluid
Chromic acid 1%	- 15 mL
Aq. O_sO_4 2%	- 4 mL
Glacial acetic acid	- 1 mL

Advantages: This fixative is mostly used for nuclear elements especially chromosomes. It is the only fixative, which permanently preserve lipids.
Disadvantages: It has poor penetration power and should be used for small pieces of tissues. The solution deteriorate rapidly and must be prepared immediately before use. The tissue fixed in Fleming's fluid should be washed for 24 hours in running tap water prior to dehydration.
- **Carnoy's fluid:** It is used for fixing chromosomes, lymph glands and urgent biopsies. The period of fixation required from ½ – 3 hours.

Composition of Carnoy's fluid
Absolute alcohol	- 60 mL
Chloroform	- 30 mL
Glacial acetic acid	- 10 mL

Advantages: It is rapidly penetrating and active fixative. Its main use is for the quick fixation of tissues for urgent diagnosis. Glycogen is preserved properly.
Disadvantages: Excessive shrinkage in caused by this solution and it is only suitable for small pieces of tissue. RBCs are hemolyzed.

   b. Cytoplasmic fixatives
   - **Flemings fluid without acetic acid:** It is recommended for mitochondria and the period of fixation is from 24–48 hours. Its formula is similar to that of Flemings fluid without acetic acid, and instead of distilled water 0.75% NaCl is used as solvent. This mixture gives superior preservation than that of Flemings fluid. Its disadvantages are similar to that of Flemings fluid. Helly's fluid and 10% formal saline are also used as cytoplasmic fixatives.
   - **Champy's fluid—formula:** This fixative is unstable, hence should be prepared fresh before use. It penetrates poorly and unevenly. It preserves mitochondria, fat yolk and lipids. Tissue must be washed overnight after fixation.

Composition of Champy's fluid
3 g/dL potassiumdichromate	- 7 mL
1% (v/v) chromic acid	- 7 mL
2g/dL Osmium tetraoxide	- 4 mL

c. Histochemical fixatives
- **Buffer formalin:** It is most common fixative used for histochemical purposes. Immersion in acetone at 0–40°C is widely used for the fixation of tissue in which it is intended to study enzymes.

■ Vapor Fixatives

Vapor fixatives were originally used to retain soluble materials in situ by converting them to an insoluble product before contacting with water or non-aqueous solvents. Various chemicals which act as vapor fixatives include aldehydes (formaldehyde, glutaraldehyde and acrolein), osmium tetroxide, chromyl chloride, ethanol, diethyl pyrocarbonate, benzoquinone, and diacetyl. The most common vapor fixative is formaldehyde, osmium tetroxide and alcohol. The most important application of formaldehyde vapors as fixative at elevated temperatures is convertion of catecholamines and 5-hydroxy-tryptamine in freeze dried tissue to produce fluorescent condensation products. Thus highly reactive vapor fixatives are able to capture and render the insoluble otherwise highly soluble, low molecular weight compounds. Monomeric vapor formaldehyde is obtained from heating paraformaldehyde.

Osmium tetraoxide at 37°C produces a vapor pressure which is sufficient to allow very rapid penetration into freeze-dried blocks of tissue and exposure for 1 hr or less is usually adequate. Ethanol vapors at 60°C has a pronounced denaturing effect on freeze-dried tissues and polysaccharides like glycogen become less soluble.

FIXATION OF SPECIFIC SUBSTANCES

1. Glycogen: A variety of glycogens occur naturally and show different degrees of polymerization. Less highly polymerized glycogens are not well fixed by routine fixatives and diffuse into the fixing fluid. This occurs in cases of glycogen storage disease where glycogen is of lighter type. In contrast, the larger molecules of more highly polymerized glycogens are retained with a wide variety of fixatives as well as alcohol containing reagents. The glycogen is preserved due to trapping in a matrix of fixed protein or due to its covalent binding to proteins.

Use of alcohols, as fixative for glycogen, is extensively practiced. Fixative include a mixture of 96% alcohol saturated with picric acid, 40% formalin and acetic acid. Other fixatives are Rossman's fluid and Gendre's fluid.

Composition of Gendre's fluid

90% Ethanol saturated with picric acid	- 80 mL
40% Formaldehyde	- 15 mL
Glacial acetic acid	- 5 mL
Fixation time is normally for a 4 hours and followed by washing in 80%, 95%, and 100% ethanol	

Composition of Rossman's fluid

100% Ethanol saturated with picric acid	- 90 mL
Neutralized common formalin	- 10 mL
Fixation time 12–24 hrs and wash well in 95% ethanol	

2. Lipids: With standard methods of fixation, lipids are largely lost from tissues during processing. Only osmium tetroxide, and chromic acid fix lipids in the true sense by making them insoluble. Phospholipids are preserved by Baker's fixative and osmium tetroxide for unsaturated lipids. For cryostat sections Elftmann's fluid is used. Fixation time is 3 days at room temperature.

Composition of Elftmann's fluid

Mercuric chloride	: 5 g
Potassium dichromate	: 2.5 g
Water	: 100 mL

3. Proteins: The fixation of tissue proteins by aldehydes mostly takes place by the formation of cross-linkages between various reactive groups in proteins. Most fixatives preserve proteins in 1 to 2 days. Glutaraldehyde fixes proteins very rapidly whereas, formaldehyde requires 24 hours. Osmium tetroxide reacts with proteins by producing cross-links and protein gels. Prolonged exposure to osmium tetroxide may result in protein breakdown.

4. Muco-substances: It includes glucose, starch, and cellulose (homoglycans) and galactose, lactose, etc. (heteroglycans). The later are composed of glycosaminoglycans like keratosulfate and sialoglycans, and glycosaminoglucoronoglycans comprising hyaluronic acid, chondroitin sulfates and heparin. Loss of mucosubstances from tissues may take place during fixation but many fixatives can prevent this.

Like basic lead acetate for acid heteroglycans, 8% lead nitrate with or without 10% formalin for connective tissue glycosaminoglucoronoglycans, formalin for proteoglycans, Carnoy's fluid and formalin alchohol mixture for heteroglycans. The most successful method for preservation of all types of mucin is freeze drying following hot formaldehyde vapors.

5. Nucleic acids and nucleoproteins: They exist in many different states of polymerization and the method of fixation includes changes in their physical state. Formalin is not a good fixative for nucleic acids and nucleoproteins because it blocks a large number of reactive groups reducing their staining properties. Precipitant fixatives like alcohol, acetic acid, and Carnoy's fluid are preferred fixatives. However, prolonged fixation in there fixatives profoundly alter nuclear proteins and extracts RNA and DNA.

6. Biogenic amines: It includes two main groups, like catecholamines, adrenaline and noradrenaline, indo/alkylamines, dopamine, DOPA (dihydroxyphenylalanine), and 5-hydroxytryptamine. Formalin with sodium acetate and potassium dichromate may fix these amines. Other fixatives includes glutaraldehyde (pH7.2–7.4)+1.5% potassium dichromate for noradrenaline and adrenaline. A more effective method of fixing biogenic amines for ultrastructural examination is the use of three stage fixation method. This includes primary fixation in a mixture of 1% glutaraldehyde, 0.4% formaldehyde, sodium chromate and potassium dichromate followed by storage for 18 hours in a mixture of sodium chromate and potassium dichromate, and finally, post fixation in 2% osmium tetroxide, sodium chlorate and potassium dichromate.

7. Enzymes: Enzyme activity is best demonstrated in frozen sections. For paraffin embedding the fixation is carried out in alcohol/acetone at 4°C. This method retained alkaline phosphatase activity. Various fixatives for specific enzyme preservation includes, formalin-sucrose-ammonia and 1–4% glutaraldehyde for cholinesterases, formaldehyde for acid phosphates and formalin + 0.1% chloral hydrate for β-glucuronidase.

Ideally, tissues should be fixed immediately and completely from the living state, but this is not possible in case of human tissues. As most tissues are removed surgically, the organ/tissue is relatively anoxic for some period because of anesthesia and the placement of surgical clamps and ligatures to stop bleeding. Furthermore, when the tissue is placed in fixative, there is a latent period before adequate penetration of the tissue. Anoxic changes occur more rapidly at room temperature than in the cold. Anoxic changes includes:
- Damage to mitochondria within 10 minutes.
- Loss of enzymes within an hour.
- Variation within the tissue as cells in the center of block suffer more anoxia due to delay in penetration of fixative.

ARTEFACTS

Though fixation preserve the tissue in as lifelike sate as possible, but fixation itself may cause certain artefacts. Artefacts are structures or features in tissue that interfere with normal histological examination. These are not always present in normal tissue and can come from outside sources. Artefacts interfere with histology by changing the tissue appearance and hiding structures. These can be divided into two categories:
- **Pre-histology:** These are features and structures that have been introduced prior to the collection of the tissues. A common example of these include ink from tattoos and freckles (melanin) in skin samples.
- **Post-histology:** Artefacts can result from tissue processing. Processing commonly leads to changes like shrinkage, color changes in different tissues types and alterations of the structures in the tissue. The majority of post-histology artefacts can be avoided or removed after being discovered. A common example is mercury pigment left behind after using Zenker's fixative to fix a section.

Artefacts and agonal changes may result in:
- Expansion and shrinkage of tissues.
- Hardening of tissue.
- Movement of unfixed material resulting in false localization of organelle.
- Diffusion of unfixed hemoglobin from RBC to periphery of block.
- Complete diffusion of certain molecules like inorganic ions, cofactors, etc. from the tissue.
- Denaturation of chromogranin releasing biogenic amines and ATP.
- False histochemical reactions due to chemical changes caused by fixation.
- Substances like histidine, tyrosine, mercaptides may get removed during the removal of the excess of fixative after fixation.
- Enzymes may get lost during fixation.
- Prolonged fixation may result in loss of certain water soluble substances.

PRESERVATION AND STORAGE OF TISSUES

Tissues fixed in formalin that are not immediately required for sectioning are often allowed to remain in the charged fixative, sometimes for several years. This results in a progressive impairment of the staining quality, although the use of buffered neutral solutions will return this effect. Another common practice is to use 70% alcohol as a preserving fluid after fixation and washing out of the fixative.

POINTS TO REMEMBER DURING FIXATION OF TISSUES

The following points must be considered before fixing the tissue in appropriate fixative.

- **Choice of fixative:** The choice of fixative depends upon (i) Nature of the tissue, (ii) The diversity of the tissue, (iii) The size of the tissue, (iv) Penetrating power of the fixative and, (v) Stain used for staining of the sections.
- **Size of the tissue:** The size of the tissue is important factor to achieve proper fixation. When fixative has the poor penetration power then use as small piece of tissue as possible. For normal fixation the tissue should not be more than 2–6 µm in thickness.
- **Hardening effect of fixative:** If the fixative have an excessive hardening effect, then do not use that fixative and select a fixative having minimum hardening effect and proper fixing quality. It is always better to fix the tissue in formalin.
- **Volume of fixative:** The volume of fixative directly influences the proper fixation of the tissue. If possible volume of the fixative should be about 30–40 times more than that of the volume of the tissue.
- **Duration of fixation:** Duration of fixation depends upon the (i) Kind of the fixative use, (ii) Rate of penetration of the fixative, (iii) Size and density of the tissue, (iv) Action of fixative on tissues. In any case the tissue must not be allowed to be left in the fixative beyond the necessary time, otherwise, it will lead to the over hardening and distortion of the tissue.

SPECIAL FIXATIVES FOR SPECIAL TISSUE SAMPLES

Special tissue	Fixative used
Biopsies	Tissues for routine processing is placed in 10% formalin. Renal biopsies or tissues for elution microscopy are to be placed in special fixative.
Bone marrows	Obtain a bone marrow kit from histology laboratory. Follow the procedural instructions included in the kit.
Muscle biopsies	Do not place specimen in fixative. If there is any delay, wrap the biopsy gently with gauze pads soaked with physiological saline.
Nerve biopsies	Do not place specimen in fixative. If there is any delay, wrap the biopsy gently with gauze pads soaked with physiological saline.
Skin biopsies	For immunofluorescent studies place tissue immediately into immunofluorescent fixative, i.e. ammonium sulfate fixative.
Testicular biopsies	Fix in Bouin's fixative for 4 hours, remove the specimen and place in 70% alcohol or tissue fixative.
Liver biopsies	For light microscopy, specimen in fixed in 10% buffered formalin within 1 minute. For transmission electron microscopy 1 mm cubes of specimens are fixed immediately in glutaraldehyde with further processing.
Urate crystals (uric acid)	Tissue for crystal identification should be fixed in 95% alcohol or tissue fixative. Special processing is required.
Lymph nodes	Do not place specimen in fixative. If there is any delay, wrap the biopsy gently with gauze pads soaked with normal saline.
Frozen sections	Do not place specimen in any fixative. If there will be a delay due to transportation, place in normal saline.
Hormone receptor assays	Submit specimen in 10% formalin.
Cytogenetic or flow cytometry studies	Special RPMI (RPMI = Roswell Park Memorial Institute) fixative is used. If there is any delay in obtaining RPMI fixative, the specimen may be placed in a sterile container with sterile saline.

EXERCISE

1. What is fixation? Describe various fixatives in detail.
2. Describe various fixatives used in histopathological processing. Explain their mode of action.
3. List considerations when choosing a fixative.
4. Describe ways of classification of fixatives.
5. Define fixatives. Give classification of fixative with example.
6. Write definition and functions of ideal fixative.
7. Discuss properties of various tissue fixatives.
8. List factors that affect quality of fixation.
9. What are common causes of poor tissue fixation?
10. Discuss histological fixatives.
11. Write about micro-anatomical fixatives.
12. What is vapor fixatives?
13. Describe methods of fixation.
14. Discuss tissue fixatives used in histopathology with composition and properties.
15. Write about simple fixatives with their advantages and disadvantages.
16. Discuss formalin as a fixative. Write different types of formalin fixatives.
17. Describe mercuric chloride fixatives. Write composition and disadvantages of Heidenhain Susa fixative, Zenker's solution, and Helly's fluid.
18. Write short notes on nuclear fixatives.
19. Describe the process of preservation and storage of tissues.
20. Describe post-fixation procedures.
21. Write properties, action and disadvantages of following fixatives:
    i. Formaldehyde
    ii. Mercuric chloride
    iii. Potassium dichromate
    iv. Osmium tetroxide
22. Describe fixation artefacts (formalin pigment, mercury pigment, chrome pigment), and method of removal.
23. What are artefacts ? Give disadvantages of formation of artefacts during fixation.
24. Describe method of fixation of testicular biopsies and lymph node.

OBJECTIVE QUESTIONS

1. Destruction of tissue by intracellular enzymes is called _____.
    a. Autolysis
    b. Lipolysis
    c. Pyrolysis
    d. None

2. The cells and tissues are preserved in a close a life like state by _____.
    a. Dehydration
    b. Clearing
    c. Fixation
    d. Infiltration

3. Zenker's fixative is a _____.
    a. Simple fixative
    b. Compound fixative
    c. None
    d. Both

4. Fleming's fluid is an example of _____.
    a. Simple fixative
    b. Compound fixative
    c. Micro-anatomical fixative
    d. Cytological fixative

5. Formaldehyde is commercially available as
    a. 30% formalin
    b. 10% formalin
    c. 90% formalin
    d. 40% formalin

6. _____ is used as fixative for enzymes to be studies by electron microscopy.
    a. Glutaraldehyde
    b. Formaldehyde
    c. Acetaldehyde
    d. Benzaldehyde

7. _____ is an example of mercuric chloride fixative.
    a. Neutral formalin
    b. Helly's fixative
    c. Bouin's fluid
    d. Flemming's fluid

8. Heidenhain's Susa fixative contain _____ as main fixative.
    a. HCHO
    b. CH_3OH
    c. O_sO_4
    d. $HgCl_2$

9. The fixative recommended for the preservation of nuclear structure is _____.
   a. Champy's fluid
   b. Helly's fixative
   c. Bouin's fluid
   d. Flemming's fluid

10. The most commonly used metallic ion fixative is _____.
    a. HCHO
    b. $K_2Cr_2O_7$
    c. O_sO_4
    d. $HgCl_2$

11. In Carnoy's fluid _____ is used as fixing agent.
    a. CH_3OH
    b. $K_2Cr_2O_7$
    c. O_sO_4
    d. $HgCl_2$

12. Fixative containing potassium dichromate is _____.
    a. Champy's fluid
    b. Zenker's fixative
    c. Bouin's fluid
    d. Formal saline

13. In 10% buffered neutral formalin _____ buffer is used.
    a. Phosphate buffer
    b. Acetate buffer
    c. Ammonia buffer
    d. Citrate buffer

14. Formalin produces acid-formalin-hematin pigment in tissues containing _____.
    a. Blood
    b. Sugar
    c. Protein
    d. Lipid

15. For hormone receptor assay submit the specimen in _____.
    a. 95% alcohol
    b. 10% formalin
    c. RPMI fixation
    d. 10% glutaraldehyde

16. _____ is not used as vapor fixative.
    a. Formalin
    b. Acraline
    c. 10% formalin
    d. None

17. Well known fixative for glycogen is
    a. Alcohol
    b. Aldehyde
    c. Mercuric salt
    d. None

18. Zenker's fixative may produce a brown to black granular deposit which gets uniformly distributed throughout the tissue, called as _____ pigments.
    a. Formalin
    b. Mercuric
    c. Hematin
    d. Bile

19. Formalin pigments are removed from sections by treatment with _____.
    a. Alcoholic solution of picric acid
    b. Acidic solution of picric acid
    c. Neutral solution of picric acid
    d. Alkaline solution of picric acid

20. Mercuric pigments are removed by treating sections with _____ solution.
    a. Iodine
    b. Picric acid
    c. Chlorine
    d. Formalin

21. Rossman's fluid is used for fixation of _____
    a. Glycogen
    b. Protein
    c. Lipids
    d. Nucleic acid

22. Osmium tetroxide fix _____ in true sense by making them insoluble
    a. Protein
    b. Lipids
    c. Nucleic acid
    d. All

23. Methacarn is a mixture of absolute methanol, chloroform and _____.
    a. Glacial acetic acid
    b. Butyric acid
    c. Carbonic acid
    d. Benzene

ANSWERS

1-a, 2-c, 3-b, 4-d, 5-d, 6-a, 7-b, 8-d, 9-d, 10-c, 11-a, 12-a, 13-a, 14-a, 15-b, 16-d, 17-a, 18-b, 19-a, 20-a, 21-a, 22-a, 23-a.

CHAPTER 5

Decalcification

INTRODUCTION

Tissues such as bones, teeth, nails, cornified tissues are hard and hence their sections are difficult to obtain. These tissues are hard due to large deposits of calcium, which create problems in section cutting. In pathological conditions, calcium deposits are also found in varying amounts in other tissues, notably those involved in tuberculous or cancerous changes. Calcium deposits are also present in large blood vessels like the aorta of elderly people.

Hence, it is necessary to remove the calcium from the hard tissues and thus make the tissue soft so that it is easy to cut thin sections of them. This is carried out by treatment with reagents which reacts with calcium to remove it by making it soluble. Such reagents are called as decalcifying agents.

The choice of the decalcifying agents depends upon three factors: The urgency of the case, the degree of calcium deposition, and the subsequent staining techniques used.

PROPERTIES OF DECALCIFYING AGENTS

An ideal decalcifying agent should have following properties:
- It should completely remove the calcium salts.
- It should not distort the cells and connective tissue.
- It should not have harmful effects on staining reactions.

The speed of the decalcification depends upon the strength, temperature and volume of the decalcifying solution in relation to the size and consistency of the tissue undergoing decalcification. An increase in the concentration of decalcifying agent or the temperature of decalcification can markedly decrease the time required.

TECHNIQUE OF DECALCIFICATION

It involves the following steps:
- Selection of tissue
- Fixation
- Decalcification
- Acid neutralization
- Washing

■ Selection of Tissue

The specimen submitted to the pathological laboratory may include bone biopsy, curettings, larger specimens, hard tissues like teeth, calcified tissues, etc.

Bone: Bone biopsy specimens vary from very small "chips" to a needle trephine to full resections of major bones or whole limb amputations. Larger specimens are generally subjected to radiography so that the area of interest can be isolated from the bulk of the specimen.

Curettings and small biopsies of bone often arrive at the laboratory in a minimal amount of fixative. They should be immediately transferred to fresh fixative and a volume ratio of about 20:1 is maintained to avoid the histological artefacts which may result from delayed fixation. The samples should be fixed for a minimum of 12–16 hours (or longer) depending upon the density of the tissue. Longer specimens, mostly include ribs, whole or parts of digits and resected femoral heads. When a specimen of bone containing the tumor is received, then it is essential to include all of the resection margins in the block to ensure that there has been complete excision of the tumor.

Similarly, in case of specimens submitted for investigation of fracture, the block must include tissue from the fracture site. As it is not possible to process the specimens immediately after receiving, they should be wrapped thoroughly and then kept in the refrigerator or cold room to avoid pre-fixation artifacts and desiccation. The specimen should be X-rayed or radiographed as soon as possible to determine the area of pathological interest and then cut into more manageable pieces using either bandsaw or handsaw. These smaller samples are then fixed in suitable fixative.

Teeth: Blocks of teeth for sectioning are usually best taken when the specimen is either completely or partially decalcified. They may then be selected with a sharp knife, thereby causing a minimum of damage and distortion of the tissue.

Calcified tissues: Calcified tissue blocks are selected from fixed soft tissue containing calcified area using a sharp knife. The selected tissue blocks should not exceed 5 mm in thickness.

■ Fixation

The choice of fixative depends upon the purpose for which it is required. For most purposes 10% phosphate buffer formalin is adequate. Mercuric chloride containing fixatives such as Zenker's or Heidenhain's Susa may give improved cellular detail. But samples fixed in mercuric chloride solutions cannot be analyzed radiographically to determine the endpoint of decalcification, due to the presence of the radio-opaque metal.

Fixation using 70% ethanol is essential for demonstration of uric acid crystals. It is very important that the fixation should be thorough before processing for decalcification. The duration of fixation depends to a large extent on the size and density of the tissue block. Dense cortical bone containing specimens requires longer time for fixation whereas porous cancellous bone samples require less time for fixation. It is advisable to restrict blocks to a thickness of approximately 3 mm, and should not be thicker than 5 mm for routine diagnostic work.

■ Decalcification

The process of decalcification involves following steps:
- The selected tissue block is suspended in decalcifying solution by means of a waxed thread. The volume of the decalcifying fluid should be approximately 50–100 times the volume of the tissue.
- The progress of the decalcification should be tested at regular intervals, usually daily.
- When the decalcification is complete the tissue is transferred directly to 70% alcohol and given several changes over 8–12 hours. This not only effectively washes out the acid, but also established the first stage of dehydration.
- The tissue is then completely dehydrated and processed according to the required embedding technique.

TESTS FOR COMPLETION OF DECALCIFICATION

The tissues should not be exposed to decalcifying fluids for longer than necessary for complete removal of calcium. Prolonged immersion beyond this stage will result in deterioration of cell and tissue morphology and quality of subsequent staining reactions. The progress of decalcification and completion can be assessed by (i) X-ray method, (ii) Chemical method, (iii) Physical method.

■ X-ray Method

It is the most satisfactory method, depending upon the availability of the facilities. But this method cannot be used when the material is fixed in mercuric chloride because this fixative renders the tissue radio-opaque. Radiographs are useful not only for determining the extent of mineralization in a bone sample, but also for the demonstration of small deposits of calcification in other tissues, as well as identifying foreign bodies, such as prosthesis and fragments of glass and metal in soft tissue samples.

■ Chemical Method

In the absence of X-ray examination, chemical test is used to detect the end point of decalcification. It involves following steps:
- About 5 mL of used decalcifying fluid is taken into a clean test tube and to it a small piece of litmus paper is added.
- Strong ammonia is added drop by drop with agitation to the tube until the litmus paper just turns blue indicating alkalinity.
- If the solution becomes turbid at this stage calcium is present in considerable amounts and tissue should be transferred to the fresh decalcifying fluid.
- If the solution remains clear then add 0.5 mL of saturated aqueous ammonium oxalate, mix and keep for 30 minutes. Any turbidity indicates the presence of trace amount of calcium, thus retreatment of tissue with fresh decalcifying fluid is necessary.
- If the solution remains clear, decalcification is completed, then proceed for the next step.

■ Physical Method

This is a very rough way of detection and completion of decalcification. It involves observation of cessation of gas bubble formation on the surface of the bone. When the decalcification is completed the tissue become soft, can easily bend, squeeze or trimmed and a sharp needle can easily penetrate through it. But these methods are not satisfactory.

DECALCIFYING AGENTS

The various decalcifying agents which can be used are
- Dilute mineral acids
- Ion exchange resins
- Chelating agents
- Electrolytic decalcification.

Dilute Mineral Acids

The most common method of decalcification is by dissolving the calcium salts in acid solutions. Various acids, which can be used for decalcification, are nitric acid, formic acid, and trichloroacetic acid.

a. **Formic acid (HCOOH):** It is widely used as decalcifying agent. It is much slower than nitric acid. It can be used as 5-10% aqueous solution with additives like formalin or a buffer. Formaldehyde is added to effect simultaneous fixation and decalcification. Time necessary for decalcification is 2-7 days.

Formic acid solution	
Formic acid	- 5 mL
Distilled water	- 90 mL
Formaldehyde (40%)	- 5 mL

Advantages: It permits excellent staining results and is used as a best decalcifying agent for routine work.

Disadvantages:
- It is not suitable for urgent surgical specimens.
- It is not recommended for dense cortical bone.
- It also causes interference in the chemical test used to control the degree of decalcification.

b. **Nitric acid (HNO_3):** It can be used as a simple aqueous solution of 5-10%. It requires 24-48 hours for decalcification.

Advantages: It is a rapid decalcifying solution which causes very little hydrolysis, provided that the tissue is not allowed to immerse in it beyond the stage of decalcification. It results in good subsequent staining. It is used for urgent biopsy specimens.

Nitric acid solution	
Nitric acid	- 5–10 mL
Distilled water	- 100 mL

Disadvantages:
- Decalcification longer than 24-48 hours causes serious deterioration of sustainability.
- Nitric acid slowly becomes yellowish due to formation of nitrous acid which gives yellowish color to tissue. It can be prevented by adding 1% urea.
- This solution is not suitable for heavily mineralized and cortical bone.

c. **Perani's fluid:** A less vigorous but useful decalcifying solution for routine purposes is Pereni's fluid. It require 2-10 days for decalcification. When fresh it is yellow, but rapidly changes to violet color.

Advantages: It does not cause hardening of tissue. It can be used as a softening agent before dehydration. It can also be used as fixative which preserve cellular components and results in good staining.

Pereni's fluid	
Nitric acid (10%) aq. Sol	- 40 mL
Absolute ethyl alcohol	- 30 mL
Chromic acid (0.5%) aq. Sol	- 30 mL

Disadvantages: It is a slow decalcifying agent for dense bone. It requires a modified test for detection and completion of decalcifications.

d. **Ebner's Fluid:** It is mostly used for decalcification of teeth, which requires 3-5 days.

Advantages: It is fairly rapid decalcifying solution and subsequent staining results are good. The excess of acid is removed by several changes of 90% alcohol for 24 hours.

Disadvantages: Nuclear staining is not as good as that obtained after formic acid decalcifications.

Ebner's fluid	
Saturated solution of sodium chloride	- 50 mL
Distilled water	- 50 mL
Hydrochloric acid	- 8 mL

e. **Trichloroacetic acid:** It has been used as a decalcifying agent for many years and is recommended for the decalcification of teeth. A 5% aq. solution of trichloroacetic acid is quicker in action than the same concentration of formic acid. It requires 4-5 days for decalcifications.

Trichloroacetic acid	
Trichloroacetic acid	- 5 g
10% formal saline	- 95 mL

Advantages: It permits good nuclear staining. The excess acid is removed by washing in 90% alcohol.
Disadvantages: It is a slow decalcifying solution and is not recommended for dense bone.

- **Citrate–Citric acid buffer (pH 4.5):** It is recommended when speed is not an important factor, because time required is 6 days.

> **Citrate – Citric acid buffer**
>
> Citric acid (7%)   - 5 mL
> Ammonium citrate (7.4%)   - 95 mL
> Zinc sulfate (1%)   - 0.2 mL
> Chloroform (preservative) few drops

Advantages: It does not damage cells or tissue constituents and permits excellent staining results.
Disadvantages: It is too slow for routine work.

Ion Exchange Resins

The principle of the method is that the calcium ions are removed from the solution by the action exchange resins, thereby increasing the rate of solubility of the calcium from the tissue. But the use of resin does not increase the rate of decalcification. A layer of resin, approximately 13 mm thick is spread at the bottom of the vessel and the specimen is allowed to rest on it. The decalcifying solution is added, the volume of the solution should be 20-30 times that of the tissue. The end point is determined by radio graphical examination. Commonly used resin is ammonium salt of sufonated polystyrene. After use resin is regenerated by washing twice with N/10 hydrochloric acid followed by washing with distilled water thrice.

The use of ion exchange resins is limited to decalcifying solutions having non mineral acid as an active constituent, mostly formic acid.

Chelating Agents

This is a very slow decalcifying solution recommended only for detailed microscopical studies where time is not an important factor. It is not suitable for urgent specimens. The most widely used chelating agent is ethylenediamine tetra-acetic acid (EDTA). EDTA is a white crystalline powder, soluble in water up to 20%. As decalcifying agent combines with calcium ions to form soluble, non-ionized compound. Deposites of iron and other metals may also be removed by EDTA. The solution is effective at neutral pH, hence staining is excellent and superior than other agents.

> **Neutral EDTA Solution**
>
> EDTA (Disodium salt)   - 5.5 gm
> 10 % Neutral formalin - 100 mL

Advantages: Tissue is not hardened, on the other hand the tissue can be easily cut. It can be used for bones, teeth or any calcified tissue. The decalcification requires 4-40 days. For checking of completion of decalcification X-ray method is more reliable when EDTA is used.

Electrolytic Decalcifications

It is based on a simple electroplating device in which the bone is attached to the anode and a current is passed through an electrolytic solution (mostly hydrochloric acid/ formic acid), forcing the calcium ions to migrate towards the cathode. The temperature should be 30-45°C.
Disadvantages: During operation heat is liberated which increases the rate of decalcification, but on the other hand, this heat causes burning of tissues, destruction or damage of tissue, swelling and hydrolysis of the tissues. Hence, this method is not used for decalcifications.

TREATMENT AFTER DECALCIFICATION

Neutralization: Various neutralizing treatment can be used to neutralize the acid after acid decalcification. After decalcification, the excess of acid from the surface of the tissue blocks is removed by blotting or quickly rinsing in tap water before transferring to the secondary fixative or a first dehydrating agent. Immersion in a 6% aqueous sodium sulfate or 1% aqueous sodium bicarbonate for a few hours will remove acid from the tissue. This avoids the contamination of the next fluid. After neutralization, tissue can be stored in 70% alcohol.

Washing: Thorough washing of the tissue before processing is essential to remove acid (or alkali used for neutralization) which would otherwise interfere with staining. Decalcified tissues for frozen sectioning should be thoroughly washed with water or stored in formal saline before being frozen.

SURFACE DECALCIFICATION

Surface decalcification is required when incompletely decalcified paraffin blocks or paraffin blocks of tissues containing unsuspected mineral deposits prevent the production of satisfactory sections.

In surface decalcification, rough trimming or cutting with a knife or needle exposes the surface of the tissue. The block is then placed in an acid solution (1% hydrochloric acid or 10% formic acid) for about 15-60 minutes. so that the exposed surface comes in contact with the acid solution. These progressive decalcifications do not have an adverse effect on the subsequent staining. After decalcification the block should be washed briefly in water, dried and properly oriented in the microtome for sectioning.

The advantages of surface decalcification is that, as only the surface layer of the tissue is treated, the process is completed in a relatively short time and artefacts due to over-decalcification can be avoided. This form of decalcification is best suited to material containing small spicules of mineralization.

FACTORS AFFECTING THE RATE OF DECALCIFICATION

There are several factors relating to strong acid/chelating agent mixtures which can be varied to either increase or decrease the rate at which specimens are decalcified.

Concentration of acid: As the concentration of the acid component increases, the speed of decalcification also increases. However, there is a parallel increase in the degree of tissue damage like hydrolysis of proteins. Conversely, decalcification is slowed with a reduction in the acid concentration. The effect varies between particular species of acids, but, in general, mineral acids are most effective at a concentration of around 10%.

Reaction temperature: An increase in temperature accelerates decalcification and a decrease slows it down, However, if the temperature is too high, the tissue can be damaged and if it is too low, decalcification will not proceed at a satisfactory rate. A suitable temperature range is 20-25°C. If necessary specimens can be stored at 4°C to prevent over-decalcification.

Agitation: Mechanical agitation probably has minimal effect on promoting the chemical exchanges between bone and fluid unless the specimens are kept on a rolling device such as a blood tube mixer.

Suspension: It is very important that all the surfaces of the tissue receive adequate exposure to the decalcifying fluid, especially if flat slices of tissue are to be treated. In order to achieve this, it may be necessary to suspend the tissue in the fluid or place some absorbent material on the bottom of the specimen container.

TIPS FOR PROPER DECALCIFICATION

The first rule: Specimens must be fixed before exposure to an acid solution. If a combination of fixative/decalcifying solution is used, the specimen should be at least partially fixed first.

The second rule: Specimens must be washed in running water before and after exposure to acid solutions, especially hydrochloric acid. The combination of formalin and hydrochloric acid can create the formation of bis-chloromethyl ether which is a known carcinogen.

- Suspend the specimen so it is not in contact with any of the surfaces of the container. This allows exposure to all of the specimen surfaces and allows the precipitated calcium salts to sink to the bottom of the container.
- Use either X-ray or chemical end-point determination techniques. Do not use probes, needles, scalpels or bending. This will cause physical damage to the specimen.
- Small specimens should not be left in the solution overnight. If decalcification is incomplete, wash it in water and return it to fixative. Wash again before returning to the decalcification solution to complete the process.
- Consider extending processing times for large specimens.
- Embed decalcified bone specimens in "hard" paraffin for additional support during microtomy.
- Embed the harder cortical bone so that it is the last surface to be sectioned and at an angle so that the knife does not contact the entire surface at once.
- Use a sharp knife or well supported disposable blade. A heavy duty blade might be necessary.
- Soak difficult specimens briefly in ice water.
- If decalcification was incomplete, surface decalcification techniques may be used. Be certain to rinse the block before it is placed in the microtome.
- Remember that bone has all of the same tissue elements as any other tissue. In order to demonstrate them effectively the specimen must be well fixed and carefully monitored.

EXERCISE

1. Define decalcification. What is the purpose of decalcification?
2. Describe selection of tissue and fixation requirements for decalcification.
3. What is decalcifying agents? What is the criteria for selecting a good decalcifying agent?
4. List criteria for selecting a decalcifying agent.
5. Describe chemical method of decalcification.
6. Describe steps of decalcification.
7. Describe the process of decalcification.
8. Give X-ray method of assessing completion of decalcification.

9. Describe methods of assessing completion of decalcification.
10. What is decalcification? Mention indications and methods of assessment of decalcification.
11. Enlist various decalcifying agents. Write advantages and disadvantages of nitric acid.
12. Give composition, action, advantages and disadvantages of various decalcifying agents.
13. Describe in brief different methods of decalcification.
14. Write a note on decalcifying agents ion exchange resin and EDTA.
15. What is electrolytic decalcification?
16. State purpose of surface decalcification. How is it done?
17. Write various points to be remembered during the process of decalcification.
18. Describe various factors affecting rate of decalcification.

OBJECTIVE QUESTIONS

1. Decalcification is the process of removal of _____ from the hard tissue.
   a. Magnesium
   b. Calcium
   c. Sodium
   d. Potassium

2. An increase in concentration of acid _____ the rate of decalcification.
   a. Decreases
   b. Increases
   c. Do not affect
   d. None

3. Rate of decalcification _____ with increase in temperature.
   a. Increases
   b. Decreases
   c. Do not affect
   d. None

4. _____ is the most accurate method of determining the extent of mineralization in hard specimen.
   a. Chemical method
   b. X-ray
   c. Physical method
   d. All

5. Saturated solution of _____ is used to determine end point of decalcification.
   a. Ammonium chloride
   b. Ammonium hydroxide
   c. Ammonium oxalate
   d. Ammonium acetate

6. Samples fixed in _____ solutions cannot be analyzed radiographically to determine the end point of decalcification.
   a. Alcohol
   b. Picric acid
   c. Formalin
   d. Mercuric

7. Generally, the thickness of the blocks used for decalcification ranges from
   a. 3–5 mm
   b. 5–8 mm
   c. 8–10 mm
   d. 10–15 mm

8. Widely used decalcifying agent is _____.
   a. EDTA
   b. Picric acid
   c. Formic acid
   d. TCA

9. Incompletely decalcified paraffin blocks which prevent the production of good section require _____.
   a. Surface decalcification
   b. Electrolytic decalcification
   c. Microwave decalcification
   d. Ultrasonic decalcification

ANSWERS

1-b, 2-b, 3-a, 4-b, 5-c, 6-d, 7-a, 8-c, 9-a.

CHAPTER 6

Tissue Processing

PRINCIPLE OF TISSUE PROCESSING

Tissue processing is concerned with the diffusion of various substances into and out of stabilized porous tissues. The diffusion process result from the thermodynamic tendency of processing reagents to equalize concentrations inside and outside blocks of tissue, thus generally conforming to "Fick's law" the rate of solution diffusion through tissues is proportional to the concentration gradient (the difference between the concentrations of the fluids inside and outside the tissue) as a multiple of temperature dependent constants for specific substances. Thus, significant variables in tissue processing are the operating conditions, particularly temperature, the characteristics and concentrations of the reagents and the properties of tissues.

During tissue processing, the tissue is subjected to a number of chemical reagents so that it becomes sufficiently hard to cut into thin slices.

■ Steps of Tissue Processing

The tissue processing using paraffin wax involves following steps:
- Selection and labeling of tissues
- Completion of fixation before processing
- Post-fixation procedures
- Dehydration
- Clearing
- Impregnation and infiltration
- Embedding.

SELECTION AND LABELING OF TISSUES

Following fixation, pieces of tissue, for the histological examination are selected from the gross specimen. A brief description of the nature of the tissue and the site of origin should be recorded.

The introduction of plastic embedding cassettes has greatly facilitated the processing of tissue and reduces the risk of possible error. When cassettes are not used, a small cardboard ticket complete with the number identifying the block is written in waterproof ink and accompany the specimen throughout its processing schedule.

COMPLETION OF FIXATION BEFORE PROCESSING

Tissues should be fixed before processing is initiated. Poorly fixed tissues are inadequately protected against the physical and chemical rigours of processing. Strategies commonly employed to ensure complete fixation of tissues include:
- Continuing fixation on tissue processor with one or more changes of the routine fixative, often at elevated temperature of 40–60°C.
- Secondary fixation of tissues in formal sublimate on the tissue processor, or in alcoholic fixative which will complete fixation whilst initiating dehydration.
- Fixing in buffered phenol-formaldehyde pH 7.0 and pH 5.5 sequence at 40°C.
- Microwave irradiation of biopsy specimens in normal saline.

POST-FIXATION PROCEDURES

On completion of fixation, tissues fixed in certain reagents must undergo special treatment.
- **Fixatives containing dichromate and chromium trioxide:** Dichromates and chromium trioxide are reduced to insoluble green-brown chromic oxide in the higher alcohols and in dioxane. Tissues must be washed for 8–12 hours in running water before transferring to 60–70% ethanol or dioxane.
- **Fixatives containing phosphate:** Phosphate salts precipitate in alcoholic solutions stronger than 70%

ethanol, dimethoxy propane, and diethoxy propane. If they are deposited within tissues the precipitate can cause sectioning difficulties. Tissues are rinsed free of fixative with water and processing is initiated in 60–70% ethanol.
- **Fixatives containing picric acid**: Tissues fixed in non-alcoholic picric acid-based fixatives are washed in repeated 1–3 hourly changes of 50–70% ethanol until the supernatant is faintly yellowish or clear. This may take 2–3 days. Specimens fixed in alcoholic picric acid fluids are washed in 80%–90% ethanol, as anhydrous conditions must be maintained. Picric acid retained in tissues can impede wax infiltration and exacerbate static electrification of ribbons during sectioning. It also has an adverse effect on stored wax embedded tissues.
- **Fixatives containing urea:** Tissues fixed in urea containing fluids are washed overnight before transfer to 4% formaldehyde solution for storage. Urea complexes with formaldehyde to form insoluble urea-polymer pigments.
- **Specific fixative requirements:** Carnoy fixed tissues are near-anhydrous and are placed directly in absolute ethanol or in alcohol-transition solvent. Heidenhain's SUSA fixed tissues are transferred directly to 95% ethanol, as trichloroacetic acid fixed collagen swells in aqueous solutions. Tissues fixed in osmium tetroxide-based fixatives are washed for 5 hours in running water and dehydration initiated in 30% ethanol. Osmium tetroxide is reduced to black osmium in ethanol.

DEHYDRATION

The aim of tissue processing is to embed the tissue in a solid medium firm enough to support the tissue and give it sufficient rigidity to enable thin sections to be cut. The most satisfactory embedding medium for routine histology is paraffin wax. It is essential that the embedding medium thoroughly permeates the tissue in fluid form and then solidifies with little damage to the tissue. The tissue is mostly fixed in aqueous fixative and paraffin wax cannot penetrate tissues in the presence of water, hence dehydration of the tissue is an essential step. This is carried out by immersing the tissue in some dehydrating agent.

Numerous dehydrating agents are available and are used in a series of increasing strength, beginning by immersing the tissue in, lower grade and then successively in higher grades. Example first in 70% alcohol, progressing through 95% and finally several changes in absolute alcohol. For delicate tissue dehydration is started with 30% alcohol.

The use of successive higher grades of dehydrating agent is essential to prevent the distortion caused by direct transfer of the tissue from aqueous fixative to absolute alcohol.

In practice, dehydration is carried out either in stoppered glass jars or in tissue processing machines. The various dehydrating fluids are ethanol, denatured alcohol, methanol, isopropyl alcohol, acetone, dioxane, etc.

■ Dehydrating Agents

Alcohols

Beside acting as dehydrant alcohols also act as secondary coagulant fixative during tissue processing.
a. **Ethanol/Ethyl alcohol ($CH_3 CH_2 OH$):** It is most commonly used dehydrating agent. It is a clear liquid, which is inflammable with pleasant odor. It is hydrophilic and therefore miscible with water in all volumes as well as with many organic solvents. It is supplied as 99.85% ethanol (absolute ethanol, high grade or standard grade) or methylated spirit which is 99.85% ethanol denatured with 2% methanol. For dehydration successive or progressive grades of alcohol is used. The dehydrating grade is determined by the nature of fixative in which tissue is fixed. If the fixative do not contain water, then tissue can be directly dehydrated with grade having the same percentage of alcohol as that of the fixative, for example if the fixative has 80% alcohol, then dehydration can be started with 80% alcohol. But if the fixative is prepared in water then dehydration is started with 30–50% alcohol.

Sl. No.	Grade of Alcohol	Time (Hours)
1.	80% Alcohol	1 hour
2.	90% Alcohol	1 hour
3.	90% Alcohol	1 hour
4.	100% Alcohol	1 hour
5.	100% Alcohol	1 hour
6.	100% Alcohol	1 hour

Disadvantages: Due to the high excise duty, it is too expensive for dehydration purposes.
b. **Denatured Alcohol/methylated spirit:** This has same physical characteristics as ethanol, but has a more pronounced odor. It consists of ethanol to which small amount of methanol is added to make the fluid unfit for consumption. The strength is normally quoted as 64, 66 or 74 over proof (OP) spirit, the diluent being water. A proof spirit is the standard and is referred to as 100°. A spirit stated as 70° would therefore be 30° UP (under proof 100°–70°). A spirit stated 160° would be 60°OP (over proof 100° + 60°). 95% alcohol is equivalent to 60°OP. The period required for dehydration may be reduced by processing at 37°C instead of room temperature.

c. **Isopropyl alcohol or 2-Propanol (CH$_3$-CHOH-CH$_3$):** It was first suggested as a substitute of ethanol. It is a universal solvent available as 99.8% (absolute) isopropanol. It is slightly slower in action and not as hygroscopic as ethanol, but a far superior lipid solvent. Isopropanol is completely miscible with water and most organic solvents and is fully miscible with melted paraffin wax. Isopropanol shrinks and hardens tissues less than ethanol and is used to dehydrate hard, dense tissue, which can remain in the solvent for extended period without harm. To minimize shrinkage, fixed tissues are transferred via 60–70% isopropanol to absolute isopropanol. It is used as a transition solvent in microwave stimulated processing.

Disadvantage: It only dissolves nitrocellulose. It cannot be used as a dehydrant in alcohol-ether-celloidin technique.

Ketones

Acetone (CH$_3$COCH$_3$): It is a clear, colorless, inflammable liquid with a characteristic pungent odor, miscible with water, ethanol and most organic solvents. It is more volatile than most commonly used dehydrating agents and is more rapid in action than ethanol or methanol. It is widely used as a routine dehydrant in automated processing schedule, due to its volatile, inflammable nature and because of its hardening effect. When speed is essential acetone is a suitable dehydrant in manual processing techniques, rapidly removed by most clearing agents. Acetone has a greater solvent action than ethanol and methanol on lipids. Due to its inflammability and volatility dehydration must be carried out quickly following successive grades of acetone, i.e. 7%, 10%, 15%. 20% 25%, 30%, 40%, 50%, 60%, 70%, 90%, absolute acetone.

Disadvantages: Prolonged treatment with acetone causes brittleness of tissue, which causes difficulty in section cutting.

Glycol Ethers

i. **Dioxane (diethylene dioxide):** It is a unique reagent which has the unusual property of being miscible with both water and molten paraffin wax. It has advantages that it has no drastic effect on the tissue, it penetrates the tissue rapidly and does not make the tissue brittle.

Disadvantages: The most important disadvantage is that, it is toxic, hygroscopic and causes shrinkage of the tissue. Its use requires carefully controlled conditions.

ii. **2-Ethoxyethanol (ethylene glycol monoethyl ether, cellosolve or oxitol):** It is used as a dehydrant preceding polyester wax embedding, for dehydration following dioxane-based fixation of hard animal tissues, and in the agar-ester wax double embedding technique. Ethoxyethanol is a colorless, nearly odorless flammable liquid, strongly hygroscopic, miscible with water and most organic solvents. Cellosolve dissolves nitrocellulose and tends to decompose on exposure to sunlight. It is rapid but non-hardening in action, and tissues can remain in it for years. To avoid severe shrinkage, tissues are transferred from aqueous fixative or washing via 60–70% ethanol into full strength cellosolve.

iii. **Polyethylene glycols (PEG):** They are water miscible polymers used to dehydrate and embed substances labile to the solvents and heat of the paraffin wax method. They are clear, viscous, slightly hygroscopic liquids or solids of low toxicity. Polyethylene glycols are miscible with most organic solvents and dissolve nitrocellulose. Dehydration is initiated in the low molecular weight liquid glycols. Tissues pass through glycols of increasing molecular weight and viscosity, and are finally embedded in a high molecular weight PEG which is solid at room temperature. Polyethylene glycol used for dehydration can be regenerated by heating at 104°C for 24 hours.

■ Test For Completion of Dehydration

To ensure complete dehydration anhydrous copper sulfate test is usually carried out. A small amount of anhydrous copper sulfate is added in final alcohol grade. If it turns blue, it indicates incomplete dehydration and thus few changes has to be given in fresh absolute alcohol. If the copper sulfate does not change to blue, it indicates complete dehydration and proceed for the next stage of clearing (Fig. 6.1).

■ Precaution During Dehydration

- Dehydration should be carried out in tightly closed containers to avoid evaporation of alcohol or entry of humidity.
- Earlier grades of alcohol should be completely drained off before putting the tissue in the next higher grade of alcohol. This can be done by keeping the tissue on blotting paper for a few seconds.
- The amount of alcohol used in dehydration should be sufficient enough to completely immerse the tissue in it.

Keep 10 mm layer of anhydrous copper sulfate at the bottom of the last jar of absolute alcohol as an indicator of water.

CLEARING

The process of dehydration leads to the saturation of tissue with alcohol. The next step is the impregnation of tissue with paraffin wax to make it firm for the purpose of section cutting. This means that paraffin has to remove the alcohol from the tissue to take its place. However, the diffusion of

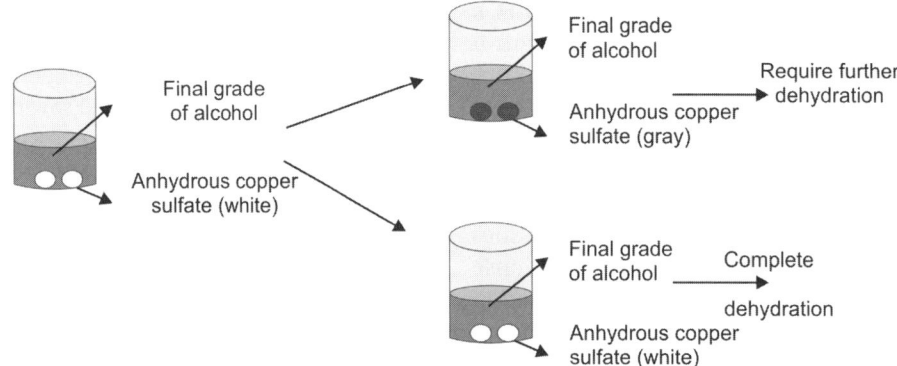

Fig. 6.1: Test for completion of dehydration

paraffin into the tissue is not possible because paraffin is immiscible with alcohol. Hence, after the dehydration, tissue has to pass through an intermediate step, in which it is placed in a reagent which is miscible with alcohol as well as paraffin. This intermediate step is called as "**Clearing**" or "**Dealcoholization**" and the agents used are called as "**Clearing Agents**".

This step is called clearing because most of the reagents used for this purpose raise the refractive index of tissue rendering it more or less transparent.

Criteria for selection of suitable clearing agents are:
- Speed of removal of alcohol
- Types of tissue processed
- Processing conditions like temperature, pressure and vacuum
- Ease of removal of molten impregnating medium
- Gentleness towards tissue
- Flammability
- Toxicity
- Cost

Most clearing agents are inflammable liquids, which warrant considerable caution during processing. The boiling point of the clearing agent gives an indication of its speed of removal by molten paraffin wax. Fluids with a low boiling point can easily removed more rapidly than fluids with high boiling point. Similarly viscosity plays important role in determining the speed of penetration of the clearing agent.

Clearing agent brings about infiltration of paraffin into the tissue and also it make them transparent. If turbidity appears on keeping the tissue in clearing agent, it indicates that tissue is not perfectly dehydrated. In such condition tissue should be removed from clearing agent and placed back in absolute alcohol for 2–3 hours to get complete dehydration. After this tissue should be kept in fresh quantity of clearing agent. The optimum time, which tissue is to be kept in clearing agent, is indicated by shine or transparency of tissue. This varies according to the nature and thickness of the tissue, and it mostly ranges from 2–4 hours. However, the tissue should not be kept for longer period in clearing agent because the tissue become hard and brittle and it will create problems during further processing of the tissue.

Clearing Agents

Various clearing agents which can be used for clearing are xylene, toluene, chloroform, benzene, cedar wood oil, clove oil, inhibisol, etc.

a. **Xylene:** Chemically, it is dimethylbenzene. It is a mixture of ortho- para- and meta-xylene. It is a colorless liquid with a pleasant odor having a specific gravity of 0.863 and boiling point of about 140°C. It is most commonly used clearing agent in histology. It is a rapid clearing agent suitable for urgent biopsies.

Advantages:
- It brings about quick removal of alcohol from the tissue and increases the infiltration of paraffin into the tissue.
- It imparts no color or ting to the tissue.
- It can be used when celloidin is used as an embedding medium.
- It makes tissue transparent and get volatilize readily in paraffin oven.
- Biopsies, and tissue blocks of 3 mm thickness are cleared in 15–20 minutes.

Disadvantages: It makes the tissue hard and brittle if it is placed in xylene for a longer period of time. It is not suitable for brain and lymph nodes. Xylene fumes should not be inhaled and thus require adequate protection from fumes.

b. **Benzene:** It is colorless, highly refractive mobile liquid with unpleasant smell. It has a specific gravity of 0.879

and boiling point 80°C. It is insoluble in water and soluble in ether, alcohol and petrol. It has similar properties to xylene.

Advantages: It can be used for cold embedding. It causes minimum shrinkage and does not make the tissue hard and brittle.

Disadvantages: It is highly poisonous and should be handled carefully. It is highly toxic and inflammable hence it is not recommended for use as a clearing agent. Also, it is possible carcinogenic agent.

c. **Toluene:** It is colorless mobile liquid having a specific gravity of 0.866. It is insoluble in water and soluble in ethanol, ether and petroleum. Its properties are similar to xylene.

Advantages: It is less damaging on prolonged exposure of tissue. It is a suitable clearing agent for automated tissue processing. Clearing time is from 15–180 minutes. Depending upon tissue type and thickness. The solvent can be used with adequate protection from fumes.

Disadvantages: It is highly inflammable and potentially dangerous.

d. **Chloroform:** It is a colorless liquid with a specific gravity of 1.489 and boiling point 61°C. It is slower in action than xylene or toluene, but causes less brittleness. Thick blocks can be processed providing that sufficient time is allowed for clearing.

Advantages: It has less or little hardening and shrinkage effect and hence it is widely used in histopathology especially with brain and bone.

Disadvantages: It has a high specific gravity and hence tissue floats on the surface of the chloroform due to which the process of clearing is not uniform. It is toxic and have a deleterious effect on the rubber and synthetic sealing rings of the vacuum impregnating bath.

e. **Cedar wood oil:** It is obtained by steam distillation of red cedar. It has a yellowish ting and has a specific gravity of 0.927 and boiling point of 237°C.

Advantages: It has a gentle action with little hardening of tissue, even after prolonged immersion. This reagent causes little or no damage to even the most delicate tissues. It is particularly valuable in research laboratory and in embryological procedures. Certain tissues, notably skin and dense fibrous tissue, benefit from treatment with cedar wood oil in that it imparts a consistency to the tissues which facilitates subsequent section cutting. Complete dehydration is not prerequisite with this clearing agent because it can accommodate some water.

Disadvantages: Due to its high boiling point it is difficult to remove oil in the wax baths, hence several changes of wax bath is required. It sometimes partially solidifies, through the formation of needle like crystals due to contamination with acetic acid. Due to its low volatility it cannot be removed by vacuum impregnation.

f. **Clove oil:** It is obtained from the clove tree by distillation of buds. It has a good refractive index and has capacity to accommodate some moisture in the tissue. It gives clearing and transparency to the tissue relatively earlier.

Disadvantages: It gives yellowish ting to the tissue and make the tissue harder earlier than the other agents. It is very expensive, hence it is rarely used as a clearing agent.

g. **Inhibisol:** It is the trade name of a clearing agent consisting of 1,1,1-trichloroethane with patented inhibitor designed to reduce its toxicity.

Advantages: It is fairly low toxic and non-inflammable. The speed of action is moderate and do not cause brittleness of the tissue.

Disadvantages: It may cause distortion of plastic processing beakers.

h. **Amyl acetate, methyl benzoate and methyl salicylate:** These are chiefly used as nitrocellulose solvents in double embedding techniques. They have low toxicity, but their strong penetrating odor necessitates good laboratory ventilation. They are ideal for manual processing as tissues may be left in them for extended periods without hardening. These esters are difficult to eliminate from paraffin wax and should be extracted from tissues with one or two brief changes of toluene or similar solvent before passing through two or three changes of wax.

IMPREGNATION AND INFILTRATION

Infiltration is the saturation of tissue cavities and cells by a supporting substance which is generally, but not always, the medium in which they are finally embedded. Tissues are infiltrated by immersion in a substance such as a wax, which is fluid when hot and solid when cold. Alternatively, tissue can be infiltrated with a solution of a substance dissolved in a solvent, for example-nitrocellulose in alcohol-ether, which solidifies on evaporation of the solvent to provide a firm mass suitable for sectioning.

Characteristics of suitable infiltration media:
- Soluble in processing fluids
- Suitable for sectioning and ribboning
- Molten between 30°C and 60°C
- Translucent or transparent or colorless
- Stable and non-toxic
- Homogeneous and capable of flattening after ribboning
- Odorless, easily to handle and inexpensive.

Requirement for Impregnation and Infiltration

- Suitable impregnating medium
- Paraffin impregnation oven
- Wax dispenser

a. **Suitable impregnation medium:** Impregnation is defined as the process of diffusion of the impregnating medium into the tissue to replace the clearing agent. Paraffin waxes are most commonly used impregnating medium. The choice of paraffin depends on the conditions under which it is to be used and the thickness of the sections required. Paraffin is of two types soft and hard. Paraffin having melting point range 50–52°C or 53–55°C is considered to be the soft paraffin whereas hard paraffin has 56–58°C or 60–68°C range. Soft paraffin should be used when relatively thick sections are required. If thinner sections (5–7 μ) are to be cut paraffin of 56–58°C melting point should be preferred. For extremely thin section (less than 5μ) best results can be achieved with paraffin of 60–68°C melting point. Choice of paraffin is also influenced by temperature. Warm temperature is better for sectioning with hard paraffin and soft paraffin requires cold temperature for better sectioning.

b. **Paraffin embedding/impregnation oven:** The oven should be large enough to accommodate an enamel jug and funnel, fitted with Whatman No.1 filter paper for the filtration of new or reclaimed wax and a number of glass containers of suitable size for the wax infiltration of the tissues (Fig. 6.2). The temperature of the oven should be adjusted between 50–60°C. The functions carried out by paraffin embedding oven are
   - Melting and storing of molten paraffin wax.
   - Infiltration and impregnation of paraffin wax inside the tissue.
   - Warming of solutions during the preparation of the reagents.

c. **Wax dispenser:** The storage and dispensing of the molten paraffin wax is facilitated by the use of a wax dispenser. This is electrically heated, temperature controlled insulated tank with an integral outlet filter, heated tap and loose fitting lid. The temperature is adjusted up to 70°C and a safety cut out device operating at 90°C prevents accidental overheating of the wax causing fire risk.

Procedure: Tissues are transferred, after clearing, to a bath of molten paraffin wax, either in an impregnation/embedding oven or in a chamber of an automatic processing machine. During this combined process, clearing agent is eliminated from the tissue by diffusion into the surrounding melted wax (infiltration) following which the wax diffuses into the tissue to replace the clearing agent (impregnation). This is carried out at a temperature of 50–60°C for 2–3 hours. This temperature of molten paraffin wax is very critical if it increases above this temperature the tissue become cooked or over hardened and greatly distorted. In order to obtain a good result, there should be at least one change in wax to completely remove the clearing agent. Inadequate impregnation leads to drying and shrinkage of the embedded tissue. In addition, during section cutting, cracks and crumbles develop if the wax inadequately supports tissues. On the other hand, excessive exposure of tissue to the high temperature of wax beyond the critical temperature will over hardened the tissue and will not give good sections. Moreover, residual clearing agent in an embedded tissue block will render the production of good sections impossible.

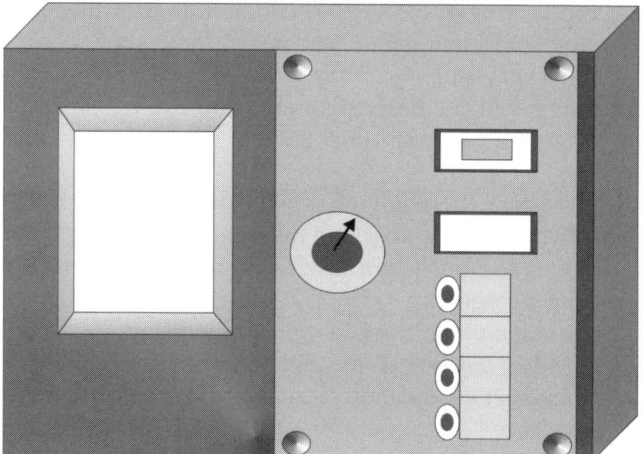

Fig. 6.2: Impregnation oven

Factors Affecting Infiltration and Impregnation

- **Impregnation time:** The time required for complete infiltration and impregnation mostly depends upon the tissue density and size of the tissue block. Table 6.1 shows the impregnation time in paraffin wax.
- **Tissue density:** Dense tissues require longer immersion in molten paraffin wax to ensure complete impregnation, therefore, structures such as bone, fibro-mass, and brain require approximately twice as long as soft tissues such as kidney or liver. The

excessive hardness of dense tissues caused by this increased exposure to hot wax is undesirable because the wax infiltration of such tissues can be obtained without undue hardening by the use of the vacuum impregnation technique.
- **Size of tissue blocks:** The amount of clearing agent carried to the wax bath depends on the surface area of the tissue block. When treating large pieces the effect of this contamination may be minimized by frequent changes of wax. The time required for thorough impregnation depends on the thickness of the tissue, a piece of 5 mm thick, for example, takes about 3 hours, whereas a piece of 10 mm thick may take up to 10 hours. Table 6.1 shows the impregnation time in paraffin wax.
- **Temperature:** At low temperatures reagent viscosities increase and diffusion rates decrease, resulting in prolonged impregnation time. High infiltration temperature cause marked tissue shrinkage and hardening which can be avoided by maintaining embedding waxes 2-3°C above their melting points. Prolonged immersion in paraffin wax at the correct temperature results in only slight tissue shrinkage though tissues such as blood, muscle and yolk may harden and become brittle.
- **Pressure and vacuum:** High pressure facilitates the infiltration of dense specimens with viscous resinous embedding media at the block forming stage, but is rarely employed for biological specimens. Positive pressures for fluid transfer that are encountered in closed system processors are probably too low to have a significant influence on tissue infiltration. Vacuum applied during dehydration, clearing and infiltration stages improves the quality of processing. Tissues, particularly lung, are deaerated, and the solvent boiling point is reduced, thus facilitating evaporation of the reagent from the molten infiltration medium. Duration of wax infiltration is dependent upon viscosity and is not reduced by the application of vacuum.
- **Agitation:** Diffusion of infiltrating medium inside the tissue can be increased by exposure of the maximum tissue surface area to the reagent. This can be achieved by agitating the medium and the tissue. During processing tissues should be loosely packed, suspended and agitated within the medium. Agitation of tissues and fluids in manual processing is achieved using rotors or magnetic stirrers. For efficient and effective infiltration the fluid volume ratio of at least 1: 50 should be maintained.

Table 6.1: The impregnation times in paraffin wax

Tissue thickness (mm)	Clearing agent used	Paraffin wax Time (Hrs)	Changes
<3	Xylene	1–5	1
	Toluene	1–5	1
<3	Chloroform	2–3	2
	Cedar wood oil	2–3	2
3–5	Xylene	2–3	2
	Toluene	2–3	2
3–5	Chloroform	3–5	3
	Cedar wood oil	3–5	3
5–8	Xylene	3–5	2
	Toluene	3–5	2
5–8	Chloroform	5–8	3
	Cedar wood oil	5–8	3

Vacuum Impregnation

The vacuum impregnation technique depends on the production of negative pressure above the specimens in the impregnating wax. The vacuum treatment is required.
- To remove bubbles from the tissue as may occur in porous tissues like lungs.
- To reduce the time of impregnation in case of dense tissue.
- To remove clearing agent more rapidly by increasing vaporization.
- In case of urgent biopsies.
- This technique is desirable for dense tissues, lung tissues and very fatty tissues.

The facility of vacuum impregnation in generally available with the automatic tissue processors. The time required for vacuum impregnation can be reduced to half by using this technique. Reduced pressure is obtained by use of vacuum.

The vacuum impregnation oven (Fig. 6.3) commonly in use consists of a flat bottomed brass vacuum chamber with a heavy glass lid resting on a thick rubber washer which provides an air tight junction. The vacuum chamber is immersed in a thermostatically controlled water jacket. Air is allowed into the chamber when the oven is under negative pressure by means of a valve fitted on one side of the chamber. The interior is connected to the vacuum pump by a small tube which is on the opposite side of the chamber.

The impregnation is carried out as follows:
- To a container of molten wax, transfer the cleared tissue and place it in the vacuum oven.
- Press the heavy glass lid firmly into position.

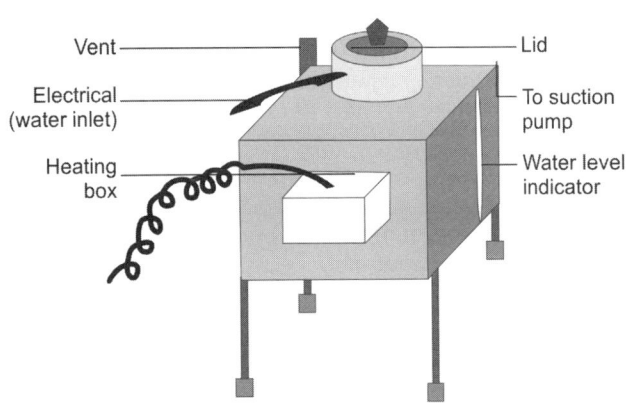

Fig. 6.3: Vacuum impregnation oven

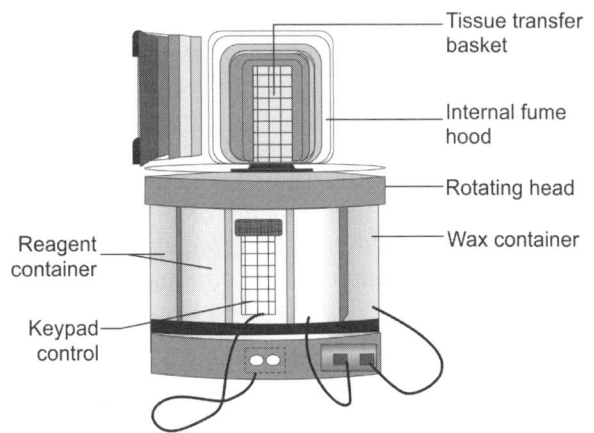

Fig. 6.4: Tissue transfer processor

- Shut the valve and evacuate the chamber with the vacuum pump to give a negative pressure of 400–500 mm on the manometer.
- At the end of the impregnation time, gradually open the screw valve to allow the pressure to return to normal.
- Embed the tissue.

AUTOMATIC TISSUE PROCESSING

In recent years, most histopathology departments, including those handling comparatively small numbers of tissue blocks have opted for the use of machines to process tissues. These machines decrease both time and labor necessary for processing tissue and produce reproducible results. The time required for processing is decreased by:
- Continuous agitation
- Application of vacuum and
- Increased temperature to improve the penetration and production of more consistent results. A variety of these machines are available. Some act on the carousel principle with tissue blocks in baskets being transferred from one container to another. Other designs have a single central chamber into which processing fluids are transferred. There are two broad types of automatic tissue processors, namely tissue transfer and fluid transfer types.

■ Tissue-Transfer Processors

These processors are characterized by the transfer of tissues, contained within a basket, through a series of stationary reagents arranged in-line or in a circular carousel plan. The rotary or carousel is the most common model of automatic tissue processor. It is provided with 9–10 reagent and 2–3 wax positions, with a capacity of 30–110 cassettes depending upon the mode. Fluid agitation is achieved by vertical oscillation or rotary motion of the tissue basket. Processing schedules are card-notched, pin or touch pad programed. Tissue transfer processors allow maximum flexibility in the choice of reagents and schedules that can be run on them, in particular, metal-corrosive fixatives, a wide range of solvents and relatively viscous nitrocellulose solutions can all be accommodated. These machines have a rapid turn around time for day/night processing (Fig. 6.4).

Day schedule for urgent specimens, tissues 2 mm, fixed in Carnoy's fluid and overnight schedule for routine processing of tissue blocks 2–3 mm, single load is given in Table 6.2. For a double load, immersion times should be. In equal weekend

Table 6.2: Processing schedules for tissue, transfer processor

Step	Duration	
	Day	Overnight
Fixative		120 minutes
Fixative		120 minutes
70% ethanol		60 minutes
90% ethanol		60 minutes
Absolute ethanol	30 minutes	60 minutes
Absolute ethanol	30 minutes	60 minutes
Absolute ethanol	30 minutes	60 minutes
Toluene or substitute	30 minutes	60 minutes
Toluene or substitute	30 minutes	60 minutes
Paraffin wax	30 minutes	90 minutes
Paraffin wax	30 minutes	90 minutes
Paraffin wax	30 minutes	90 minutes
Paraffin wax (under vacuum)	30 minutes	30 minutes
Embed		
Total Time	4.5 hours	16 hours

processing tissues are held in fixative, or preferably 70% ethanol until Sunday.

■ Fluid-Transfer Processors

In the fluid-transfer units processing fluids are pumped to and from a retort in which the tissues remain stationary. There are 10–12 reagent stations with temperatures adjustable between 30–45°C. 3–4 paraffin wax stations with variable temperature settings between 48–68°C and vacuum-pressure options for each station. Depending upon the model these machines can process 100–300 cassettes at a time. Agitation is achieved by tidal action. Schedules are microprocessor programed and controlled. Vacuum-pressure cycles coupled with heated reagents allow effective reductions in processing times and improved infiltration of dense tissues (Fig. 6.5).

Fluid transfer processors overcome the main drawbacks of the tissue-transfer machine. Tissues are unable to dry out within the sealed retort and reagent vapours are vented through filters or retained in a closed loop system. Processors are provided with alert systems and diagnostic programs for troubleshooting and maintenance.

Most of the automatic tissue processors are designed to operate a 24 hours schedule, although same are made to operate a one hour schedule for fast processing or a 7 day schedule for slow processing (Table 6.3). There is a mechanism that allows the delay of actual starting time for

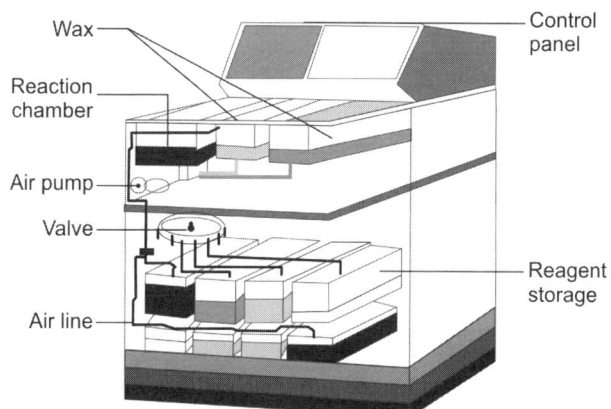

Fig. 6.5: Fluid transfer processor

24 hours. The machines also do incorporate a number of safety devices. A cut out device automatically comes into operation when the processing cycle is completed with the tissue bucket in the second wax bath until it is removed by hand. Another safety device operates when the wax in the first wax bath has solidified. In this case the transfer mechanism will transfer the tissue containers straight to second wax bath. Also, in the event of a power failure or fuse being blown, a battery operated alarm bell located in a strategic position in the laboratory goes off.

Table 6.3: Processing schedules for a fluid-transfer processor
Rapid (30 minutes) day schedule for endoscopic or needle biopsy. Overnight schedule for routine lightly fixed specimens P/V pressure vacuum option

Steps	Day			Overnight		
	Time	Temp (°C)	P/V	Time	Temp (°C)	P/V
Fixative				3.0 hours	35	
Fixative				1.5 hours	35	
70% ethanol	15 minutes		on	1.0 hour	40	
90% ethanol	15 minutes	40	on	1.0 hour	40	
Absolute ethanol	15 minutes	40	on	0.5 hour	45	on
Absolute ethanol	15 minutes	40	on	0.5 hour	45	
Absolute ethanol	15 minutes	40	on	0.5 hour	45	
Absolute ethanol	15 minutes	40	on	1.5 hour	45	on
Toluene or subst	15 minutes	40	on	0.5 hour	50	
Toluene or subst	15 minutes	40	on	1.5 hour	50	on
Paraffin wax				0.5 hour	60	on
Paraffin wax	15 minutes	60	on	0.5 hour	60	on
Paraffin wax	15 minutes	60	on	1.5 hours	60	on
Paraffin wax	15 minutes	60	on	1.5 hours	60	on
Embed						
Total Time (exclusive of fluid transfer time)	2.75 hours			15.5 hours		

Tissue Containers

Special containers made of either stainless or plastic are provided. Some containers are designed with one, two four or six divisions and are supplied with close fitting lids and with a choice of mesh size. Special baskets for curetting and fragmentary tissue are available. Plastic containers are of value when processing tissues fixed in solutions containing mercuric chloride.

Changing of Solutions

No hard and fast rules can be laid down as to the frequency with which fluids should be changed. It depends upon the number and size of the tissue processed. The fluid used in complete dehydration and clearing tends to become contaminated with fluid carried over from the previous vat by the tissue. Hence more than one are kept in a series, 100% alcohol, 3 times and xylene, 2 times. After using them for 2 to 3 days the last solution in the series are replaced by fresh solution of 100% alcohol and xylene and the previously used ones are moved forward while the first one is discarded. Other solutions are changed once a week or earlier with an average workload. Multiple processing machines, such as the Shadon 'Duplex' when used fully loaded require more frequent changes of fluid than the single processors.

Precautions to be Taken During Automatic Tissue Processing

- Beakers and wax baths must be filled to the correct fluid level and located in their fasteners.
- Any spillage of fluid should be wiped away.
- Accumulation of wax must be removed, particularly from the beaker covers.
- Wax bath thermostats are set at a satisfactory level, usually 2–3°C above the melting point of wax.
- Particular attention should be paid to the fastening of the processing baskets on the machine some machines are prone to shed baskets with disastrous results.
- Care must be taken in setting the timing mechanism when loading tissues.
- The paraffin wax baths should be checked to ensure that the wax in molten electric plugs may inadvertently be removed.
- Most tissue processing machines have facilities for setting a delay period before processing commences this period should be carefully checked.
- Baskets and metal cassettes should be clean and wax-free.

Processing Schedule for Automatic Tissue Processor

The processing schedule used in automatic tissue processors varies according to the types of tissue, the nature of the work, the clearing reagent used, and personal preference. Some of the examples of processing schedule are given in the Table 6.4.

MANUAL TISSUE PROCESSING

In some instances, it is desirable that arrangements are maintained for the occasional treatment of tissues by a manual processing method. It is found necessary in the following circumstances:

- For large tissue slices which would require resetting of the machine processing schedule.
- For speed of processing.
- On occasions of electrical power failure or processing machine breakdown.

Table 6.4: Showing some example which gives good results

Step	Schedule 1 Reagents	Time	Schedule 2 Reagent	Time	Schedule 3 Reagent	Time
1.	80% alcohol	2 hours	70% alcohol	2 hours	70% alcohol	2 hours
2.	95% alcohol	1 hour	90% alcohol	3 hours	90% alcohol	2 hours
3.	95% alcohol	1 hour	100% alcohol	3 hours	96% alcohol	2 hours
4.	100% alcohol	1 hour	100% alcohol	3 hours	100% alcohol	2 hours
5.	100% alcohol	1 hour	100% alcohol	3 hours	100% alcohol	2 hours
6.	100% alcohol	1 hour	Toluene	0.5 hours	100% alcohol	2 hours
7.	Xylene	1 hour	Toluene	1 hour	Chloroform	2 hours
8.	Xylene	2 hours	Paraffin wax	3 hours	Chloroform	2 hours
9.	Paraffin wax	2 hours	Paraffin wax	3 hours	Chloroform	2 hours
10.	Paraffin wax	2 hours	Paraffin wax	0.5 hours	Paraffin wax	2 hours
11.	Paraffin wax	2 hours			Paraffin vacuum bam	0.5 hour

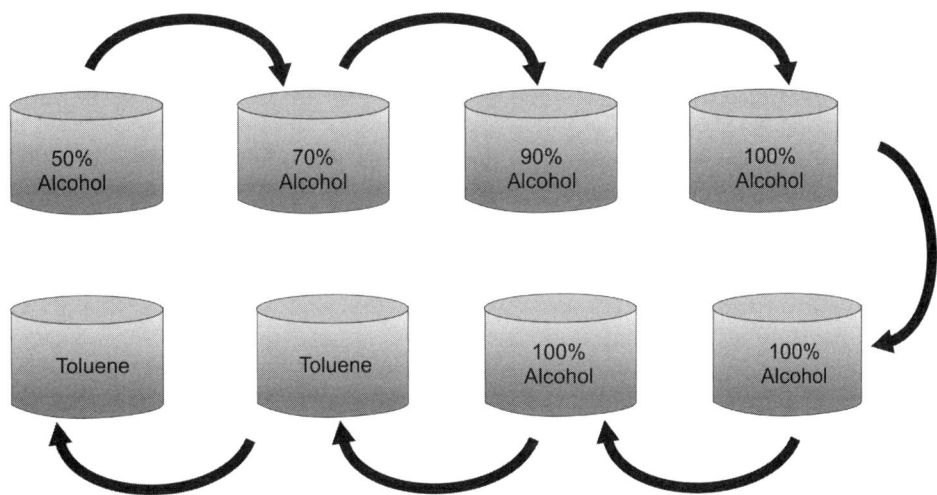

Fig. 6.6: Arrangement for dehydration and clearing tissue manually

- Very large or thick tissue blocks.
- Requirement for a non-standard processing schedule.
- For delicate materials.
- Hard, dense tissues.
- Resin embedding.

The advantage of manual tissue processing is its flexibility the tissue is treated for optimum duration in each fluid. A further advantage of manual processing is the use of fluids which are flammable volatile or costly and are unacceptable in automated techniques. The acetone as a dehydrants can be used in manual which in not recommended for automated technique. If a single block is to be processed keep the tissue in a single container and change the fluid. It required minimum bench space. When the tissues are to be processed regularly by manual means a permanent arrangement of containers allows fewer possibilities of error and great speed (Fig. 6.6). Tissue cassettes used for automatic techniques can be used for manual processing. In all steps of processing the volume of fluid is important. If good results are required the volume of fluid must exceed that of the tissue by at least a factor of 50.

Agitate tissues frequently to assist rapid transfer of fluid. Instead of absolute alcohol 74°OP spirit can be used as a dehydrating agent.

Though manual processing can be time consuming and inconvenient, care must be exercised so that tissues are left overnight in reagents that will cause minimal harm. Tissues are processed in tubes and agitated on a rotor. Reagents are pipetted, or decanted through a fine sieve. Multiple specimens or large blocks are economically processed in large lidded jars of processing fluids. Table 6.5 and 6.6 shows manual tissue processing.

■ Embedding

Having been completely impregnated it is necessary to obtain a solid block containing the tissue for getting very thin/fine sections of the tissue. Embedding can be defined

Table 6.5: Manual processing of large, thick, hard, well fixed tissue blocks using terpene transition solvents. Other terpenes such as terpineol or limonene-based solvents can be substituted for the cedarwood oil

Stage	Duration
70% ethanol	3 hours
90% ethanol	6–24 hours
95% ethanol, 2 changes, over	6–24 hours
Absolute ethanol-cedar wood oil 1:1	3–6 hours
Cedar wood oil, 2 changes over	6–24 hours
Toluene or chloroform or substitute, 2 changes, each	0.5-1 hour
Paraffin wax, 4 changes, each	1-1.5 hours
Total time	29 hours-5 days

Table 6.6: Manual processing: One and two day schedules for well fixed tissues processed using a magnetic stirrer

Step	Duration	
	Tissue thickness	
	1–2 mm	3–4 mm
70% ethanol	20 minutes	1.5 hours
90% ethanol	20 minutes	1.5 hours
Absolute ethanol	20 minutes	1.5 hours
Absolute ethanol	20 minutes	1.5 hours
Absolute ethanol	20 minutes	1.5 hours
Chloroform or substitute	20 minutes	
Chloroform or substitute	20 minutes	
Methyl salicylate		Overnight
Paraffin wax	20 minutes	1.0 hour
Paraffin wax	20 minutes	2.0 hour
Paraffin wax		1.0 hour
Paraffin wax under vacuum	20 minutes	0.5 hour
Total Time	2 hours	1.5 days

as the reinforcement of suitable solidifying medium in the tissue. Various embedding media used for this purpose are paraffin wax, ester wax, water soluble waxes, cellulose nitrate, synthetic resins, carbowax, gelatin, paraplast, etc. But most commonly used embedding medium is paraffin wax.

Embedding Media

1. **Paraffin waxes:** Paraffin wax is a polycrystalline mixture of solid hydrocarbons produced in the cracking of mineral oils. Wax hardness (viscosity) depends upon the molecular weight of the components and the ambient temperature. High molecular weight mixtures melt at high temperature than waxes comprises of low molecular weight fractions. Paraffin wax is traditionally marketed by its melting point which ranges from 39–68°C. In order to produce ribbons of sections, it is necessary to select a wax of suitable hardness at room temperature. Waxes of melting point 54–58°C are satisfactory for routine purposes.

   Tissue—wax adhesion depends on crystal morphology of embedding medium. Small, uniform sized crystals provide better physical support for specimens through close packing. Crystalline morphology of paraffin wax can be altered by incorporating additives which result in a less brittle more homogeneous wax with good cutting characteristics.

   Advantages: It is most popular due to ease with which large numbers of tissue blocks can be processed in comparatively short times with the minimum of supervision. In addition, sectioning and later staining presents fewer difficulties than other media.

   Disadvantages: On prolonged heating of wax 10–20°C above the melting point, some waxes undergo oxidation producing yellow tinge and soap like consistency.

   Modified paraffin waxes: The properties of paraffin wax are improved for histological purposes by the addition of some substances to the wax:
   - To improve ribboning: prolonged heating of paraffin wax at high temperature or use microcrystalline wax.
   - To increase hardness: add stearic acid.
   - To decrease melting point: Add spermaceti or phenanthrene.
   - To improve adhesion between specimen and wax: Add 0.5% ceresin, 0.1–5% beewax, rubber asphalt, bayberry wax, etc.

2. **Alternative embedding media:** Although, paraffin wax is extensively used as an embedding medium for large numbers of tissue blocks and is ideally suited for automation, in some circumstances, it is not the technique of choice due to following reasons:
   - The impregnating medium is not sufficiently hard and fails to provide adequate support.
   - The tissue is adversely affected by heat.
   - The use of dehydrating and clearing agents destroy or distort the tissue or tissue components.
   - The adhesion between paraffin wax and the tissue is inadequate, resulting in the breaking away of the tissue from wax during sectioning.
   - Sectioning of whole organs like lungs or brain.
   - The crystalline structure of paraffin wax is unsuitable.
   - Very thick or thin sections are required.
   - Hard and dense tissues are inadequately supported.

Because of the above reasons, alternative media are used for embedding. Various alternative embedding media, which satisfy some of the above criteria are water soluble waxes, ester wax, polyester wax, microcrystalline wax, acrylic resin, epoxy resins, agar, gelatin, celloidin, etc.

Aqueous Media

Agar: A high melting point and low gelling temperature of agar make it ideal for double embedding of multiple small tissue fragments. Agar is generally unstained by overnight stains, but will stain with alcian blue.

Gelatine: It is used for simple embedding in a similar manner to agar. However, the low melting point of gelatin (35–40°C) makes it unsuitable for double embedding. It is used in the whole organ sectioning method. In phospholipids and enzyme studies, tissues may be infiltered and embedded in gelatin and the resulting blocks sectioned on a freezing microtome.

Sodium carboxy methyl cellulose (CMC): It is used as an embedding medium for whole body sectioning techniques, frozen tissues are transferred from coolant directly into 5% CMC briefly placed under vacuum to remove trapped air, then frozen to a solid block for sectioning.

Polyvinyl alcohol (PVA): It is a highly polar, water soluble medium suited particularly for histochemical studies of lipids and enzymes. Tissues are infiltered at elevated or room temperature through ascending series of aqueous PVA-glycerol solutions and embedded in 15% aqueous PVA.

Water Soluble Media

Several water soluble waxes are commercially available and they are polyethylene glycols and their fatty acid esters. They are dense, crystalline substances with melting point of 35–50°C. They are less elastic, denser and harder than paraffin waxes.

Advantages:
They are completely soluble in water at room temperature.
- Their adhesive properties are superior than paraffin wax, and their ribboning and sectioning properties are within range.
- The tissue processed and embedded in them are more softer than paraffin wax.
- Many lipids and enzymes can be demonstrated in tissue by this method.
- It is possible to directly embed the tissue after fixation.

Disadvantages:
- The greatest difficulty encountered with these waxes is at the floating out stage. Once the sections come into contact with the floating out fluid, the impregnating medium dissolves, causing disruption of the tissue and disintegration of the tissue at the surface.
- Handling and storage of processed tissue is difficult because the medium is hygroscopic.

Water Tolerant Media

- **Ester wax:** It is a mixture of diethylene glycol distearate, glyceryl monostearate and polyethylene glycol. It is a dense, white, slightly brittle substance with a melting point of 45–47°C. It is harder than paraffin wax at room temperature. The wax is miscible with 95% alcohol, acetone and clearing agent xylene. It has fine crystalline structure.

Advantages: The consistency of the wax improves on storage and sections can be easily cut after 36–48 hours. It can give sufficient support to undecalcified bones.
A section up to a thickness of 5 µm can be easily cut.
Disadvantages: It is about eight times more expensive than paraffin wax.
- **Polyester wax**: It is a dense white substance and also called as polyester wax 90/10, having composition
  - 400 polyethylene glycol distearate   - 90 g
  - Cetyl alcohol   - 10 g

It has a melting point of 38°C and is miscible with 95% ethanol, acetone, ether, esters and hydrocarbons and common clearing agents. It require 36–48 hours for complete impregnation.

Advantages:
- Its main advantage over paraffin and ester waxes is its low melting point, which reduces tissue hardening, shrinkage and eliminates the need for infiltration ovens.
- The wax is water tolerant, almost opaque and sections easily.
- No electrification of ribbon occurs during sectioning.
- The sections of 2 µm or more can be cut at room temperature between 10–22°C.

Disadvantage: It provides less support to the tissue. The tissues are often left soft due to lower processing temperature. It is hygroscopic and should not be allowed to come into direct contact with water/ice.

Hydrophobic Media

Cellulose nitrate (celloidin): Celloidin is an amorphous, slightly yellowish substance also called as collodion and parlodion. A slightly different formulation is called as LVN (low viscosity nitrocellulose). It is completely insoluble in water and is dissolved in 50 : 50 diethyl ether : ethanol. Clearing agents are not required and no heat is used. After impregnation, tissues are embedded in a thick solution of cellulose nitrate and blocks are stored in alcohol.

Advantages:
- It causes less shrinkage of the tissue.
- It provides improved cutting qualities of large blocks of dense tissue such as bone.
- Thick sections of the brain can be obtained easily with less shrinkage and distortion.
- It is a good embedding medium for eyes.

Disadvantages:
- It has low penetration power, so require long time about 2–4 weeks for complete impregnation.
- It is difficult to cut thin sections (less than 10 µm).
- It does not give ribbon of sections.
- The medium is highly inflammable and inconvenient to store.

Other Embedding Media

- **Paramat and paramat extra:** Paramat is the blend of paraffin wax with plastic polymers. When plastic polymers are added to paraffin the elasticity of the final block increases as compared with paraffin alone. It also improves tissue penetration, easy ribboning of sections, reduces the tendency of crumble and improve overall results with fibrous tissue. Recently, a very small amount of dimethyl sulfoxide (DMSO) has been added to paramat which increases the penetration of the tissue resulting in more homogeneous matrix to support the specimen. This mixture is called paramat extra. Paramat is soluble in xylene and gives sections of 4 µm thickness.
- **Paraplast:** It is in the form of handy pellet having melting point from 53–56°C. It can cut to 2 µ thick and gives excellent ribbon continuity.
- **Peel away paraffin embedding wax:** It is a new polymer paraffin having a low melting point which is used for routine histological work. It is more translucent and small dermatological and biopsy specimens can be seen and sectioned with ease. It requires less time for deparaffinization and infiltration.

iv. **Polyfin:** It is a mixture of highly refined paraffin and copolymer alloys in the form of wax pellet. Polyfin provides optimal tissue support and gives exceptional clarity. It has low a melting point (55°C) which reduces the tissue distortion caused by excessive heat during processing.

■ Moulds For Embedding

A variety of moulds are available for 'Blocking Out' or embedding the tissue in paraffin wax (Fig. 6.7).

- **Leuckhard embedding boxes:** These are convenient moulds for large specimens. They consist of two L-shaped pieces of metal, usually brass, formed in a variety of sizes. They are arranged on a glass or metal plate to form a mould of the desired size. When the embedding wax solidified, the moulds are removed and the blocks are separated from the base.
- **Plastic ice trays:** These have been used with one block being embedded in each compartment. When set, the wax blocks are easily removed by flexing the plastic tray. This may be facilitated by smearing the inside of the mould with a little glycerol/liquid paraffin.
- **Plastic embedding cassettes:** These are disposable products available in a variety of sizes and colors. A flat portion of the cassettes has a matt surface which can be used to label the block either with a graphite pencil or automated block labeling machine.
- **Plastic embedding moulds:** They are available in five sizes from 8 × 8 mm cutting area to 22 × 40 mm. After solidification of the block the plastic mould is peeled away and discarded. The block is clamped directly into the chuck of the microtome.

■ Tissue Embedding Center

For routine processing of large numbers of tissues of small and moderate size mostly tissue embedding center system is used. This system does not require further trimming of the block. This center includes a molten wax dispenser, together with hot and cold plates. A base mould of suitable size for the specimen is placed on the hot plate, and the tissue is positioned carefully. The plastic cassette is placed in position and the paraffin wax poured in until it reaches the top.

After cooling on the cold plate the base mould is easily detached, leaving the embedding tissue ready for cutting. No trimming is necessary and the wax filled plastic cassette serves as a block holder. Some embedding centers are provided with temperature controlled electrically heated forceps which are convenient and reduce fire hazards (Fig. 6.8).

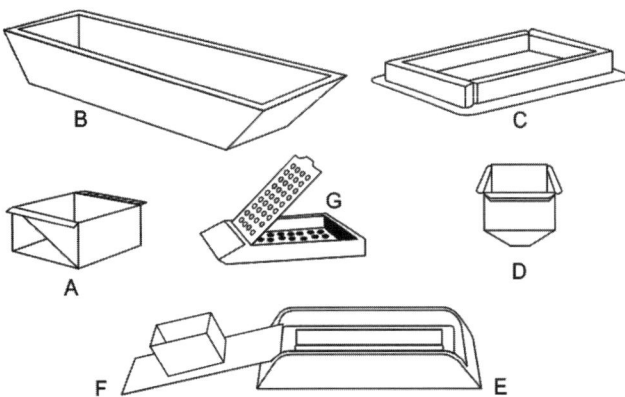

Fig. 6.7: Embedding moulds: (A) Paper boat; (B) Metal boat mould; (C) Dimmock embedding mould; (D) Peel-a-way disposable mould; (E) Base mould used with embedding ring (F) or cassette bases (G)

PARAFFIN WAX EMBEDDING

The various steps involved in the embedding with paraffin wax using L-moulds are as follows:

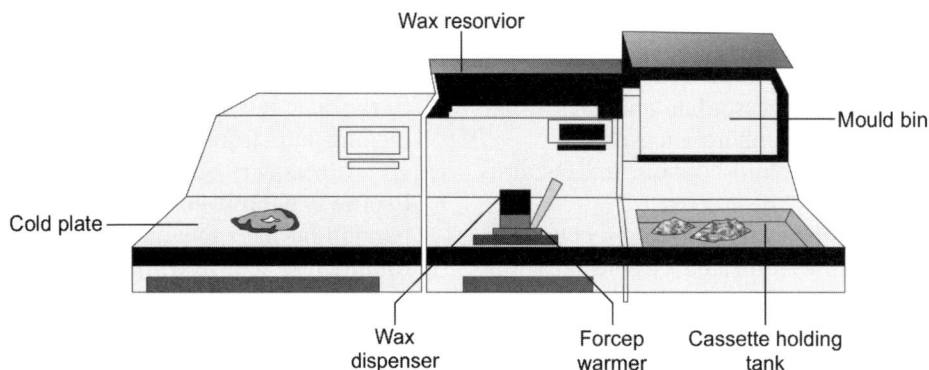

Fig. 6.8: Tissue embedding center

- The L-moulds should be adjusted on a glass plate so that it should form a rectangular cavity between them. Now fill this cavity with molten paraffin wax up to half cm. height.
- Place the impregnated tissue and orient it according to the plane of section needed inside the cavity.
- Pour the remaining molten paraffin wax up to the top of the cavity (Fig. 6.9).
- With the help of a warm blunt forcep remove the air bubbles by moving the forcep slowly around the tissue.
- Fix the label carrying all the details of the tissue on one side of the mould.
- Blow air gently on the mould. This results in formation of a thin film on the surface of the wax.
- Now gently immerse the mould in cold water rapidly. The mould should be immersed by slightly tilting the glass plate to avoid sudden contact with water, otherwise cracks will appear in the block, (or refrigerate it).
- After complete cooling, remove the L-moulds and glass plate and store it in a cool place in a small paper bag until used for sectioning.

Orientation of tissue in the block: Correct orientation of tissue in a mould is the most important step in embedding. Incorrect placement of tissues may result in diagnostically important tissue elements being missed or damaged during microtomy. In circumstances, where precise orientation is essential, tissue should be marked or agar double embedded. Usually tissues are embedded with the surface to be cut facing down in the mould (Fig. 6.10). Some general considerations are as follows:

- Elongated tissues are placed diagonally across the block.
- Tubular and walled specimens such as vas deferens, cysts and gastrointestinal tissues are embedded so as to provided transverse sections showing all tissue layers.
- Tissues with an epithelial surface such as skin, are embedded to provide sections in a plane at right angles to the surface (hairy or keratinized epithelia is oriented to face the knife diagonally).
- Multiple tissue pieces are aligned across the long axis of the mould, and not placed at random.

Precautions:
- The wax to be used must contain no trace of the clearing agent.
- No dust particles must be present in paraffin wax.
- Immediately after embedding the wax must be rapidly cooled to reduce wax crystal size.

Table 6.7 shows general embedding faults.

STORAGE OF PARAFFIN BLOCKS

When not needed paraffin wax blocks are stored by two methods:

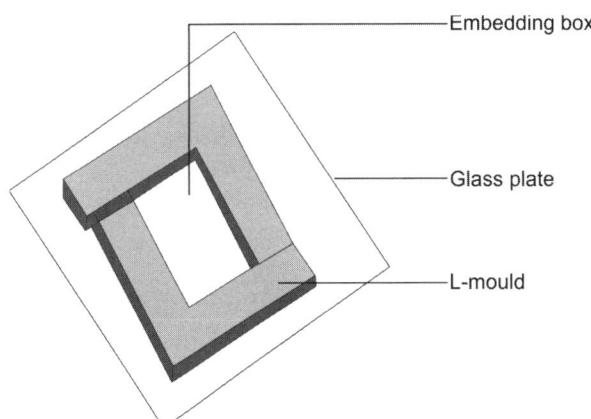

Fig. 6.9: Embedding of the tissue in L-moulds

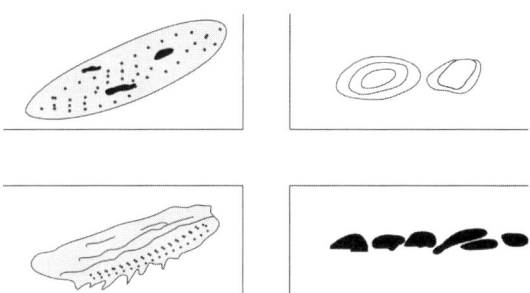

Fig. 6.10: Orientation of tissue in the block

Table 6.7 General embedding faults with causes and remedies

Sr. No.	Fault	Cause	Remedy
1.	Fluffy white spot or patches in block	• Slow cooling of block • Impurities of clearing agent left in the block	Re-embed the tissue
2.	Sharp peaks at the surface	• Sudden immersion of embedding container in cold water without keeping the upper surface above the water	Re-embed the tissue
3.	A depression in the center of upper surface of the block	• The container is not deep enough • Tissue is embedded too high • Paraffin is very hot	Re-embed the tissue

Contd...

Contd...

Sr. No.	Fault	Cause	Remedy
4.	Air space in the block	• Use of very hot paraffin and very cold water for cooling	Adjust desired temperature of paraffin and water
5.	Water trap in block	• Block is immersed in water before formation of thin film on the surface	Re-embed the tissue
6.	Fractures appear in the block	• Block was cooled too rapidly • Paraffin is poured in two layers	Re-embed the tissue

- Keep the blocks either in thick paper bags or in clean wooden boxes having a cotton cloth lining and protected from dust.
- Keep the blocks in a mixture of equal volume of 40% alcohol and glycerin in well-stoppered bottles.

CELLOIDIN AND LOW VISCOSITY NITROCELLULOSE EMBEDDING

The celloidin and the low viscosity nitrocellulose are both forms of cellulose nitrate of which the low viscosity nitrocellulose (LVN) is of less viscosity. The LVN, because of its low viscosity, penetrates more readily and may be used in higher concentrations than celloidin. It gives a much harder block and allows thinner sections to be cut.

Fixed and dehydrated tissues are impregnated with increasing concentrations of celloidin of LVN dissolved in a mixture of absolute alcohol and ether. Clearing agents are not utilized and no heat is required in the process. As a result, distortion of the tissues is minimal.

Impregnations:
- After completion of the dehydration transfer the tissue to a mixture of equal parts of absolute alcohol and ether. This is to speed up the impregnation process.
- Transfer the tissue to 2% solution of celloidin or 8% solution of LVN for 4–7 days.
- Transfer the tissue to 4% solution of celloidin or 16% solution of LVN for 4–7 days.
- Transfer the tissue to 8% solution of celloidin or 24% solution of LVN for 2–3 days.

Embedding:
- Fill the special embedding mould upto the half way mark with 8% celloidin or 24% LVN, place the tissue in position with surface to cut uppermost.
- Fill the mould with more of the embedding solution.
- Place the mould in a desiccator containing ether vapours.
- When all the air bubbles have been removed by the ether vapor, place the tissue with the surface to be cut facing downwards in the mould. This will prevent any air bubble from being trapped beneath the tissue.
- Keep the mould to a second desiccator containing chloroform vapor to harden the celloidin or LVN to the desired consistency. The desired consistency is determined when the thumb pressed on the block leaves no impression.
- Transfer the block from the mould into pure chloroform. The block slowly sinks to the bottom of the solution.
- Finally, transfer the block to 75% alcohol until required for cutting.

Advantages of celloidin and LVN:
- There is a considerable minimization of shrinkage of the tissues, mainly due to the absence of heat in the process.
- Both celloidin and LVN improve cutting qualities of large block of dense tissues as a result of the reduced hardening and plasticity of the medium.
- They give superior cohesion to tissue layers of different consistency.
- They are very useful for the preparation of sections of brain.

Disadvantages:
- The processing time is long and tissues such as the brain can take up to three weeks to process.
- Thinner sections up to 10 μm are difficult to cut.
- Serial sections are difficult to produce.
- There is storage problem.
- Celloidin and LVN are highly explosive if they left for drying.

GELATIN EMBEDDING

Gelatin is a chemically modified form of collage, a protein that is insoluble and which is distinguished by its high content of glycerin and hydroxyl proline. The collagen used in gelatin is identified as a form of organic matter in the bones of cattle and from the white connective tissue fibers in the skin of cattle and pigs.

Gelatin is an embedding medium finds its main use as a supporting medium for frozen sections. Generally, the tissue from which frozen sections are to be cut is not embedded, the freezing itself provides sufficient support for sectioning. But when frozen sections are to be prepared from tough or friable tissues, a supporting medium is required to prevent the tissue from fragmenting. This is where the gelatin is very useful. After embedding, the blocks of tissues are put in formalin to harden.

Advantages: One major advantage of gelatin as an embedding medium is the absence of dehydration at any time in the process thus avoiding distortion of the tissue by shrinkage.

Disadvantages: However, because gelatin cannot be removed from the tissue and since it is capable of taking up both acidic and basic dyes, it very often gives the poor microscopical picture. Also, thin sections are not easily cut while ribboning of the sections is difficult.

Embedding solutions:

Solution A: Gelatin   : 12.5 g
             Distilled water   : 87.5 mL
             Phenol crystals   : 1.0 g
Solution B: Gelatin   : 25 g
             Distilled water   : 75 mL
             Phenol crystals   : 1.0 g

Solution A and B is prepared by heating distilled water to 37°C. Dissolve the phenol in warm distilled water. Add gelatin and incubate at 37°C until the gelatin is dissolved. Filter through surgical gauze. Bottle and label.

Solution C: Formalin   : 5 mL
             Distilled water   : 95 mL

Method:
1. Place the tissue (not exceeding 3 mm in thickness) in solution A for at least 12 hours at 37°C.
2. Transfer to solution B for at least 12 hours at 37°C.
3. Using Leukhart's embedding mould, embed the tissue in solution B. Allow to cool and then trim.
4. Transfer the trimmed block to solution C for 18–24 hours.
5. Cut sections as for frozen section.

PLASTIC EMBEDDING

More recent developments in the formulation of plastic resins have begun to alter the way sections are embedded. For electron microscopy, that require ultrathin sections, paraffin is simply not suitable. Paraffin and nitrocellulose are too soft to yield thin enough sections. Instead, special formulations of hard plastics are used, and the basic process is similar to that for paraffin. The alterations involve placing a dehydrated tissue sample of about 1 mm^3 into a liquid plastic which is then polymerized to form a hard block. The plastic block is trimmed and sectioned with an ultramicrotome to obtain sections of a few hundred angstroms.

Table 6.8: Light and electron microscopy preparations

Process	Light microscopy	Electron microscopy
• Sample size	• 1 cm^3	• 1 cm^3
• Fixative	• Formaldehyde	• Glutaraldehyde
• Post-fixation	• None	• Osmium
• Dehydration	• Graded alcohol	• Tetraoxide
• Clearing agent	• Xylol/toluene	• Alcohol/acetone
• Embedding material	• Paraffin	• Propylene oxide
• Section thickness	• 5–10 µ	• Various plastics 60–90 nm
• Stain	• Colored dyes	• Heavy metals

The Table 6.8 presents a comparison of paraffin embedding with the typical plastic embedding for TEM.

Softer plastics are also being used for routine light microscopy. The average thickness of a paraffin sectioned tissue is between 7–10 µ. Often this will consist of two cell layers and, consequently definition for cytoplasmic structures. With a plastic such as polysciences JB-4 it is possible to section tissues in the 1–3 µ range with increased sharpness. This is particularly helpful if photomicrographs are to be taken. With the decrease in section thickness, however, comes a loss of contrast, and thin sections (1µ) usually require a phase contrast microscope as well as special staining procedure. The sharp image make the effort worthwhile. The soft plastics, which can be sectioned with a standard steel microtome blade, do not require glass or diamond knives, as with the harder plastics used for EM work.

RESIN EMBEDDING

In case of some specific tissues like renal, bone marrow or lymphoid tissues, greater cytological and nuclear details are required, which can be provided by 3–5 µm paraffin sections. To get such thin sections materials harder than paraffin wax are required to provide adequate support to the tissues in the cutting phase.

Embedding tissues in resin meets the above requirements. These agents are readily available, relatively inexpensive, easy to prepare and handle. It requires less time for infiltration and provide thin sections. Ideally, resins should demonstrate stability, uniform polymerization, water solubility and should be degradable and non toxic and produce minimum artifacts. Unfortunately, none of the resin media currently available which can meet all these demands. Excessive shrinkage is common problems.

The tissues are fixed in commonly used formalin and mercuric based fixatives and then dehydrated with ethanol and acetone if required and cleared with propylene oxide.

Impregnation is carried out by the progressive replacement of fixative or dehydrants with resin. With more viscous resin impregnation is best performed under vacuum.

Epoxy resins (*Araldite or Epon or Spur*): An epoxy resin is a substance which contains the – C – C – groups and is also capable of polymerization to form 3–D irreversible structure. Epoxy compounds are hard resins from which 0.5–1 µm thick sections can be cut using either a glass or diamond knife.

Araldite embedding solution:
- Araldite stock solutions: Araldite 10 g, epson 10 g, and hardener 15 g
- Mix thoroughly using mechanical shaker. It is stable for 3 weeks.
- A working solution is prepared by adding 2 g accelerator to every 100 mL stock solution and mix thoroughly.

Acrylic resins (Methacrylates): Methacrylates rapidly infiltrates fixes, dehydrates tissue at room temperature. These resins are more suited for hard materials like undecalcified bone. Methacrylates are the soft resin from which 0.5–2 µm thick sections can be readily obtained using carbide, glass or diamond knives. Different types of acrylic resins available are butyl methacrylate, glycol methacrylate, etc.

DOUBLE EMBEDDING

Double embedding methods such as agar-paraffin embedding, are used when tissues require external support or particular pre-embedment orientation. Paraffin wax double infiltration methods provide hard tissues with additional support provided by substances such as agar or nitrocellulose, with the convenience and ease of wax microtomy.

- **Agar-Paraffin wax double embedding:** Double embedding in agar-paraffin is a reliable and convenient method of handling minute and friable tissue fragments such as curettings and endoscopic biopsies, which can be lost during tissue processing. It also overcomes the difficulty of manipulating small tissue fragments during embedding and facilitates correct orientation and identification of tissues for histochemical and immunohistochemical control tissues.

Reagents required

Agar (technical or microbiological grade)	: 1.5–3.0 g
Distilled water	: 90 mL
37% formaldehyde solution	: 10 mL

Method: Dissolve the agar in distilled water using a boiling water bath, autoclave or microwave oven. Add formaldehyde and mix well. Distribute 20 mL aliquots into screw capped bottles. Store at 4°C. For use melt the agar as previously indicated. Cool to 50–60°C and hold in a 60°C oven. Loosen container caps before remelting agar. Embed tissues by pipetting agar solution over tissue fragments correctly oriented on a clean, flat surface or membrane filter.

- **Agar-Ester wax double infiltration:** Double infiltration of tissues in agar and ester wax aids thin serial sectioning of chitinized tissues at 0.5–1.0 µm and is a possible alternative to pine resin-beewax paraffin wax used to support plastic vascular prostheses for sectioning. The fine crystalline nature and hardness of ester wax improves tissue-wax adhesion and provides adequate support for thin serial sectioning.

Reagent required: 5% aqueous agar cellosolve.

Method: Infiltrate fixed tissues in 5% aqueous agar solution for 1 hour orientate tissues in an agar filled mould. Allow the agar to set. Trim the block. Pass the block, though the following series, 30 minutes in each solutions: 30%, 50%, 70% ethanol, 90% ethanol plus cellosolve, 2:1, the same 1:2; pure cellosolve, 3 changes; cellosolve plus ester wax 1;1; pure ester wax at least 2 changes, the last overnight. Embed as usual and cool rapidly.

RE-EMBEDDING

For re-embedding follow the following steps:
- Trim the paraffin block carefully as close to the tissue as possible without injury to the tissue.
- Immerse the trimmed tissue block in the fresh infiltrating bath for 30–60 minutes.
- When all the paraffin is melted completed, re-embed the tissue.

EXERCISE

1. What are the major steps of tissue processing involved in the "Paraffin wax technique"? Explain in detail.
2. Enumerate four major steps in paraffin wax technique and describe in detail infiltration and impregnation technique.
3. Give the significance of the following in the preparation of histological specimen—fixation, embedding dehydration and rehydration.
4. Why is it necessary to dehydrate the tissue? Describe the procedure of dehydration and test for completion of dehydration.
5. What is dehydration of tissue? How is it carried out for paraffin or celloidin embedding method?
6. Enlist various dehydrating agents. Write their action, advantages and disadvantages.

7. Write in detail process of dehydration of tissue.
8. What is meant by clearing of tissue? Why is it necessary to clear the tissue?
9. What are clearing agents? Enlist and mention their advantages and disadvantages.
10. What is tissue processing? Enlist various steps of tissue processing using paraffin wax and describe each step in brief.
11. Write notes on:
    i. Ethanol as dehydrating agent
    ii. Cedar wood oil as clearing agent
12. Explain the process of infiltration and impregnation.
13. What is vacuum impregnation? Describe the procedure of vacuum impregnation with their advantages and disadvantages.
14. Describe the apparatus and procedure for vacuum impregnation.
15. Describe the process of celloidin impregnation and embedding with the advantages and disadvantages of celloidin.
16. Describe automatic tissue processor.
17. Explain the construction and working of automatic tissue processor with neat labeled diagram. Write precaution to be taken during processing.
18. What is embedding? How gelatin is used as an embedding medium?
19. Write one of the example of processing schedule used in manual tissue processing.
20. What is the importance of manual tissue processing? Describe the process in short.
21. Describe different embedding media used by histopathology technique.
22. Explain use of paraffin wax as embedding medium. What are disadvantages of it? Write causes of using the alternative embedding medium.
23. Enumerate different types of moulds with a brief description of each.
24. Describe various steps involved in technique of embedding.
25. What are different faults encountered during the process of embedding? Write their causes and remedial measures to be taken.
26. Write short notes on :
    i. L-moulds
    ii. Dehydration
    iii. Rehydration
    iv. Embedding
    v. Clearing
    vi. Wax dispenser

OBJECTIVE QUESTIONS

1. The process by which water from tissue is removed is called _____
    a. Clearing   b. Fixation
    c. Infiltration d. Dehydration

2. A mixture containing ethanol to which small amount of methanol is added to make the fluid unfit for consumption
    a. Denatured spirit   b. Methylated spirit
    c. Proof spirit   d. All

3. Generally successive _____ grades of dehydrating agent is used
    a. Higher   b. Lower
    c. Absolute   d. None

4. _____ is used to ensure completion of dehydration.
    a. Anhydrous copper sulfate
    b. Anhydrous zinc sulfate
    c. Anhydrous potassium sulfate
    d. Anhydrous sodium sulfate

5. Step after dehydration is _____
    a. Fixation   b. Clearing
    c. Infiltration   d. Embedding

6. The process of clearing is also called as _____
    a. Dealcoholization   b. Dechlorination
    c. Dehydration   d. None

7. The most common clearing agent used in histopathology laboratory is
    a. Propylene   b. Toluene
    c. Benzene   d. Xylene

8. _____ is the saturation of tissue cavities and cells by a supporting medium.
    a. Infiltration   b. Embedding
    c. Clearing   d. Mounting

9. Vacuum infiltration is the impregnation of tissues by a molten medium under _____ pressure.
    a. Increased   b. Reduced
    c. Atmospheric   d. None

10. _____ is the polycrystalline mixture of solid hydrocarbons produced during refining of coal and mineral oils.
    a. Paraffin wax   b. Bee wax
    c. Carbowax   d. All

11. _____ is an example of aqueous embedding medium
    a. Gelatin   b. Carbowax
    c. Polyethylene glycol d. Ester waxes

12. Polyethylene glycol is an example of:
    a. Water miscible media
    b. Aqueous media
    c. Water tolerant media
    d. Water immiscible media

13. Celloidin embedding technique is mostly used for sectioning of _____ tissues.
    a. Hard   b. Soft
    c. Very soft   d. Adiposed tissue

14. _____ is used for plastic embedding.
    a. Agar
    b. Gelatin
    c. Araldite
    d. Carboxymethyl cellulose

15. Elongated tissues are placed _____ across the block.
    a. Diagonally   b. Vertically
    c. Horizontally   d. None

16. Tubular and walled specimens are embedded so as to provide _____ sections showing all tissue layers.
    a. Longitudinal   b. Transverse
    c. Vertical   d. Elongated

17. When tissue require external support or pre-embedment orientation _____ technique is used
    a. Double embedding   b. Double clearing
    c. Double dehydration d. Double fixation

18. Leuckhard embedding boxes are two _____ pieces of metals.
    a. U-shaped   b. C-shaped
    c. V-shaped   d. L-shaped

ANSWERS

1-d, 2-b, 3-a, 4-a, 5-b, 6-a, 7-d, 8-a, 9-b, 10-a 11-a, 12-c, 13-b, 14-c, 15-a, 16-b, 17-a, 18-d.

CHAPTER 7

Microtomy and Section Cutting

Microtomy: The embedded tissues are then subjected to section cutting. This involves the technique of microtomy which yields thin sections of the tissue for microscopic examination of the internal structure.

Sections are prepared on an instrument known as a microtome of which various types are available. Common features of all the microtomes are that they are having firm support for knife and tissue block and a feed mechanism designed to advance the specimen a predetermined number of micrometers on each cutting stroke. The thickness of the sections produced during microtomy may range between a fraction of one micrometer (ultramicrotomy) to several hundred micrometers. The most common range is 3–8 μm.

MICROTOMES

Depending upon the time of work, the nature of tissue preparation and embedding medium and other factors, there are many types of microtomes. Generally there are seven types of microtomes namely:
- Rotary microtome
- Rocking microtome
- Sliding microtome
- Base sledge microtome
- Freezing microtome
- Cold (cryostat) microtome
- Ultra thin microtome.

Rotary, rocking and sledge microtomes are widely used for paraffin wax embedded material while the sliding microtome is used principally for sectioning cellulose nitrate embedded tissue.

■ Rotary Microtome (Fig. 7.1)

It is the excellent and most popular microtome generally used for preparation of serial sections. They are named 'rotary' because the feed mechanism is actuated by turning a wheel on one side of the machine. The knife is fixed, edge upper most and the object move against the knife according to the thickness of the section, rising and falling vertically. It consists of following parts:

- **Heavy base:** It is the lowermost part of the microtome on which all other parts are present.
- **Central axis:** There is a central axis having an arrangement in its front to fix the block holder.
- **Knife holder:** On the front part of the heavy base there are two broad grooves in which knife holder is fit which can be moved. The screws are provided on this holder to the adjust the angle of the knife.
- **Knife or razor:** It is mounted on the razor or knife holder with the help of screws. The knife can be adjusted to the desired angle by moving the knife holder.
- **Block holder:** It is a short, wide rod having the expanded circular head on which paraffin tissue block is fixed. This is fixed in the space, with a simple clamp operated by screws.
- **Drive wheel:** It is a circular drive wheel with a handle which drives the central axis forward. It is provided with a lock. One rotation of the drive wheel produces a

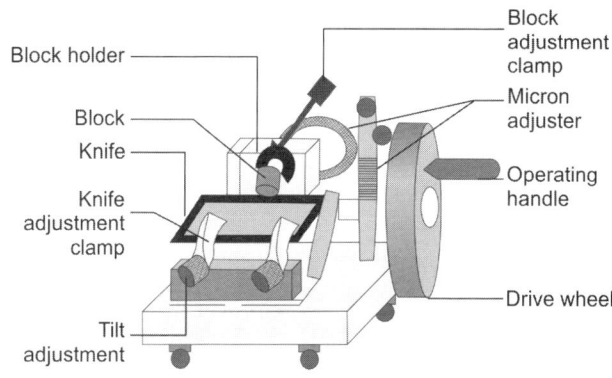

Fig. 7.1: Parts of rotary microtome

complete cycle of downward cutting stroke, an upward return stroke and activation of the advance mechanism. One complete rotation will remove a section of known thickness from the face of the block.
- **Micron adjuster:** It is present on the posterior part of the heavy base. It is connected to the advance mechanism by a shaft. It has an adjustment lever, which gives the sections of desired thickness.

The rotary microtome is easily adapted to an electrically driven mechanical drive acting on the external operating wheel. This helps in preparing multiple sections from a single block. It is mostly used for paraffin wax embedded material and well-suited for producing serial sections. But it is not suitable for cutting cellulose nitrate blocks as in the sliding microtome.

■ Rocking Microtome

They are most simplest of all the microtomes. The knife is fixed, with the edge uppermost, and the object moves against rigid knife in the arc of a circle, producing a slightly curved surface on top of the block. This cutting stroke is spring operated and somewhat less controllable than with other microtome. It is simple to operate and used for paraffin embedded tissue. During operation, it produces jerk ' rock' noise, hence the name 'rocking' (Fig. 7.2).

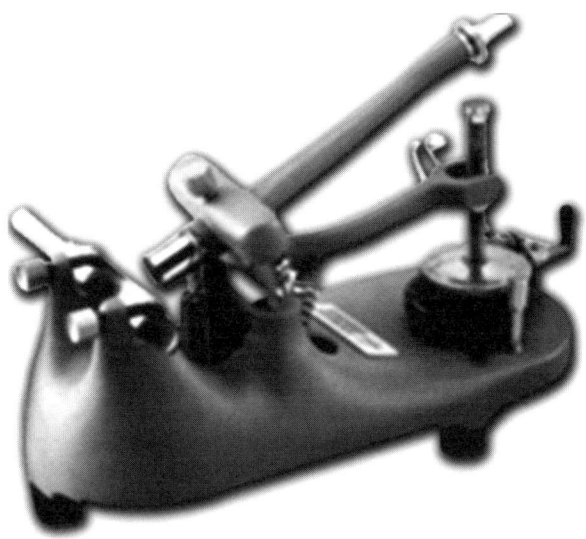

Fig. 7.2: Cambridge rocking microtome

■ Sliding Microtome

It is mostly used for cutting tissue embedded in cellulose nitrate (celloidin), hence are also called as celloidin microtome. The difference between the sliding microtome and other microtomes is that the block remains stationary while the microtome knife moves during the process of sectioning. The main feature of sliding microtome is the ease with which it cuts sections from tissue block (Fig. 7.3).

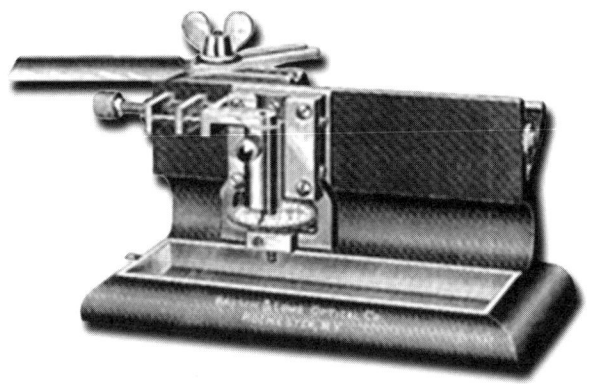

Fig. 7.3: Sliding microtome

■ Base Sledge Microtome

It is a rigidly constructed machine, readily used for sectioning specimens embedded in all types of embedding medium. It consists of a fixed knife beneath which travels the tissue block mounted on a heavy sliding base containing feed mechanism. This base/sledge is moved to and fro on runners against the knife to produce sections. The feed mechanism is either automatic or manual. It is mostly used for specimens which are often large and hard. They are particularly suitable for cutting bone and teeth (Fig. 7.4).

■ Freezing Microtome

These are designed for the preparation of 'frozen' sections of fixed or unfixed tissues, usually without preliminary embedding. The tissue is fixed to this microtome. In the process of

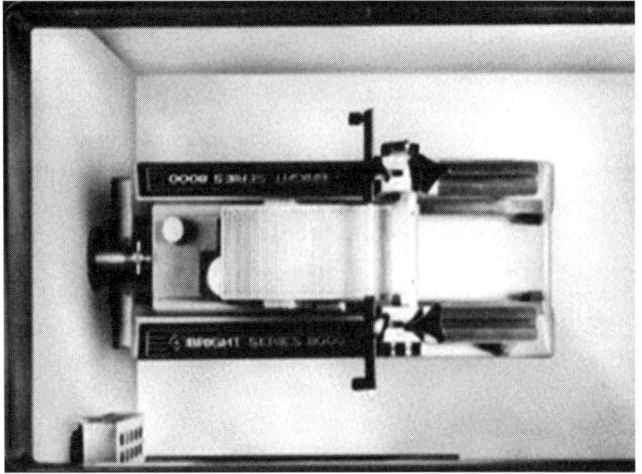

Fig. 7.4: Base sledge microtome

section cutting, the knife moves in a horizontal plane and simultaneously the tissue is frozen by liquid, compressed carbon dioxide. For every next section, the tissue is moved ahead so that the number of sections we get is very less. It is a clinical microtome which is mostly used in hospitals to obtain tissue sections which are immediately or urgently required for observation.

■ Cold Microtome/Cryostat

It is used for cutting frozen sections of a tissue. Unembedded soft specimens are generally cut in the frozen state which gives necessary firmness to the tissue. This method is useful for rapid histopathological diagnosis during an operation. It is also useful to examine the sections of structure or a substance that would be destroyed in the routine preparation of sections.

■ Ultra Microtome

These are instruments especially designed for preparation of the very thin sections necessary for examination with an electron microscope. They differ from the conventional microtome in the finess and precision of the feed mechanism which is actuated either by mechanical means or by electrically controlled thermal means to give a thickness range of 5–100 nm (0.005–0.1µm) and specially prepared knives (usually plate-glass) are used to cut the very thin section of tissue embedded in a hard synthetic resin.

■ Saw Microtome

Saw microtomes will cut sections of very hard material such as undecalcifed bone, glass or ceramics. The samples, commonly embedded in resins, are moved extremely slowly against a diamond coated saw rotating at approximately 600 rpm. Sections of 20 µm or greater are possible, providing the saw blade is in perfect condition. Very thin sections are not possible.

■ Vibrating Microtome

Originally conceived as a microtome which could produce high quality sections of fresh, unfixed material from animal or botanical sources and to replace the hand microtome. The name of the instrument derives from the high speed vibration produced in a safety razor blade to provide the cutting power. The amplitude of vibration is adjusted by altering electrical voltage applied to the 'knife'. Different degrees of vibration are required to produce sections from varying densities of material. To prevent tearing, soft material is cut whilst immersed in a fluid which also aids in dissipating heat produced at the vibrating edge of the razor as it cuts.

■ Hand Microtome

The successful use of a hand microtome is limited to sectioning intrinsically rigid botanical material. It is difficult to obtain a thin, even sections of animal tissues.

MICROTOME KNIVES

The production of thin sections of tissues depends upon properly sharpened knife. It is one of the most important components of the microtome and require constant care and maintenance. Microtome knives are made from high grade steel tempered to a specific harness for its propose. They are available in various types and sizes according to the microtome and embedding medium used.

■ Knife Profiles

Knives are identified by their profile. There are four basic types of profile (Fig. 7.5)

Strongly planoconcave/biconcave	-	Profile A
Planoconcave	-	Profile B
Wedge shape	-	Profile C
Plane-shaped	-	Profile D

- **Strongly planoconcave:** One surface of the planoconcave knife is straight whilst the other is hollow ground. The bi-concave knife has two hollow ground surfaces. Both knives are extremely sharp and are used for cutting soft, celloidin embedded material or foam compounds. These knives are not suitable for relatively hard materials, which cause the edge to vibrate and produce the phenomenon known as chattering. To obtain the best result the knife should always be oblique to the object when cutting sections.
- **Planoconcave:** This knife is similar to a profile A knife but has a thicker back. It is used for cutting sections from material which is too hard to cut with a profile A knife but can also be used for softer materials embedded in paraffin wax. This profile knife is also suitable for cutting the softer components (stalks, leaves) of fresh botanical

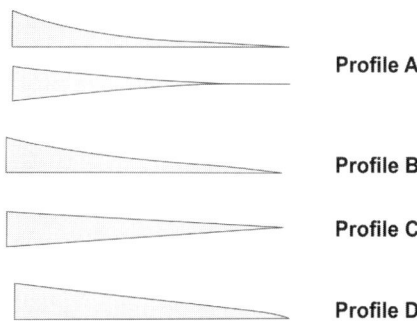

Fig. 7.5: Microtome knife profiles

specimens. This knife should be positioned obliquely to the material being sectioned.
- **Wedge shape:** The wedge-shaped knife has more rigidity than profile A or B knife and can therefore be used for cutting harder materials. Because of the extra thick nature of the wedge at the tip this type of knife cannot be ground as sharp as profile A and B knife. Commonly used for cutting sections from paraffin wax embedded material, frozen sections, cryostat sections, and synthetic resin embedded material. This knife can also cut soft plastics, rubber, wood and some textile fibers. With this style of knife the cutting plane is transverse to the object.
- **Plane-shaped:** This knife will cut hard and tough material as it has greater stability than any of the other profile knives. As only one bevel provides the cutting edge this knife is the least sharp of all of the profiles. It is commonly used for cutting synthetic resin blocks, hard materials embedded in paraffin wax, large wax blocks and the various substances used in industry.

■ Types of Microtome Knives

- **Steel knives:** Steel microtome knives are manufactured from high quality carbon or tool grade steel which is heat treated to harden the edge. The steel should be free from impurities, contain anti-corrosives and be rust-resistant. The best knives are those that are fully hardened. Those which are only surface hardened lose the cutting edge very quickly once the hardened area is removed through repeated re-sharpening.
- **Non-corrosive knives for cryostats:** These are manufactured from hardened, heat treated stainless steel free from all impurities and containing 12 to 15% chromium.
- **Disposable blades:** Disposable microtome blades are essentially refined, thickened razor blades. When held in a specially adapted knife holder the blades consistently produce high quality sections and have replaced conventional microtome knives in many instances. All disposable blades are manufactured from high quality stainless steel, although there are different grades according to the thickness of the blade. The edge of disposable blades can be coated with platinum or chromium to enhance strength and prolong cutting life. Teflon coated blades are particularly suitable for use in cryostats as these offer reduced cutting resistance and minimal friction. The smaller, thinner disposable blade also reaches cryostat chamber temperature more rapidly than a conventional knife minimizing time delay during blade exchanges or temperature adjustments. Disposable blades need to be held rigidly in a special holder to prevent vibration during the cutting stroke.

These knives consistently produce high quality sections virtually free from compression.
- **Tungsten carbide:** Knives manufactured from high quality tungsten carbide are non corrosive, practically non magnetic and 100 times harder than hardened tool steel. The knives have excellent resistance to wear, but are brittle because of their extreme hardness and should be handled carefully. Up to 30,000 serial sections of undecalcifed bone embedded in methacrylate per sharpening has been reported.
- **Glass knives:** The cutting edge of glass knives used for conventional sectioning is parallel to on surface of the glass ('Ralph knives' with edges of 25 or 38 mm) whilst in those used for ultramicrotomy it is across the thickness of the glass. A commercial glass knife maker is recommended to ensure consistency and reproducibility of the knife edge. Glass knives are hard, but brittle and care is required with their handling. These knives deteriorate with storage due to changes in the 'flow' or 'strain' of the glass after fracture and from oxidation impurities remaining in the hardened glass after manufacture. Knives should thus be prepared immediately before use.
- **Diamond knives:** Diamond knives are manufactured from gem quality diamonds without flaws. Although, this makes them very expensive the knives are extremely durable, because of the hardness factor of the diamond, and are used primarily for cutting very thin, resin sections.
- **Sapphire knives:** These knives are manufactured from one piece of solid sapphire artificially produced from an alumina monocrystal under computer controlled thermal conditions. Sapphire is harder than tungsten carbide or glass which ensures high durability of the cutting edge for all types of material. The only restriction when using a sapphire knife is block size as the knife edge is limited to 11 mm. A special knife holder is required.

■ Knife Handles and Backs

Most microtome knives are provided with a detachable handle with screws on one end of the blade (Fig. 7.6).

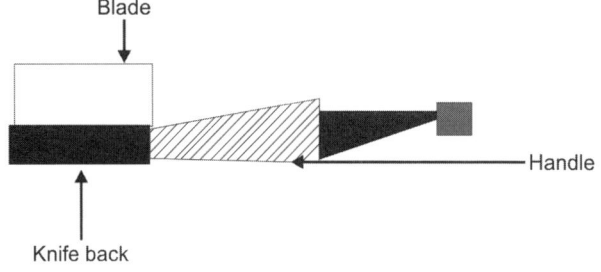

Fig. 7.6: Knife, knife handle and knife back

Care of Microtome Knife

It is the most important and integral part of the microtome which require constant care and maintenance. If properly used, it can give a long period of service. There are three common ways of runing the edge of the a microtome knife which are:
- Trying to cut hard object
- Careless storage of knife
- Improper handling during sharpening.

Following care should be taken during using knife
- Do not cut hard object like undecalcified bone with the knife (use decalcified bone).
- Do not cut the tissue in the center of the knife this will cause uneven wearing of the knife.
- Store knife properly in knife box after cleaning with a cloth moistened with xylene.
- Before using the knife, clean it properly to remove rusty spots or dust if any present on it.
- Keep the knife always in the knife box when not in use.
- Applying grease to the knife if it is not in use for longer period of time, to avoid corrosion of the knife.
- Keep the knife box in an airy place, do not lock it in a wooden cabinet.

Knife Sharpening

Sharpening of microtome knives may be carried out either by manual means or on automated machines. The results should be equally satisfactory if correctly performed, although manual sharpening requires more skill, experience and time.

Requirement for Knife Sharpening

It includes abrasive surfaces, supporting surface, lubricants, abrasive powder, abrasive stones, and handles and backs.
- **Abrasive surface:** Mostly knife sharpening require slabs of stones having a different range of abrasive properties. Though these abrasive blocks give satisfactory results, but have a number of disadvantages like they are expensive, sharpening results surface wear, and have insufficient surface area.
- **Supporting surfaces for abrasives:** It is recommended to use the separate abrasive powder for knife sharpening. A number of different surfaces may be employed for supporting the abrasive powders and lubricant. Any perfectly flat, rigid surface can be used as supporting surface.

Glass plates: Half inch glass plate having flat, smooth surface can be used as a surface.

Metal plates: Metal such as copper, bronze, aluminium, cast iron, can be used as a surface plate for knife sharpening.

Other materials like plastic, wood can be used if the glass or metal plates are not available.

Lubricants: Use of lubricants during knife sharpening perform functions like:
- They act as coolants.
- Fine metal particles are allowed to flow away from the knife.
- They reduces the tendency of the stone's pores to become blocked with metal particles.
- **Types of lubricants:** Aqueous lubricants which can be used are 1% liquid soap, 10% liquid detergent, 50% glycerol, 10–30% soluble oil. Non aqueous lubricants includes use of lubricating oils, or oil thinned with paraffin. Use of dialap fluid is recommended.
- **Abrasive powder:** Abrasive powders are the fine dust particles of substances which are applied to the surface of the supporting surface for the formation of the abrasive surface for knife sharpening. The various abrasive powders which can be used are diamond, carborandum, alumina, magnesium oxide, chromium oxide, etc.
  - **Diamond:** The ideal abrasive is diamond dust for the final polishing of the knife. It is available in various particle sizes, and it has advantages that it do not undergo wear during sharpening.
  - **Carborandum/silicon carbide:** This is available in various particle sizes. Particles breakdown readily with prolonged action of knife sharpening. 2F, 3F, and 4F grades of particles are mostly used.
  - **Alumina (aluminium oxide):** Alpha, gamma alumina is mostly used in the final stages of sharpening. They are available in various particle sizes.
  - **Magnesium oxide:** It is used due to its tendency to aggregate and cause scoring. It has smaller and softer particle size than alumina and suitable only for the final polishing stages.
  - **Chromium oxide:** It is sometimes used instead of alumina, particularly on the softer metal plates.
  - **Abrasive stones:** The small carborandum stones or Yellow Belgian water stones or Arkansas stones or Aloxite stones can be directly used for coarse sharpening. They have coarse and smooth sides. The coarse side is used for coarse sharpening and smooth side is used for fine sharpening. But these stones are not used for final sharpening of the stones.

Yellow or Blue Belgian Stones

The Belgian coticule stones offer a combination of honing properties resulting in an incredible smooth and sharp edge. The blue stone is around the 4000-5000 grit while the yellow is around the 8000-10000 grit level.

Stones can be used as slurry, wet or dry. Each will give a different stage and result. The yellow coticule contains about 35-40% of garnets and the blue has around 30% of garnet content. Belgian whetstones will sharpen any kind of steel and this includes stainless steel and high speed steel (HSS), such as knives, chisels, scissors, axes, adzes, draw knives, straight razors and much more. The stone is non-porous and is used with water only. The blue side of his combostone is very uniform a true 4000-6000 grit. The yellow side is the perfect 8000 grit when used with slurry and a true polisher when used with water only or dry around the 10000 grit. Very uniform with a small 1 inch natural occuring crack which does not affect anything and will never hurt or damage the edge.

■ Methods of Knife Sharpening

The various steps of knife sharpening are as follows:
- **Examination of knife edge:** Before starting knife sharpening, the edge of the knife should be examined under a dissecting microscope, both in vertical and horizontal position. Gross irregularities in the edge should be visible in the horizontal position, whilst in the vertical position any rounding of the edge is seen as a ribbon of reflected light.
- **Process of sharpening:** It consists of two parts honing and stropping. It can be done mechanically or by automated knife sharpeners. The process of removing nicks and irregularities from the knife edge is called as honing and the process of giving final polishing to the edge of the knife is called stropping.

Honing

It includes grinding of the knife on a special stone. The stone is called hone which is usually a rectangular block of stone mostly of yellow Belgian water stone or Carborandum Stones or Arkansas Stones or Aloxite stone.

Technique of honing (Fig. 7.7): It involves the following steps:
- With the help of a xylene soaked cloth clean the knife.
- Keep the hone on a table of suitable height and place a damp cloth under the hone.
- Remove any dirt or dust from the surface of the hone and apply a suitable lubricating oil (coconut oil) or soap water.
- Now keep the knife on the hone at one end, such that the cutting edge of the knife is away from you.
- Push the knife diagonally forward by applying sufficient pressure so that the cutting edge of the knife just touches the surface of the hone.
- Just before reaching the other end of the hone, turn over the knife on its back without lifting it so that the cutting edge is now facing towards you.
- Pull back the knife towards you in a diagonal stroke.
- Repeat the procedure and observe the knife edge under the microscope (50×) from time to time to check the progress of honing.
- The edge will be seen to be fine but regularly serrated. The serrations are due to the abrasiveness of the hone and can be removed by the polishing action of subsequent stropping.

Stropping

It is mostly done to remove the wire edge (serrations) caused by the friction of knife steel on the hone during honing. Whether the sharpening is done by hand or automatic sharpeners, the final polishing is done on a strop (Fig. 7.8). Strop is mostly made of leather. Strops are of two types rigid or flexible. The rigid strop is a leather strop which is stretched over a solid wooden block. Flexible

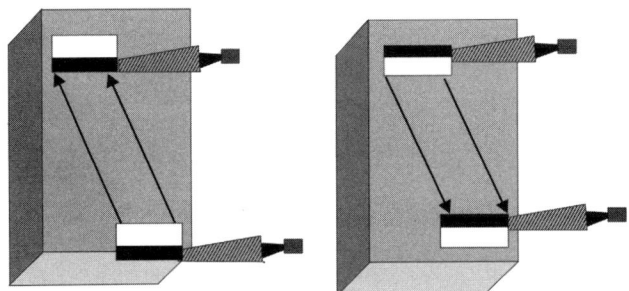

Fig. 7.7: Technique of honing

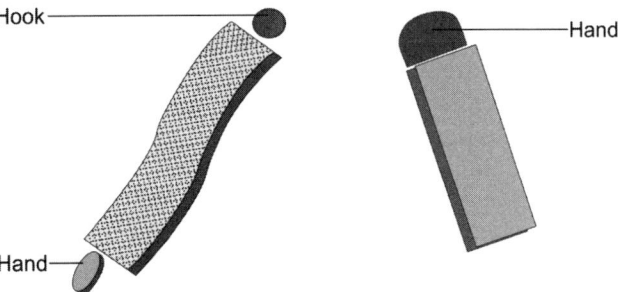

Fig. 7.8: Flexible strop; rigid strop

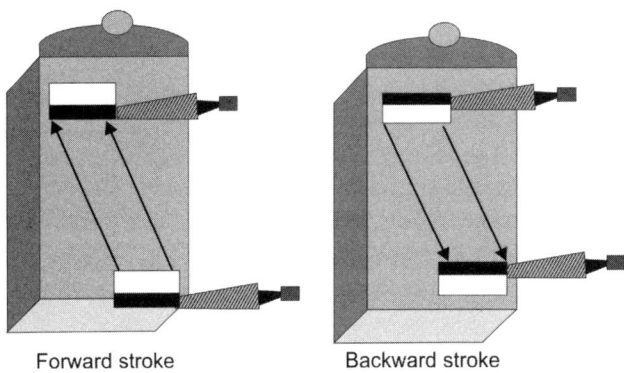

Fig. 7.9: Stropping

strop consists of two leather belts joined together. One leather is impregnated with a fine diamond dust which is used for coarse stropping whereas the other leather is a pig skin, which is used for the fine stropping. Flexible strop is provided with a hood and a handle for attaching it on the immovable object and handling respectively. The strop should be occasionally cleaned with mild soap solution or strop paste. The soap solution should be massaged on the leather cleaned with cloth, and dried overnight.

Technique of Stropping (Fig. 7.9)

- The knife which is to be sharped should be thoroughly cleaned before stropping.
- The rigid strop is then placed on the bench, cleaned with mild soap solution and then with water. Finally, it is properly cleaned with a soft, lintless cloth and dried overnight.
- The knife is placed at one end of the strop and is pushed diagonally forward.
- Apply and maintain the pressure on the knife just sufficient to keep the edge in contact with the surface of the strop.
- Just before reaching the other end of the strop turn over the knife on its back so that the cutting edge is now away from you.
- Pull back the knife steadily along the strop towards you.
- Repeat the procedure for 20 to 30 double strokes, rhythmly and steadily and observe the edge of the knife under the microscope.
- A well-sharpened knife has a sharp, smooth, and even edge and is without irregularities.

SECTION CUTTING

Equipment required for section cutting

- Floating water bath
- Hot plate or drying oven
- Fine pointed forceps
- Small brush
- Scalpel
- Clean cloth
- Slides
- Section adhesive
- Blotting paper.

Floating Water Bath

Water bath used in histopathological laboratory is mostly thermostatically controlled. The temperature of water bath should be maintained at 45°C when the melting point of the paraffin wax used for block making is about 56°C. Sometimes, a trace of detergent is added to water to help in the flattening of the sections.

Hot Plate/Drying Oven

The drying of sections on the slides recommended to take place at a temperature as low as 37°C but this is not practically possible because the time required for drying of sections at this temperature is very much. Hence, mostly the drying of sections is done on a hot plate. It looks quite easy though this requires great care and precaution, otherwise it may lead to the distortion of the tissue.

Slides

The most commonly used slides are those having size 76 mm × 25 mm. Slides are available in different thickness, but mostly 1.0 to 1.2 mm in thickness slide are preferred as they get easily fit into the staining racks and are not fragile.

Section Adhesives

During the staining procedure most of the tissue sections remain adhered to the slide if they are properly dried on to the slides. But section tends to become detached from the slide due to:

- Prolonged immersion of sections in alkaline medium or solutions.
- Fixation of tissues in powerful protein coagulation fluid like Bouin's fixative.
- Techniques which require prolonged immersion like, immunocytochemistry.

Hence, section adhesive should be used. Mostly section of brain, spinal cord, blood clot, decalcified tissue, etc. requires use of section adhesive.

Types of Adhesive

Various adhesives which can be used as section adhesive are albumen, gelatins, starch, cellulose, sodium salicylate, and resins.

- **Albumen:** It is used in many histopathology department routinely. Due to the uptake of dyes by this medium, background staining may appear. Egg albumen, bovine albumen, or human albumens may be used with glycerol to prevent complete drying. Sodium salicylate is used as preservative. Mix and agitate the ingredients, and filter through coarse filter paper.

Mayer's Glycerol albumen	
Fresh egg white	- 50 mL
Glycerol	- 50 mL
Sodium salicylate	- 1 gm

- **Gelatin:** It provides a firmer attachment of sections than albumen, but has the same faults as that of albumen. A 0.5% solution of gelatin in distilled water with preservative is quite satisfactory as section adhesive. Before use, the solution should be gently heated to melt the gelatin.
- **Starch:** It provides greater adhesion than gelatin. It has the disadvantage of staining with the dye. As it is a carbohydrate its use is not recommended when these substances are to be investigated, for example, By the PAS reaction. Boil the mixture of strach, water and HCL for 5 minutes. After cooling add 0.1 g of thymol as preservative.

Starch	- 3 g
Boiling water	- 60 mL
Conc. HCl	- 0.5 mL

- **Cellulose:** It is an effective adhesive in the form of 1% solution. It has the advantage of albumen and starch adhesive in that it does not take up stains with commonly used staining solutions.
- **Sodium silicate:** It has a strong adhesive property and is used in the ratio of 1:10 dilution. It has little or no tendency to staining with most dyes and adhesion is not affected by the use of mild alkaline solutions. But it has disadvantages that it undergo blackening in the silver impregnation technique of staining and red staining in methyl green-pyronin technique.
- **Resins:** Epoxy resins like araldite can be used when greatest possible adhesion is required. This resin diluted 1:10 with acetone, should be painted onto clean slides immediately, before use. Araldite is little affected by most of the fluids used for treatment of the sections, but it may take up stains with many dyes.

Technique of Section Cutting

The process of section cutting involves the following steps:
1. Microtome setting
2. Trimming of the block
3. Mounting of the block to the block holder
4. Orientation of block on the microtome
5. Knife adjustments
6. Section cutting
7. Attaching sections to the slides.

Microtome Setting

- Make sure that the microtome is clean before beginning to section. Loose paraffin can be brushed into a waste container, but paraffin attached to the microtome must be wiped from the surface with xylene. It may be necessary to remove the microtome knife holder, and clean the holder and holder groove.
- Lift the microtome cover to check how far forward the tissue feed mechanism has advanced. If the tissue feed mechanism has advanced beyond the half-way point, lower the microtome arm all the way down, and rewind the crank handle on the left side of the microtome (turn it clockwise) until the mechanism is fully retracted.
- If the mechanism had been advanced to its maximum (i.e. the cone or post-like wedge is to the far right of the inclined plane), then it will be necessary to re-engage the gears by pulling on the spring loaded lever which is located behind the feed mechanism. If the gears are not engaged, the feed mechanism will not advance the tissue into the knife edge.
- Adjust the section thickness to its desired setting by turning the thickness control knob at the back of the microtome (on the old Model 820). When the correct knob is turned, the numbers in the thickness indicator window will change. On the newer versions of the Model 820 A/O (American Optical) microtomes, the thickness is adjusted by rotating a wheel next to the thickness indicator window. Most routine sections are cut at a thickness somewhere between 6 and 10 microns. It is generally better to cut sections as thin as possible, therefore, it is advisable to start at 6 microns and move up to thicker sections only when necessary (when you are unable to get sections at a lower setting). It is sometimes possible to cut sections thinner than 5 microns, depending on the tissue and the sharpness of the knife.

Trimming of the Block

Trimming is the process by which paraffin block is given correct shape. The paraffin block should be held against the light so that outside of the material can be seen clearly. It is then slowly trimmed with the help of a sharp knife or blade or scalpel by removing a little wax at a time. The trimming process should continue till tissue lies in the center of a rectangle with the central axis of material parallel to the long side of the block. The surface of the block which is to be cut should be lightly trimmed to expose the tissue. The opposite face, which is to be attached to the block holder, should be trimmed flat and parallel to the first. The side of the block, which is kept parallel to the cutting edge of the knife should be trimmed, leaving 2–3 mm of wax between the edge and the tissue. The remaining two sides should be trimmed such that only a minimum of wax is left between the edge and tissue (Fig. 7.10).

Mounting of the Block to Block Holder

After trimming a block, it is to be mounted on a block holder, which is inserted in the jaws of the microtome. Block holder is made up of metal, wood or plastic. It consists of two parts a disc with a rough surface and a cylindrical rod (Fig. 7.11).

Disk of block holder is first covered by a layer of molten paraffin wax, with the help of a heated spatula. The wax on the disk is properly spread and block is mounted on disk applying a slight pressure by forefinger in vertical direction. The whole operation of fixing the block should be done as quickly as possible. The block holder and the block should be allowed to cool by leaving them on the table. Identification tag is attached to the block holder. Figure 7.12 shows faults encountered during mounting.

After trimming, the block should be cooled with ice for a moment. This cooling helps in easy production of flat sections. The moisture is then removed by blotting.

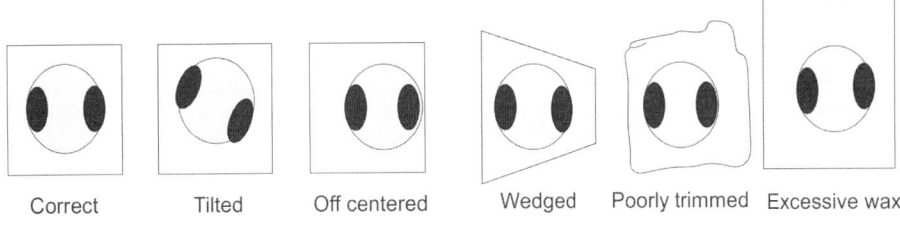

Fig. 7.10: Trimming of the block

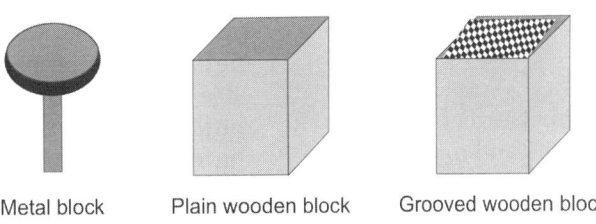

Fig. 7.11: Block holders

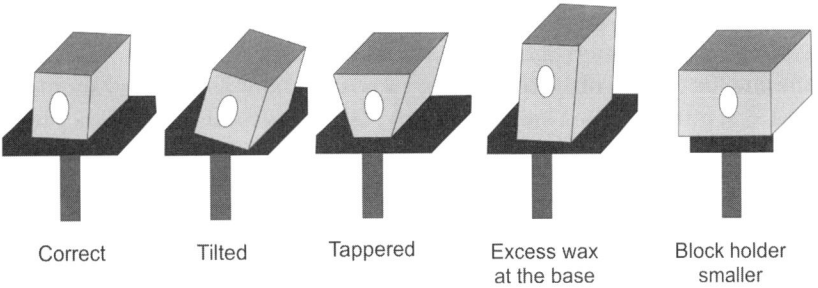

Fig. 7.12: Mounting of the block

Orientation of Block on Microtome

Insert the paraffin tissue block into the chuck of the microtome, and tighten it into position. Develop a standardized orientation for the placement of the block in the chuck (e.g. writing on the embedment ring located on the right side or on the left side) so that a block can be returned to its exact location if it becomes necessary at a later time to cut additional sections from that block. Under most circumstances, it is best to arrange the block to be exactly parallel to the knife edge. This can be accomplished by adjusting the three leveling screws on the sides and bottom of the chuck.

Knife Adjustments

Replace the microtome knife holder onto the microtome. Insert the microtome knife into the holder and tighten the clamp screws. It is a good practice to begin using a newly sharpened knife on one end of the knife, as that area becomes dull, then the knife position can be moved toward the other end. Adjust the height and tilt or angle of the knife.

Height of the knife: When the knife is at its proper height, the knife edge is several millimeters above the jaws of the knife holder clamps. This brings the edge into a proper relationship with the vertical movement of the tissue feed carrier mechanism. If the knife edge is too high, it will strike the lower edge of the paraffin block. It is not necessary to change the knife height unless knives of different widths are used. The height is adjusted with height adjusting screws located at the bottom of the microtome knife holder. The knife holder must be removed from the microtome to adjust these screws.

Tilt or angle of the knife: The optimal angle of the knife depends on the sharpness of the knife and the hardness of the tissue specimen. There is no easy way to determine the angle. It must be determined by "trial and error" even though the microtome knife holder may have angle markings on their sides. For most applications, the optimal angle is approximately 20° off the vertical. At this setting, a ribbon is typically formed, compression of the tissue section is also minimized. The angle is formed by the cutting edge between the center line of the knife and the vertical plane of the face of the tissue block (Fig. 7.13). A properly tilted knife leaves a clearance angle of about 5–10° between the back cutting facet of the knife and the face of the block so that only the knife edge strikes the face of the tissue block.

A. **Correct tilt:** Knife edge strikes the tissue block first, shoulder facet clears the face of the block.
B. **Insufficient tilt:** Knife too vertical, shoulder of cutting facet strikes the tissue block first instead of the knife edge.

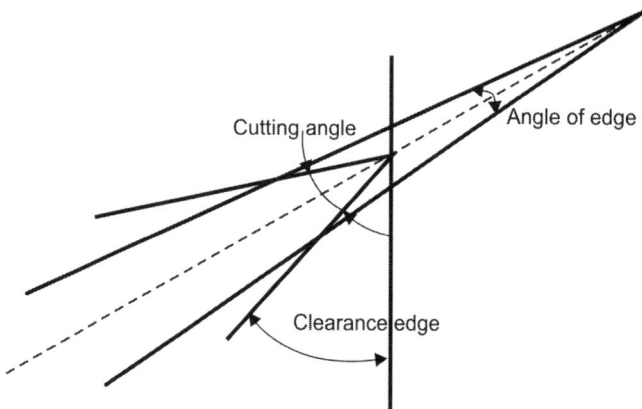

Fig. 7.13: Angles during cutting of sections

C. **Excessive tilt:** Knife too horizontal, knife edge strikes the tissue block first, but chisels through rather than cuts through the block. After the clamps of the knife holder are tightened to hold the knife, the angle adjustment is made with the tilt "wing" screws on the side of the microtome knife holder. Do not over-tighten any of the screws of the microtome; finger tight is tight enough. Unlock the brake of the microtome. With the right hand holding the rotary handle, rotate the handle clockwise until face of the tissue block is at the level of the knife edge. Simultaneously, with the left hand, slide the microtome knife holder toward the face of the block until it almost touches the face of the tissue block; tighten the knife holder to the microtome. Slowly completely rotate the handle to determine if the block just clears the knife edge. Make final adjustments with the crank handle or the tissue feed knob on the left side of the microtome. If the block clears the knife edge, the microtome is ready to begin sectioning.

Cutting Sections

- To section, turn the rotary handle (with your right hand) in a clockwise direction at a moderate and rhythmical pace.
- As sections are cut, they should adhere to one another at their edges collectively, they will form a ribbon. Friction due to sectioning of the paraffin generates enough heat to "melt" the sections together. These sections can be "controlled" with a fine-tip paint brush or some other apparatus (i.e. dissecting needle or forceps). Brushes are preferred over other items because there is less chance that they will nick the knife (do not touch the knife edge even with the brush hairs because this will also create small nicks in the knife).

- To get the ribbon started, hold the first few sections down with a brush. Once the first few sections have formed a ribbon, then place the brush under the ribbon to support it off the knife edge. When a sufficient number of sections have been cut, the rotary handle should be locked with the brake, and 2 brushes should be used to detach the ribbon from the knife and transport it to the appropriate location (ribbons can be stored for extended periods if they are kept cool and undisturbed). It is generally unwise to cut ribbons with more than 10–15 sections in them.
- If it is necessary to put multiple sections on each slide, the tissue block will need to be trimmed down with a razor blade. It is important that the tissue is entirely surrounded by paraffin and that the upper and lower edges of the block are parallel to each other and to the knife edge. If the edges are not parallel, a straight ribbon is not obtained.

Factors Affecting Production of Good Sections

- **Fixation and embedding:** Animal and human tissues are too soft when fresh to be cut thinly. Some form of pre-treatment is required to harden the tissue to facilitate cutting thin sections. This consists of either freezing or embedding tissues in a medium which offers support for cutting.
- **Sharpness of the knife edge:** A sharp unblemished knife edge is essential for smooth and even sections.
- **The correct clearance Angle:** Necessary to prevent compression in cut sections. The correct clearance angle is also important to reduce friction as the knife edge passes through the block. The clearance angle is the angle between the knife edge bevel and the block. Various angles have been recommended between 2 and 4 degrees for paraffin sections and between 5 and 7 degrees for resin or frozen sections being most effective. Determining the exact angle is largely a matter of trial and error (Fig. 7.14).
- **Cutting angle:** If the angle of bevel (cutting angle) is too great it can cause compression in the cut section. If the angle is too fine the edge of the knife can vibrate causing chatter in the section. A balance between these extremes will provide the best results. Generally, the sharper knife will have a finer cutting angle.
- **The hardness of the embedding compound:** This reflects the thickness at which sections can be cut. It is difficult to cut very thin sections from soft embedding compounds. The following is a guide to the thickness

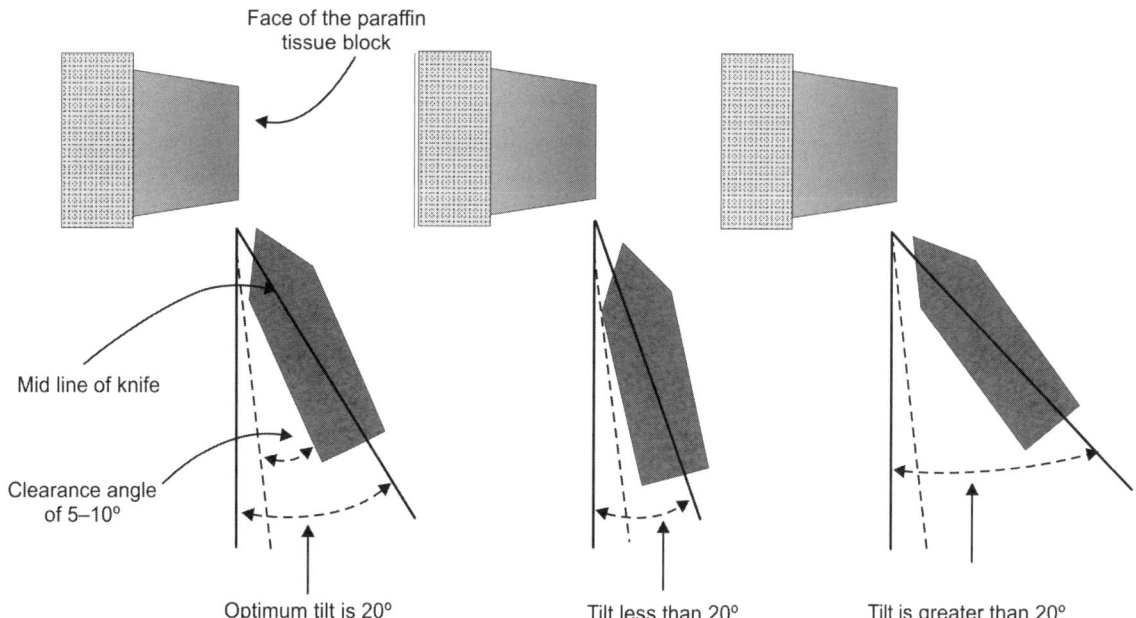

Fig. 7.14: Tilt of the microtome knife

Table 7.1: Faults and remedies in paraffin wax sectioning

Sl. No.	Cause	Remedies
1.	*When ribbon and consecutive sections are curved*	
	• Knife is blunt in one area • Horizontal edges of the block not parallel • Surplus area of wax at one side	• Sharpen the knife • Retrim the block • Trim away excess of wax
2.	*When alternate thick and thin sections are obtained*	
	• Wax too soft • Block or knife loose • Insufficient clearance angle • Mechanism of microtome faulty • Knife is blunt	• Cool wax with a knife or use high m.pt. wax • Tighten block and knife • Slightly increase the clearance angle • Check for fault • Sharpen the knife
3.	*Thick and thin zones parallel to knife edge (chattering)*	
	• Tissue is too hard • Knife or block loose in the holder • Excessively steep knife angle • Wax too hard	• Treat the tissue with mollifex/phenol during processing • Tighten them • Reduce the clearance angle • Use soft wax
4.	*Sections scored or split vertically*	
	• Nick in the knife edge • Hard particle in tissue block • Hard particle on knife edge • Hard particle in tissue	• Use different part of knife edge or re-sharpen knife • Re-embed the tissue • Clean knife edge with xylene • Decalcify the tissue
5.	*Sections fails to form a ribbon*	
	• Wax is too hard • Debris on knife edge • Knife angle too steep or too shallow • Knife edge is too dull • Upper and lower edges of the block are not parallel to the knife edge • Temperature of the microtome knife is too cold • Sections are too thick • Rate of sectioning is too slow	• Use low m. pt. Wax or apply a thin layer of the low m. pt. Wax on the block • Clean knife with xylene • Adjust the optimum angle • Resharpen knife or move to a better part of the knife • Trim the block edges to be parallel to the knife edge • Warm the knife • Cut thinner sections • Section more rapidly
6.	*Sections get attached to the block*	
	• Insufficient clearance angle • Debris on the block edge • Static electricity charges on the ribbon • Knife edge is too dull • Paraffin is too soft • Knife angle is too vertical	• Increase clearance angle • Trim edge with scalpel • Cool the microtome • Resharpen knife or move to a better part of the knife • Cool the block or, if possible, the room • Flatten out the angle
7.	*Sections roll up on the cutting*	
	• Knife is blunt • Tilt of knife is great	• Sharpen the knife • Decrease tilt of the knife
8.	*Sections get stick to the knife*	
	• Knife angle is too vertical • Knife edge is dirty, especially due to the buildup of paraffin on both cutting sides of the knife • Knife edge is too dull • Too much static electricity	• Adjust the knife angle • Use a brush or a cloth moistened with xylene to wipe off the knife • Resharpen knife or move to a better part of the knife • Increase room humidity, make short ribbons or discharge knife by frequently grounding it, or attach a "grounding wire" to the microtome knife clamp

Contd...

Contd...

9.	Crooked or uneven ribbon	
	• Upper and lower edges of paraffin block are not parallel to each other and to the knife edge: • Paraffin on one side of the block is harder than the other	• Retrim the block to make all edges parallel • Retrim block or re-embed block
10.	Excessive compression of sections	
	• Blunt knife • Bevel of knife too wide	• Sharpen the knife • Sharpen the knife to restore the bevel
11.	Sections crumble out	
	• Impregnation is not complete • Clearing is improper • Knife is blunt • Wax too soft	• Reimpregnate • Return to clearing step • Sharpen the knife • Re-embed in hard wax

at which sections can be obtained from different embedding media ranging from soft (gelatin) to hard (resin):
- Gelatin: 50 to 200 μm
- Ice: 5 to 20 μm (frozen section)
- Paraffin wax: 1 to 15 μm
- Paraffin wax/resin mixtures: 0.5 to 2 μm
- Resin: 0.05 to 1 μm

Faults and remedies in paraffin wax sectioning is given in the Table 7.1.

ATTACHING THE SECTIONS TO SLIDES

During sectioning, the sections become compressed and wrinkled and must be flattened before they can be attached to slides. This is generally accomplished by floating the sections (while still surrounded by the paraffin) on warm water that is 5–10°C below the melting point of the paraffin (generally 45–50°C). The temperature should not melt the paraffin as this can cause shrinkage, tearing and displacement of the tissue. The sections must then be attached to glass slides to provide them with solid support during the staining process. A protein adhesive must be spread onto the glass slide and immersed in the warm water to cause the tissues to adhere to the slides. Dirty glass slides can diminish tissue attachment to the slides; therefore, pre cleaned slides should be used.

■ Equipment and Reagents

Hot water bath or hot plate, 5% gelatin stock solution containing several crystals of thymol per 100 mL (must be refrigerated when not being used on a regular basis), microscope slides and coverslips and resin mounting media.

■ Method of Attaching the Sections to Slides

- **Water bath method:** Water used for this method must be clean and free from bubbles and dust. The temperature of the water should be maintained about 10°C below the melting point of the wax. To the warm water in the water bath, add 5 mL of a 5% gelatin solution for every liter of water added (Fig. 7.15).

  A short ribbon of sections is gently lowered on to the surface of the warm water using a camel hair brush or fine forceps. Slightly drag the ribbon this will produce sufficient tension in the ribbon and remove some folds from the sections. To obtain flat sections with correct orientation, floating out with the shiny surface towards the water is essential. When the ribbon comes to rest on the water, remaining wrinkles and folds can be removed by teasing apart using forceps or seeker. Complete flattening and expansion of the section is achieved after several minutes on the water surface. When the section becomes flat and expanded a clean glass slide is dipped obliquely into the water as close to the sections as possible. The slide is then slowly withdraw, allowing its surface to touch the edge of the section. Now completely remove the slide with attached sections from water. The

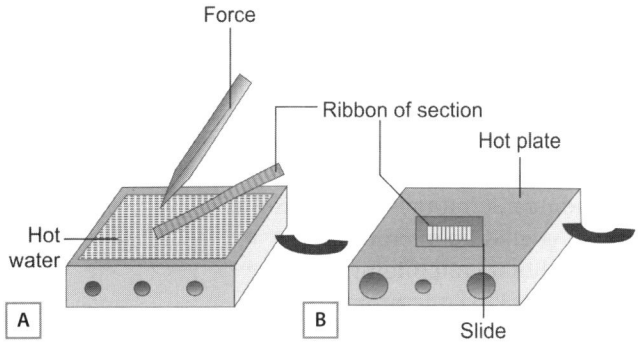

Figs 7.15A and B: (A) Water bath method; (B) Hot plate method

Table 7.2: Section mounting problems and remedies

Sl. No.	Problems	Causes	Remedies
1.	Sections fall out of the slide	Slides too greasy Slides not dried Too much albumen Paraffin melted during spreading	Remove grease Use completely dried slides Remove excess of albumen Cool sections
2.	Air bubbles under the sections	Due to air trapping Insufficient spreading of sections	Remove air Spread sections completely
3.	On drying tissue detaches from the slide	Sections dries from the edges inward Trapping of water under tissue Excess water left on the slide	Dry sections properly Remove trapped water Soak the water with blotting paper

sections are adjusted to a suitable position on the slide with a mounted needle. Drained off excess of water. Write identification number using a diamond pencil and place the slide in an incubator or hot plate (45–50°C) for at least 1 hr to dry the sections thoroughly.

- **Hot plate method:** In this method, a clean, grease-free slide is placed on a warm hot plate and flooded with distilled water. A section or short ribbon is laid on the water surface. Creases are removed by stretching the surrounding wax carefully with mounted needle. The warm water flattens the sections. After complete flattening of the slide, the slide is removed from the hot plate, labeled and dried (Fig. 7.15).

Problems and Remedies Encountered during Mounting of the Sections

Problems faced during the process of mounting is given in Table 7.2 with the remedial measures.

EXERCISE

1. Write a note on types of microtome.
2. Enlist various types of microtomes and describe in detail rotary microtome.
3. Write a note on microtome knife.
4. Write a note on care of microtome knife.
5. What is stropping? Describe the process of stropping.
6. Types of strops and their use.
7. Describe in short, section cutting, methods of sharpening and care of microtome knives.
8. Describe various faults encountered during section cutting, causes, and remedial measures to be taken.
9. Describe the frozen section technique with its advantages and disadvantages.
10. How will you obtain frozen sections?
11. Write a note on cryostat.

OBJECTIVE QUESTIONS

1. The technique by which tissues are cut into thin sections is called as _____.
   a. Necroscopy
   b. Microscopy
   c. Biopsy
   d. Microtomy

2. Microtome in which knife is fixed and object moves against knife _____ microtome.
   a. Rotary
   b. Rocking
   c. Base sledge
   d. All

3. Microtome in which block remains stationary while knife moves during processing.
   a. Rotary microtome
   b. Rocking microtome
   c. Base sledge microtome
   d. Sliding microtome

4. Sliding microtome is also called as _____.
   a. Celloidin microtome
   b. Rotary microtome
   c. Rocking microtome
   d. Ultramicrotome

Microtomy and Section Cutting

5. _____ helps to give section of desired thickness.
   a. Drive wheel
   b. Knife
   c. Micron adjuster
   d. Block holder

6. Frozen sections of a tissue are cut by using _____.
   a. Rotary microtome
   b. Rocking microtome
   c. Base sledge microtome
   d. Cryostat

7. Microtome which gives very thin sections necessary for examination with electron microscopy is _____.
   a. Freezing microtome
   b. Rotary microtome
   c. Rocking microtome
   d. Ultramicrotome

8. Saw microtome is used to cut sections of _____.
   a. Very soft tissue
   b. Undecalcified bone
   c. Spongy tissue
   d. Decalcified tissue

9. _____ profile knife is used to cut hard and tough material.
   a. A-profile
   b. B-profile
   c. D-profile
   d. None

10. Very thin resin sections are cut with _____ knives.
    a. Diamond
    b. Glass
    c. Steel
    d. All

11. Grinding of knife on a special stone is called.
    a. Honing
    b. Stropping
    c. None
    d. Both

12. _____ is mostly done to remove the wire edge caused by friction of knife steel on the hone during honing.
    a. Rubbing
    b. Stropping
    c. Grinding
    d. Crushing

13. Strop is a belt made up of _____.
    a. Cloth
    b. Plastic
    c. Wood
    d. Leather

14. Mayer's glycerol albumen is used as _____ in histopathology laboratory.
    a. Mounting media
    b. Clearing media
    c. Section adhesive
    d. Ringing media

15. _____ solution of cellulose is used as section adhesive.
    a. 1%
    b. 2%
    c. 3%
    d. 4%

16. The process by which paraffin block is given a correct shape is
    a. Honing
    b. Stropping
    c. Cutting
    d. Trimming

17. Optimum tilt angle mostly adjusted during section cutting is
    a. 20°
    b. 10°
    c. 30°
    d. 40°

18. A properly tilted knife leaves a clearance angle of about _____ between the back cutting facet of the knife and the face of the block.
    a. 5–10°
    b. 10–15°
    c. 15–20°
    d. 20–25°

19. After section cutting flattening and expansion of the section is achieved by _____.
    a. Water bath
    b. Incubator
    c. Oven
    d. Refrigerator

20. Curved ribbon of sections is obtained due to _____.
    a. Blunt knife
    b. Loose knife
    c. Nick in the knife edge
    d. Electrified knife

21. Due to _____ sections get split vertically
    a. Blunt knife
    b. Loose block
    c. Nick in the knife edge
    d. Soft wax

22. Due to _____ sections get rolled up on cutting.
    a. Blunt knife
    b. Low tilt angle
    c. Too hard wax
    d. Soft wax

23. Due to incomplete impregnation _____ result during section cutting.
    a. Section roll up
    b. Curved ribbon
    c. Compressed sections
    d. Sections crumble out

24. _____ causes formation of alternate thick and thin sections during section cutting.
    a. Block or knife loose
    b. Improper clearing
    c. Hard wax
    d. Blunt knife edge

25. If the cutting edge is too fine the edge of the knife can vibrate causing _____ in sections.
    a. Chatter
    b. Compression
    c. Expansion
    d. Split

26. The knife used in ultramicrotomy are mostly made of _____.
    a. Glass
    b. Steel
    c. Wood
    d. Plastic

27. In _____ microtome a binocular dissecting microscope is mounted over the blade.
    a. Freezing
    b. Rocking
    c. Ultra
    d. Sliding

ANSWERS

1-d, 2-d, 3-d, 4-a, 5-c, 6-d, 7-d, 8-b, 9-c, 10-a, 11-a, 12-b, 13-d, 14-c, 15-a, 16-d, 17-a, 18-a, 19-a, 20-a, 21-c, 22-a, 23-d, 24-a, 25-a, 26-a, 27-c.

CHAPTER 8

Frozen Sections and Cryostat

PRINCIPLE OF FROZEN SECTIONS

The principle underlying cutting frozen sections is that when the tissue is frozen the water within the tissue turns to ice and in this state the tissue is firm, in which ice acts as embedding medium. Thus, the tissue becomes harder by reducing the temperature and soft by increasing the temperature. For section cutting of fixed tissue requires a block temperature of some what about $-10°C$ or warmer. The fixed tissue block contains more water, hence after cooling the tissue becomes harder than an unfixed tissue block. The temperature of the tissue block can be altered during section cutting by either using thermomodules (cryostat) or the freezing microtome. Sections can be prepared for histological examination in a few minutes by the frozen section technique.

■ Applications

- For the demonstration of lipids, which get dissolved by the reagents used in the paraffin wax and cellulose nitrate methods.
- To get sections of unfixed tissues for the demonstration of substances like enzymes.
- For the demonstration of tissues like brain and spinal cord.
- In fluorescent antibody techniques.
- For the preparation of sections of materials like tendons which gets flattened after paraffin embedding.
- It is a very rapid method.

■ Advantages

- In surgical pathology where a section is required and a diagnosis is to be made in few minutes, during the course of an operation.
- It preserves morphological, biochemical and immunological properties of cell and tissues.
- It eliminate problems associated with standard practices of chemical fixation and embedding.

■ Disadvantages

- It is impossible to prepare ribbons of frozen sections.
- It is not possible to get thin sections of tissues.
- It caused damage to the structure of tissues during sectioning.
- Tissue may get damaged during freezing.
- The tissue blocks is required to keep in special low temperature cabinet.

THEORY OF FREEZING

When pure water is cooled, large hexagonal ice crystals form as a result of homogeneous and heterogeneous nucleation and subsequent growth of ice crystal nuclei. The transformation of water into ice crystals occurs at a temperature of $0°C$ and a pressure of 1 atmosphere. Where a very high rate of cooling exists, cubic rather than hexagonal ice crystals will form. These are far smaller and produce less distortion on formation. If the rate of cooling is increased further to within the order of $10^4 °K/sec$ small volumes of water can be solidified without the formation of ice crystals at all. This solid form of ice, known as vitreous ice, exists in a temperature dependent, irreversible phase transition with cubic ice, hexagonal ice and water. The critical temperatures at which these phase transitions occur have only been accurately determined for pure water, but the values of intracellular water are considered to be significantly higher (Fig. 8.1).

The formation of large, hexagonal ice crystals as the result of slow freezing occurs firstly in the less concentrated extracellular fluid. This produces an osmotic difference between the extracellular and intracellular fluid which results in a loss

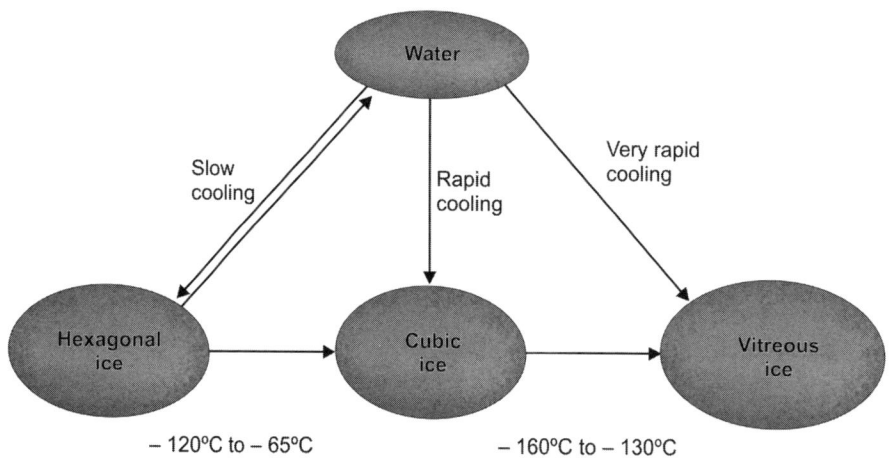

Fig. 8.1: Formation of ice from

of intracellular water and the subsequent shrinkage of the cell as the osmotic balance returns. The increased ionic concentration within the cell ruptures membranes and denatures the protoplasm. The eventual formation of ice cell within the cell, when residual intracellular fluid freezes, may then mechanically fracture the cell. These effects are collectively known as ice crystal artefacts.

The damage produced by ice crystals depends upon the size and type of crystal formed during the freezing process. Large hexagonal ice crystals will produce major structural damage to cells and tissue whilst smaller cubic ice crystals cause less cellular damage. Ideally an extremely rapid cooling rate should be used as this will produce vitreous ice without cell damage. The aim when freezing the sample, therefore, is to limit ice crystal formation as much as possible through control of the cooling rate. Factors which affect the cooling rate of the sample include:
- The absolute temperature of the cryogen.
- The heat capacity of the cryogen.
- Extent of contact between cryogen and sample.
- Degree of heat exchange between cryogen and sample.
- Diffusion of heat through the sample.

Freezing of the specimen will require selection of an appropriate cryogen and procedures which maximize the heat exchange between cryogen and specimen. The cooling rate attainable is particularly influenced by specimen size. Above a critical specimen size optimal freezing will only occur to a certain depth and the cooling rate in the deeper parts of the sample will be slow enough to allow the formation of hexagonal ice crystals with subsequent tissue damage. It is possible to reduce the level of ice crystal formation through the use of cryoprotectants which reduce the rate of ice crystal nucleation through freezing point depression.

CRYOPROTECTANTS

Cryoprotectants are thought to increase viscosity at sub zero temperatures, thereby decreasing the mobility of water molecules. The constrained water molecules are prevented from forming ice crystal nuclei and ice crystal formation is inhibited.

Cryoprotectants in common use include non-penetrating agents such as polyvinyl pyrrolidone (PVP), dextran, hydroxyethyl starch and sucrose or penetrating agents such as dimethyl sulfoxide (DMSO), glycerol, ethylene glycol and dimethyl formamide (DMF). Of these a solution of 0.5 mol/L sucrose in 3.5 mol/L DMSO allowed to infiltrate the sample at room temperature prior to freezing is highly recommended.

CRYOGEN SELECTION

A number of cryogens with differing absolute temperatures and levels of heat transfer efficiencies at the sample-cryogen interface are available. Selection requires consideration of the degree of acceptable ice crystal damage in addition to convenience, availability and cost.
- **Liquid nitrogen (–196°C):** Produces rapid freezing although overcooling can cause cracking and brittleness. A layer of gaseous nitrogen can form at the sample surface, reducing the heat transfer considerably. The use of talc to coat the sample may overcome this effect.
- **Liquid nitrogen—isopentane (–150°C):** The use of a second liquid such as isopentane or hexane which is super cooled by immersion in liquid nitrogen is very effective in reducing freezing artefact. This combination has been recommended for histochemistry although the

preparation is somewhat lengthy for rapid diagnostic procedures.
- **Electric cryobath — isopentane (-60°C):** Commercial thermoelectric cryobaths which cool isopentane or hexane have the advantage of easier preparation and although the cooling rate is not as rapid, freezing artifacts are minimal.
- **Carbon dioxide gas (-70°C):** Freezing attachments which connect to a cylinder of carbon dioxide rapidly freeze a sample by heat exchange from the expanding and vaporizing gas. These attachments are simple and efficient for routine work, but freezing artefacts are produced.
- **Solid carbon dioxide (-70°C):** The use of solid chunks of carbon dioxide (dry ice) held against the specimen can be effective and is acceptable for routine freezing.
- **Solid carbon dioxide—hydrocarbon slurry (-79°C):** Pellets of solid carbon dioxide are mixed with isopentane, hexane, acetone or ethanol to form a slurry. The specimen may be either plunged directly into this mixture or into a container of pure hydrocarbon cooled in the hydrocarbon-carbon dioxide slurry.
- **Aerosol Sprays (-50°C):** Commercial aerosol freezing sprays containing gases, liquefied under pressure are a simple and convenient method for freezing specimens for general routine work. However, the heat transfer is slow and uneven, making it prone to freezing artefact.
- **Thermoelectric Cooling (-40°C):** This type of cooling employs the Peltier effect which relies upon the use of two metal conductors. When a current is passed between the two conductors, heat is absorbed at the junction so a sample in contact with this surface will undergo heat transfer and freeze. This type of cooling device is employed as part of the stage of some freezing microtomes.
- **Refrigerated contact (-30°C):** The use of a compressor driven refrigeration coils to cool a solid metal block of aluminium or insulated cabinet forms the basis of the freezing techniques employed in most cryostats. The cooling rate is slow but the method is simple.

FREEZING MICROTOME

There are various types of freezing microtomes which are simple in design and operation. In these microtomes, the knife usually passes over the surface of the block in contrast to the paraffin microtomy where the opposite applies. The block holder, knife holder micron adjuster, and drive wheel are similar to that of the other microtomes. Sections of 5 to 10 μm can be obtained. An anti-roll plate is used to produce flat sections. It consists of a place of plastic sheet or a piece of glass slide with two narrow strips of sellotape attached to its vertical edge. The plate is carried in a holder which is fitted to the microtome so that the strips of sellotape resting on the knife face, acts as spacers between plate and knife. The gap is sufficient to prevent the sections from cutting as they are cut. After each section is cut the anti-roll plate is slowly moved back and the section removed from the knife (Fig. 8.2).

METHODS OF CUTTING FROZEN SECTIONS

The freezing microtome is used mainly in the sectioning of hard or dense tissues such as cartilage and bone, or for cutting large sections of neurological tissue. Sections less than 5 μm in thickness can be difficult to obtain.

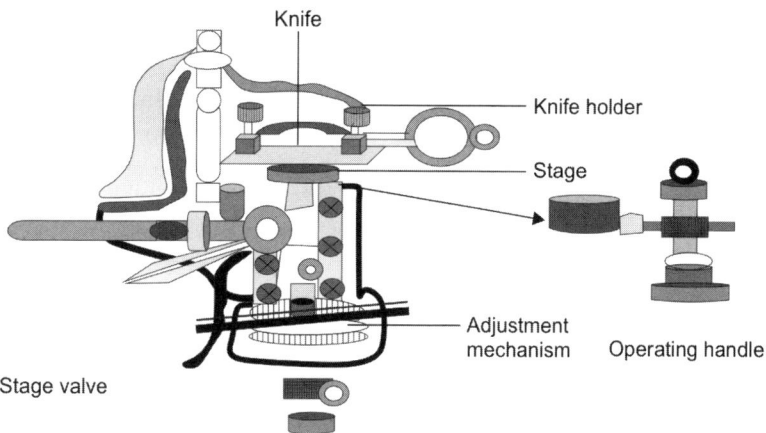

Fig. 8.2: Freezing microtome

Fixation of Tissue

A suitable block of fresh tissue is selected and trimmed with a sharp scales so that its sides are parallel. The block should be about 5 mm thick. The tissue can be directly used for section cutting or can be fixed with 10% formalin or formal alcohol. After receiving the tissue from the operation theater, it is transferred to a beaker or test tube and is boiled for 30–60 seconds along with the fixative. It in then washed with distilled water.

Infiltrating Media

Sections of certain fixed tissues such as liver, spleen and brain have a tendency to shatter on cutting. This is particularly so for the 20–40 µm sections often required for neuropathology. In order to reduce the brittleness of these tissues a specimen can be infiltrated with a protective medium. Various media have been utilized including 30% sucrose in 10% formalin, 1% gum acacia in 30% sucrose, 10% glycerol in 4% formaldehyde with 2% dimethyl sulfoxide and an aqueous glycerin-gelatin mixture. All of the infiltrative methods, however, are time consuming, taking from several hours to several weeks.

Gelatin infiltration method
Reagents required:
1. Gelatin 16 g
2. Glycerin 15 mL
3. Distilled water 70 mL
4. Thymol one crystal

Dissolve the gelatin in distilled water and add glycerin. Store at 4°C (thymol acts as a preservative) and melt in a 37°C water bath for use.

Method

1. Fix tissue in 10% formalin overnight.
2. Wash thoroughly in running water for 6–8 hours.
3. Impregnate in gelatin-glycerin mixture at 37°C for 6 hours.
4. Transfer tissue to fresh gelatin-glycerin mixture, embed in a suitable mould and allow to set at 4°C.
5. Trim block and harden the gelatin-glycerin by fixing in 10% formalin overnight or until ready for sectioning.

Mounting Tissue

The tissue is placed in a drop of water in the center of a previously cooled block holder with the cutting surface uppermost. The block should have cutting surface uppermost. The block should be parallel to the knife edge.

- Holding the block with one hand turn on the CO_2 gas slightly. Release more CO_2 in short basket until the block is frozen and get attached to the block holder (Table 8.1).
- When the tissue becomes sufficient frozen insert the block holder with tissue in the microtome object clamps.
- Orient the tilt and angle so that the face of the block is in the plane of sectioning and the block edge is parallel to that of the knife.
- Make appropriate arrangements and move the knife edge in a way that it just touches the block.
- Set the section thickness control and the automatic advance mechanism.
- Wipe off the surface of the knife, knife edge and antiroll plate and keep them clean.
- Position the anti-roll plate according to the manufactures instructions. Tighten the clamp on the object holder securely.
- Set the feed mechanism to the desired thickness (10 to 15 µm).

Section Cutting

- Pull the stage holding knife forward to allow about 5 mm clearance between block and knife edge.
- Release the drive wheel lock and make the block face in contact with the knife.
- Turn the wheel, a fraction of a turn at a time, to advance the tissue until the knife begins to cut the sections.
- Continue until a complete section is obtained.

Table 8.2 shows faults during section cutting.

Mounting of Frozen Sections

- Mounting of frozen sections should be done carefully. The sections are not rigid as that of paraffin sections and hence should handled differently.

Table 8.1: Sectioning temperature guidelines for fresh tissue. Add 5°C to 10°C for fixed tissue.

Tissue type	Temp (°C)	Tissue type	Temp (°C)	Tissue type	Temp (°C)
Uterine curettings	–7	Kidney	–15	Cervix	–20
Brain	–10	Lung	–16	Ovary	–20
Liver	–10	Muscle	–16	Prostate	–20
Spleen	–10	Connective tissue	–16	Gut	–20
Testis	–10	Skin	–16	Bone marrow	–20
Thyroid	–10	Heart	–18	Skin with fat	–25
Lip	–13	Pancreas	–20	Breast	–30
Lymph node	–15	Uterus	–20	Omentum	–35

Table 8.2: Troubleshooting the cryostat freezing procedure

Fault	Causes
Cracks appear in frozen tissue	Freezing too rapidly or specimen is overly large
Specimen detaches from microtome stub	Insufficient embedding medium, or excessively vigorous block facing
Tissue advances, but will not section	The knife is loose in its holder, specimen stub is loose in its mount, incorrect knife angle, anti-roll plate extending too far or tissue is unfrozen
Sections buckle or roll	The anti-roll plate has insufficient clearance or is incorrectly aligned, section thickness is too thin or knife is dull
Tears in section	The specimen is over frozen, knife edge is damaged or unclean
Sections thaw when cut	Incorrect cabinet or knife temperature
Frost appears on the knife	Cryostat lid has been open too long
Section adhere to the anti-roll plate	Insufficient anti-roll plate clearance, tissue or grease stuck to anti-roll plate, incorrect cabinet or knife temperature
Sections skew to one side	Debris on knife edge, a nick in the knife, blunt knife edge, or a damaged anti-roll plate
Section detaches from slide	Fixed tissue sectioned, no slide adhesive used, fatty specimen, excessively vigorous handling
Section shows horizontal splits	The specimen was too cold when sectioned

- Lift the sections from the knife edge with a fine camel hair paint brush.
- Place the section in a petridish of distilled water.
- Lift the sections directly on the slide, smoothen and flatten the section with a brush and proceed to the next step of staining.
- No adhesive is needed for sections of unfixed tissue.

■ Storage of Frozen Sections

The suitability of cryostat sections for short- or long-term storage will be determined by the stability of the component under investigation, which is in turn regulated by the initial fixation procedure. Fixatives such as Zamboni's or PLP are highly recommended.

Fixed, slide mounted cryostat sections can be stored temporarily in an airtight plastic container at 4°C with limited loss of enzyme or antigenic activity. Unfixed sections for fluorescence microscopy may also be stored temporarily in this manner with little deterioration. Longer term storage, however, requires lower temperatures of –80°C or less. Sections should be wrapped in aluminium foil and placed in an airtight container. One of the problems associated with long term storage is desiccation and denaturation of various components. Pre-treating sections with 6% polyethylene glycol, dimethyl formamide, sucrose or other cryoprotectants can prevent this change. Alternatively, wet freezing at –80°C in a glycerol-sucrose mixture is recommended.

■ Storage of Frozen Tissue

A tissue sample selected for storage must be representative of the specimen, contain no necrotic areas, pose no infectious hazard and be no more than 3 mm in thickness. Once selected the sample should be frozen immediately and not be allowed to thaw before storage.

Frozen tissue must be stored below –70°C using a low temperature freezer or liquid nitrogen storage unit. The lower temperature (–196°C) provided by liquid nitrogen is preferred as very little degradation occurs below –130°C. Short-term storage at –20°C is possible but not advisable. Avoid storing tissue in a cryostat chamber as the defrosting cycle will produce thawing and refreezing of the sample. All samples must be enclosed in a protective layer of foil or plastic wrap and sealed in an airtight container to limit desiccation.

The need for high-quality unfixed tissue samples stored in an appropriate manner is particularly important in immunocytochemistry and molecular biology. Procedures such as polymerase chain reaction (PCR) require preservation of intact DNA, mRNA or proteins with cellular preservation being of little importance. In contrast, immunochemistry and quantitative cytometry require retention of tissue morphology and cellular integrity.

■ Cryostat

The best method of preparing sections of unfixed tissue is by a cryostat. This consists essentially of a moicrotome housed in a deep freeze cabinet, maintained at a temperature of approximately –15°C to –30°C. Sections of fresh tissue can be cut on standard freezing microtomes, but cannot be handled satisfactorily. This applies particularly to fluorescent antibody techniques or certain histochemical enzyme methods to obtain satisfactory sections, which can be transferred directly from the microtome knife to a slide or coverglass. The tissue, microtome knife and surrounding atmosphere must all be

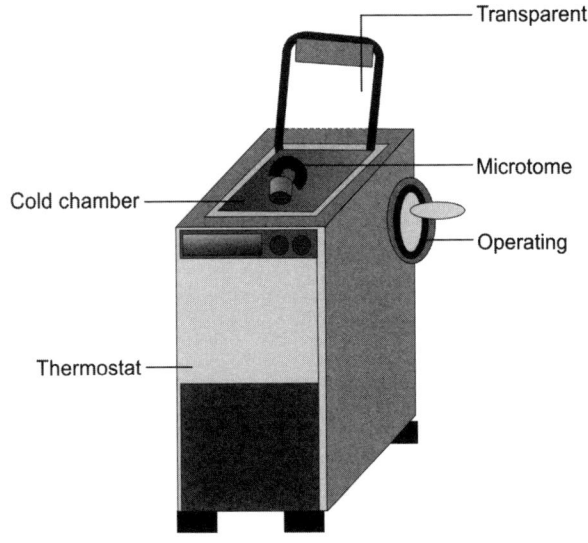

Fig. 8.3: Cryostat

at low temperature. These conditions are achieved by the use of a cryostat. Cryostats are usually provided with a rapid freezing attachment and attachment of block to block holder.

Cryostat Sectioning Procedure

- Select a representative piece of tissue trimmed to no longer than 2 cm × 2 cm × 4 mm. The 4 mm thickness is particularly important to minimize freezing artefact.
- Place the tissue on a chuck with a base of OCT compound (or similar).
- Quickly freeze the tissue with either:
  - Liquid nitrogen with or without isopentane bath,
  - Solid carbon dioxide-isopentane slurry or
  - Cryostat quick-freeze facility. If these methods are not available use solid carbon dioxide contact or aerosol cryospray.
- Secure the specimen chuck in the microtome (microtome should be in a locked position) and ensure the microtome advance mechanism is in the start position.
- Release the microtome lock and advance or retract the chuck position until the knife edge just touches the block. Roughly trim the superficial surface of the block in small steps (15–25μm) until an even, full face is achieved. Remove tissue debris from the knife with a soft brush or tissue paper.
- Position the anti-roll plate, check the thickness setting and automatic advance selector. Allow the cryostat and or specimen to reach the optimum cutting temperature.
- Cut sections using a slow even motion, except for hard tissue, which requires a firmer stroke. The sections should glide smoothly under the anti-roll plate. Alternatively, a soft brush can be used to keep the section flat as it glides out on the knife surface.
- With the section sitting flat on the knife surface, lower a clean labeled slide onto the section. It is best to rest one edge of the slide on the knife surface about 2cm beyond the section and gently lower the other end towards the section. When the slide is about 1 mm from the knife the section will lift onto the slide from the knife surface.
- Fix the slide rapidly in a fixative of choice, unless the staining procedure precludes fixation.
- Wash the slide briefly in running water and proceed with the staining procedure desired.

Fixation of Cryostat Sections

With the frozen section firmly attached to the glass slide the decision to fix sections of fresh tissue will depend upon the diagnostic urgency, potential infectiveness and the staining procedure to follow. A number of fixatives are recommended for routine use with frozen sections. These are formal acetic alcohol, formal alcohol, Carnoy's fluid, neutral buffered formalin, acetone, and Zamboni's fixative.

Zamboni's Fixative: Reagents Required

- **Solution A:** Saturated picric acid (store at 4°C).
- **Solution B:** Add 100 g paraformaldehyde to 400 mL distilled water, heat to 60°C and slowly add 1–3 drops of 1 mol/L sodium hydroxide, and stir till clear solution obtained.
- **Solution C:** Dissolve 3.31g sodium dihydrogen orthophosphate, 33.7g disodium hydrogen orthophosphate in 1 liter distilled water.
- **Method:** The working solution is prepared by mixing 150 mL solution A, 100 mL solution B and 750 mL solution C.

Advantages of Cryostat Sections

- Speed of preparations.
- Demonstration of soluble and diffusible substances.
- Thin sections.
- Serial sections possible.

Disadvantages of Cryostat Sections

- Damage to the tissue by freezing (ice crystal artefact).
- More difficult to section fixed tissue.
- High cost of equipment.

EXCERCISE

1. Write various purposes of using frozen section technique.
2. Enlist various conditions during which frozen sections are required.
3. Write advantages and disadvantages of frozen section technique.
4. Describe the theory of freezing.
5. Define cryoprotectants and cryogens.
6. Describe various cryogens used in freezing microtomy.
7. Describe various components of freezing microtome.
8. Describe method of cutting a frozen section by freezing microtome.
9. How are free floating sections mounted?
10. Describe H and E staining of frozen sections.
11. Describe polychrome methylene blue staining of frozen section.
12. What is cryostat? Describe its components.
13. State the purpose of anti-roll plate.
14. Describe cryostat sectioning procedure.
15. What is the difference between freezing microtome and cryostat?
16. Describe various difficulties which might arise during section preparation using cryostat and their possible causes.
17. Write advantages and disadvantages of cryostat sections.

OBJECTIVE QUESTIONS

1. _____ microtome is used to cut thin sections of tissues at low temperature.
    a. Base sledge
    b. Freezing
    c. Rocking
    d. Electron

2. A ribbon of sections is impossible to obtain with _____ microtome.
    a. Rocking
    b. Electron
    c. Freezing
    d. Rotary

3. One of the disadvantages of freezing microtome is _____.
    a. Damage to structure of tissue
    b. Damage to microtome
    c. Damage to knife
    d. Damage to drive wheel

4. The transformation of water into ice crystals occur at _____.
    a. 0°C
    b. 10°C
    c. –20°C
    d. –50°C

5. The important function of cryoprotectant is _____.
    a. To decrease temperature
    b. To increase pressure
    c. To increase viscosity
    d. To decrease surface tension

6. Polyvinylpyrrolidone (PVP) is an example of _____.
    a. Embedding media
    b. Dehydrating agent
    c. Infiltering media
    d. Cryoprotectants

7. Liquid nitrogen and carbon dioxide are examples of _____.
    a. Cryogen
    b. Mutagen
    c. Coating fixative
    d. Dehydrant

8. Anti-roll plate is used to produce _____.
    a. Thin sections
    b. Flat sections
    c. Thick sections
    d. Curled sections.

ANSWERS

1-b, 2-c, 3-a, 4-a, 5-c, 6-d, 7-a, 8-b.

CHAPTER 9

Staining

INTRODUCTION

As tissues and their constituent cells are usually transparent and colorless, different structures cannot be easily distinguished from each other when examined with the conventional light microscope. Successful histological techniques used for the distinction of tissue components commonly causes two changes in the tissues, either an alteration of contrast or an alteration in color.

Changes in tissue contrast can be brought about by microscopical methods, such as phase contrast or the use of polarized light. These make parts of the tissue gray or black. More often, histological staining methods depend on the production of colors in the tissues by dye—staining, which modifies the wavelength of the light that has been passed through the stained tissue, thereby imparting color into the tissue and its cells.

Successful staining methods are both specific and sensitive. Specific or selectivity is the ability to discriminate between individual tissue components and to color one or a few of these, leaving others unstained. Sensitivity is the capacity of the stain to demonstrate a tissue substance in low concentration. A satisfactory staining method is one which combines high sensitivity with high selectivity.

PRINCIPLE OF STAINING

In all staining methods, the important questions to ask are:
- Why do any tissue components stain?
- Why do stained components remain stained?
- Why are all components not stained?

Why do Any Tissue Components Stain?

The most important principle behind this is the dye-tissue or reagent-tissue affinities. When a tissue component has a high affinity for a certain dye, than the component becomes intensively stained. Affinity is also those attractive forces (coulombic, hydrogen bonding, etc.) which binds the dye to the tissue.

Hydrophobic Bonding

A major contribution to dye or reagent-tissue affinity when using organic reagent or dyes from aqueous solution is hydrophobic bonding. It involves the tendency of hydrophobic groupings (like phenylanine, tryptophan, side chains of proteins or biphenyl and naphthyl groupings of reagents and dyes) to come together to form hydrophobic bonding, example: staining of elastic fibers (made up of the non-polar protein elastin) by dyes bis-azo-dyes staining of fats by Sudan dyes.

Van der Waal's Forces

These are the most general of the dye–tissue attractive forces. Attractions are polar forces, which become stronger as the polarizability of the molecule increases, e.g. staining of elastic fibers with basic dyes like orcein or acid dyes.

Coulombic Attractions

The most important reagent tissue interactions are the coulombic attractions or electrostatic bonds. These arise due to the electrostatic attractions of unlike ions such as colored cations of basic dyes and anion of tissue structures like DNA and RNA. The amount of dye ion able to enter given tissue will depend not only on the signs of the charges on the dye and tissue, but also on their magnitude for example, staining of glycogen by periodic acid Schiff's procedure.

Hydrogen Bonding

This is a localized bond formed when a hydrogen atom is between two electronegative atoms like oxygen or nitrogen, though H is only covalently bonded to one of them example:

$$>C=O \cdots H-O, \quad \begin{matrix}H\\H\end{matrix}>N-H\cdots O\cdots H, \quad \begin{matrix}H\\H\end{matrix}>O\cdots H-O$$

Hydrogen bond is denoted by dotted line. It is important to note that water, being made of O–H groups, have extensively hydrogen bonded both to itself forming clusters important for hydrophobic bonding. H bonding plays an important role in non-aqueous solvents, e.g. staining of glycogen with alcoholic solution of carmine stains.

Covalent Bonds

Covalent bonds formed between tissue and reactive stains are also important in biological staining, e.g. action of mordant dyes in which dye is attached to tissue via metal - tissue covalencies, dye – metal ion + tissue groups.

Why do Stained Components Remain Stained?

It is found that the processing fluids like dehydrating agent, clearing agent and mounting media are substances for which the stain has a lower affinity, or/and in which these stains dissolve very slowly. At the same time due to different chemical interactions between dye and tissue different types of complexes are formed like precipitation of lead sulfide, hemosiderin pigments, crystals of silver and gold in metal impregnation, mordant dye–tissue complex, etc. have negligible solubility in any of the solvents for processing thus the tissue retain the stains.

Why are the Stains Not Taken Up into Every Part of the Tissues?

Affinity

When we stain a tissue, then some part of the tissue takes up stain whereas the other parts/components do not take up the stain. This is mostly due to the dye–tissue affinities and number of binding sites. for example, Nonionic Sudan dye will have an affinity for a fat droplet but not for proteins, basic Schiff's reagent have an affinity for DNA, etc. Negatively charged acid dyes will have higher affinities for those tissue structures having cationic charges like proteins but will have lower affinities for structures carrying negative charges (nucleic acids). Thus, positively charged cytoplasmic components will take up negatively charged acidic dyes.

Rate of Dye Uptake

Progressive dying methods are rate controlled, in which selectivity of the stains depends on the use of a short period of dying in which only fast staining tissue structure acquire color. But if the period of staining is prolonged then other components also get stains. For example, Staining of mucin with Alcian Blue or colloidal iron. Some fast diffusing dyes (picric acid) are able to penetrate all the acidic components and give rise to two—colored contrast. If three or more acid dyes are used, then they will have different rate of diffusion in the different structures example: Red blood cells stains slowly, collagen fibers rapidly and mucin fibers intermediate.

Rate of Reaction

The staining also depends upon the rate of reaction between the dye and tissue structure. The reactive dye will selectively stain the structure example: Periodic acid oxidation step of periodic acid Schiff staining.

Rate of Reagent Loss

Selective loss of stain from tissues is also important and is used in differential or regressive staining. For example, Staining of muscle with iron hematoxylin, mitochondria by acid Fuchsin, etc. In such procedure, all structures are first stained non-selectively, and then are extracted in a solvent. The dye will be first lost from easy to stain/destain structures like collagen fibers. The slow-to destain/stain structures like A and Z bands of muscles, mitochondria, etc. retains the stain longest.

TYPES OF DYES AND STAINS

There are two main types of dyes used in histology, i.e. natural and synthetic dyes.

Natural Dyes

They are obtained from the natural sources, e.g. carmine and hematoxylin. Carmine is obtained from cochineal, the dried bodies of the female insect, dactylopius cacti. Carminic acid is obtained by boiling cochineal in water and extracting with benzene. Hematoxylin is extracted from the wood of a small tree, hematoxylin campechianum. It is one of the most widely used dye in histology.

Synthetic Dyes

These are large group of organic compounds that were originally produced from coal in the coal gas industry mostly petroleum oil. The primary products include hydrocarbons, such as benzene, toluene, and naphthalene or phenols, and cresols. A large group of synthetic dyes is derived from benzene. Benzene itself is colorless. In order to obtain colored compounds from benzene it is necessary to introduce certain chemical changes and colored bearing groups in benzene called as **auxochrome.** There are three main groups of chromophore namely: The quinonoid ring usually para and sometimes ortho, azo-coupling and nitro groups.

A compound containing chromophores are known as **chromogens** which can color tissues and textiles, however, the resulting colors are not 'fast' and can be easily removed by washing in simple solutions. To convert chromogens into a true dye it is necessary to introduce an ionizing group called as an **auxochrome.** Auxochromes increases the intensity of the color. They are either basic or acidic and are the part of the dye that determining the staining action of the whole molecule. Important basic auxochromes are amino group ($-NH_2$) and aniline ring ($C_6H_5 - NH_2$) and acidic auxochromes include the sulfonic group ($-SO_3$), the carboxyl group ($-COOH$), and hydroxyl group ($-OH$). The greater the number of auxochromes that a dye contains better is the strength of the dye.

Some dyes contain an additional chemical group called **modifiers** which have the effect of altering the color of the dye. These may be methyl ($-CH_3$), or ethyl ($-C_2H_5$) and have the effect of making the color of the dye deeper. For example, If the hydrogens of the basic amino auxochromes are replaced by methyl or aryl groups, the dye becomes bluer (crystal violet is an example with multiple modifying groups). Thus, a dye is made up of an organic compound that is colored by a chromophore and ionized by an auxochromes and final color altered by modifier. For example, **Quinonoid dyes:** Basic and acid fuchsin, crystal violet, aniline blue, eosin, thionin, methylene blue, neutral red, and hematein and carminic acid etc.
Azodyes: Orange G, congo red, trypan blue, etc.
Nitro dyes: Picric acid, aurantia, etc.

CLASSIFICATION OF DYES OR STAINS

When the dyes go into the solution, they ionize giving either positively charged dye ion (cationic) or negatively charged dye ion (anionic) with either chloride ions or sodium ions respectively. Thus, depending upon their ionizations stains are classified into acidic, basic, neutral and amphoteric stains (Table 9.1).

- **Acidic stains:** They are the stains in which the acidic component of the dye molecule is colored and base being colorless usually sodium. They are used for staining the basic components of the tissue structures like cytoplasmic components like, cytoplasm, mitochondria, endoplasmic reticulum, etc. for example, Acid fuschin.
- **Basic stains:** These are stains in which the basic component of the dye molecule is colored and the acidic being colorless usually chloride. For example, Rosaniline. They usually give stains to the acidic components of the cell like nucleus, DNA, RNA, etc.
- **Neutral stains:** They are molecules which are formed by the interaction of an acidic and a basic dye. Both the cation and anion contain chromophoric groups and there is a colored dye in both parts of the dye molecule. They are soluble in alcohol and water. Example: Romanowsky dyes formed by interaction of polychrome methylene blue and eosin. These stains are widely used for staining of the blood.
- **Amphoteric stains:** These are dyes which are cationic in nature below a certain pH (isoelectric pH) and anionic above it. For example, Hematin is amphoteric dye with isoelectric pH of 6.5 (Table 9.2).
- **Colorless leuko dyes:** Some dyes can easily be reduced, due to which the chromophore is destroyed resulting in loss of dye properties. Such dyes can become recolorized by oxidation and are called leuko dyes. It is used in vital staining technique.

Table 9.1: Ionization of basic, acidic and amphoteric dyes

Dye	pH								Type
	3	4	5	6	7	8	9	10	
Crystal violet	+	+	+	+	+	+	+	+	Basic dye
Orange G	-	-	-	-	-	-	-	-	Acidic dye
Hematin	+	+	+	+	-	-	-	-	Amphoteric dye

Paraquinoid   Orthoquinoid   Azo–Coupling   Nitro

Table 9.2: Nature of tissue components

Basic (+)	Acidic (−)	Amphoteric
Collagens Red blood cells Eosinophil granules Leukocytes Granules	• DNA, chromatin • RNA • Myelin • Cartilage • Mucous • Mast cell • Granules	Cytoplasm Muscle

Table 9.3 gives a classification of dyes and chemical composition.

TYPES OF STAINING PROCESSES

Several types of staining processes are used to give tissues contrast or color these are:
- Vital staining
- Staining by elective solubility
- Staining by chemical production of colored compounds in tissue
- Metallic impregnation
- Metachromatic staining
- Fluorescent staining
- Progressive and regressive staining
- Direct and indirect staining

■ Vital Staining

Living cells can be stained by dissociation in the staining fluid (Supra-vital staining) or by injection of the dye into the living organism (intra-vital staining). These methods are not used for fixed sectioned tissues. Vital staining helps to demonstrate cytoplasmic structures by the phagocytosis of particles of dyes into the cytoplasm or by the staining pre-existing cellular components. The nuclear membrane of the living cell is impermeable to dyes, and hence, it is not possible to stain the living nucleus, vital staining of reticule endothelial by try pan blue is an example.

■ Staining by Elective Solubility

Mostly the stains, combine with tissues by simple solution in tissue fluid. In such case aqueous stains are not suitable because it gives different staining. Substance that dissolve in tissues are called as lysochromes. Lysochromes are lipid-soluble and are used for staining lipids in sections. Fat droplets can be electively colored by stains in 70% alcoholic solution of the stain. The amount of staining depends upon the partition coefficient of the stain in presence of the two solvent.

■ Staining by Chemical Production of Colored Substances

In tissues some staining techniques use pale or colorless solutions which reacts with tissue components to produce colored compounds. The resulting end products are either

Table 9.3: Chemical classification of dye

Sl. No.	Chromophore	Structure	Cationic dye (Basic)	Anionic dye (Acidic)
1.	Quinonoid ring	Triarylmethane Hematein Xanthene Thiazine Oxazine	Rosaniline dye Crystal violet Pyronin Thionin Methylene blue Crystal violet Celestine blue	Acid fuschin Aniline blue Hematein Eosin Phloxine
2.	Azo-group	Azure Monoazo Diazo	Neutral red Safranin Bismarck brown	Azocarmine Orange G Tartrazine Congo red Biebrich scarlet
3.	Nitro group			Picric acid Martius yellow

true dye or colored chemical products that are not dyes. Histochemical techniques involve chemical reactions which are highly specific, for example, Schiff's reagent used in the PAS reactions, and Feulgen reaction, in which straw colored solution is converted into a purple dye and parts reaction for iron in which colored compound potassium ferric ferrocyanide in formed which is not dye.

Metallic Impregnation

Some metallic compounds can be reduced by tissues to the metallic state, producing an opaque, usually black, deposit for example solution of ammonical silver is readily reduced to metallic silver. Tyrosine derivatives like melanin, phenolic compound present in specific cells of intestinal glands have a capacity of reducing ammonical silver. Such cells are called as argentaffin cells and other cells which cannot reduce ammonical silver are called argyrophil cells. Metallic impregnation is also used to demonstrate fibrils, pigments, spirochetes and fungi.

Metachromatic Staining

Certain tissue components combine with dyes to produce a color different from the color of the original dye and different from the color produced in the rest of the tissue. Such dyes are called metachromatic dyes. A substance that can alter the color of a metachromatic dye is a chromotrope. Orthochromatic tissues are the tissues that do not cause metachromasia. The most important metachromatic tissue components are cartilage, connective tissue, epithelial mucins, mast cell granules, and amyloid. The dyes that are metachromatic are mainly thiazines such as toluidine blue and thionin.

Thiazing dye (thonin)

Fluorescent Staining

Mostly histological stains are colored solutions that cause color reactions which are visible in day light or ordinary artificial light. Fluorochromes are quinonoid dyes with the usual chromophores and auxochromes, which behave as acidic or basic dyes, but have the capacity of altering ultraviolet (UV) light into visible light when combines with tissues. Thus, fluorescent staining is similar to ordinary color dying, but the tissues are recognized when it combines with fluorochromes by the use of ultraviolet (UV) light and not by day light.

Progressive and Regressive Staining

A progressive staining technique is one in which the different elements in the tissues are colored in sequence and at the end of the correct time in staining solution a satisfactory differential coloration of the tissues is achieved. A regressive staining technique is one in which the tissue is first over stained and then destained or differentiated by removing excess stains from unwanted parts of the tissue. Regressive staining is now commonly employed. This is because it is difficult to obtain sufficiently intense progressive staining of one part of a cell without staining of other cell structures. By differentiation it is possible to remove stain from more lightly stained sites, still leaving a strong enough staining of other structures to give selective and clear detailed, e.g. Gram's staining, H and E staining, etc.

Direct and Indirect Staining (Mordant Staining)

Many of the aniline dyes (like methylene blue, eosin) stain tissues perfectly if they are placed in a simple aqueous or alcoholic solution of the dye. This is known as direct staining. Many stains, like hematoxylin, require an additional intermediate substance known as a mordant before satisfactory combination with the tissues to take place. These are indirect stains. The dye and the mordant unite to form a colored lake, which then combines with the tissue to form a tissue-mordant-dye complex which is insoluble in ordinary aqueous or alcoholic solvent, allowing subsequent counter, staining. In histological technique the dye and mordant are either used together (e.g. hematoxylin with potassium alum in Ehrlich's hematoxylin) or the mordant many be used first before the tissue is passed into the staining solution (e.g. preliminary iron alum bath before Heidenhain's hematoxylin). Iron, aluminium and chromium compounds are mordants which combine with basic stains.

Tissue + Dye ⟶ Tissue—dye (direct staining)

Tissue + Mordant + Dye ⟶ Tissue—Mordant—Dye (Indirect staining)

Table 9.4 shows list of dyes/stains with their major uses.

Table 9.4: List of dyes or stains with their major uses

Dyes/stain	Major uses
Acid fuchsin	Stain for connective tissue and erythrocytes; and proteinaceous material in liver. Cain's method for mitochondria
Acridine orange	Pickett's fluorescence method for fungi fluorescent against a dark background. For differentiation of nucleic acids and cytology
Alcian blue 8GX	Acid mucopolysaccharides, cell walls, Cartilage granules. As a carbohydrate and mucosubstance stain in different pH levels. Movat's method for connective tissue stain. Monroe/Frommer method for pituitary staining. AB/PAS/OG method for human adenohypophyseal cytology
Alizarin red S	Minute bone and fetal ossification in mammalian embryos. Used with toluidine blue for distinction of bone and cartilage in mammalian embryos. Used with alizarin red for calcium deposits
Aniline blue	Used with biebrich scarlet for staining collagen, reticulum, muscle, plasma, and nuclei. All connective tissues. Used as a counterstain with red nuclear dye
Auramine O	Staining paraffin sections of infected tissue. Acid-fast organisms exhibit fluorescence
Azocarmine G	Alpha, beta, and all D-cells of the islets of langerhans and in all animals
Azure A	A nuclear stain. Cell granules McNeal method for leukocytes
Azure B	Distinction of cellular RNA and DNA in botanical tissue. Negri body stain, Malarial parasites
Azure II	Morphological details of marrow cells, nuclei, and bacteria
Basic fuchsin (Rosaniline)	Gram-positive/negative bacteria. A pituitary stain
Basic green 4 (Malachite green)	In microbiology, distinction of diphtheria and other bacteria. A vital stain for onion epidermis
Biebrich scarlet (Ponceau BS)	Used with picric acid/aniline blue for staining collagen, recticulum, muscle, and plasma. Luna's method for erythrocytes and eosinophil granules. Guard's method for sex chromatin and nuclear chromatin
Bismarck brown Y	PAP for staining smears. Nuclei and granules. Mucin and calciform cells of intestine, cartilage and embryo
Brilliant cresyl blue	Platelets and reticulum of immature red cells. Counterstained with Wright's stain
Carmine (Alum lake)	Glycogen stain. Elastic fibers in blood vessels, nuclei, and collagen
Cresyl fast violet, (Cresyl violet acetate)	Vogt's method for nerve cells. A neurological tissue stain. Nissl substance and PAS-positive material. Powers and Clark method for spinal cord and brain with formalin or Bouins fixed
Crystal violet	Gram-positive/Gram-negative bacteria, and filaments. Holzer's method for glial fibers (nerve). Amyloid in pathological human tissue. Determining chromatin and nucleoli in plant tissue
Eosin Y	Maximow's method for morphological details of marrow cells; a constituent of Wright Stain for elastic fibers in blood; as a eosin-phloxine counterstain
Erythrosin B (erythrosin extra bluish)	Maximow's method for morphological details of marrow cells; a constituent of Wright Stain for elastic fibers in blood; as a eosin-phloxine counterstain
Fast green FCF	Lillie modification of Masson's for cells, cytoplasm, muscle, and collagen; Guard method for sex chromatin
Fluorescein Isothiocyanate	Culing's method for fluorescent antibody staining for demonstration of specific antigens
Giemsa	Thin film stain for differentiation of types of leucocytes; Rickettsiae, bacteria, and inclusion bodies. May-Grunwald/Giemsa for bone marrow stain. Pinkus' acid orcein-giemsa for connective tissue staining
Giemsa	Same as above; prepared ready-to-use
Hematoxylin	Weigert's iron hematoxylin for nuclear stains. Gill's hematoxylin for nuclei and nuclear chromatin
Indigo-carmine	A stain for Negri bodies; used with acid fuchsin. Used in picric acid in contrast to basic fuchsin. In plant cytology
Light green SF, Yellowish	Grocott's method for fungi. Dahl's method as a bone and calcium stain. McManus' method for glycogen. Fraser-Lendrum method as a connective tissue stain

Contd...

Contd...

Methyl green	Myeloperoxidase stain; used with bismarck brown for mucin and calciformcells of intestine, cartilage of trachea, and embryonic tissue; used with toluidine blue for differentiating between diphtheria and other bacteria
Methylene blue	For use in acid-fast bacteria, acid-fast baccilli, and as a rickettsia stain. Cain's method for mitochrondria. For staining Negri bodies in nerve cells
Methyl violet 2B	Highman's method for amyloid and nuclei staining. Used with crystal violet and bismarck brown Y for staining metachromatic granules of diphtheria organisms
Nigrosin, WS	For staining the central nervous system. For the negative staining of bacteria; used in place of India ink
Nile blue A	A fat and lipid stain; differentiation of melamines and lipofuchsins. Staining for phospholipids
Orange II	Kalter's method used with fast green FCF, safranin O, and crystal violet for quadruple staining of tissues. Orange G substitution for better contrast
Orange G	For staining fibrin, keratin, collagen, and erythrocytes. Staining alpha, beta and gamma cells. For staining nissl substances and PAS-positive material
Phloxine B	For staining inclusion bodies and nuclei. Thomas's method for malarial parasites. For staining hemaglobin and hemosiderin. For staining keratin, prekeratin and mucin. A beta cell stain counterstain for hematoxylin
Pyronin Y	Cudder's method combined Gram/Pappenheim stain for gonorrheal pus. Kurnick's method used with methyl green which stains liver cells. For staining protein in the diazosulfanilic acid technique; a substitute for azure A. Can be used for pyronin B
Safranin O	Prussian blue method for hemosiderin. Weigert's iron hematoxylin with methachromic dyes which stain nuclei and granules. A alkaline phosphate stain. Flemming's method for staining chromatin and nuclear elements
Sudan black B	A stain for fat in animal tissue. A stain for chromosomes, golgi, and leukocyte granules
Toluidine Blue O	Alizarin red/toluidine blue for distinction between bone and cartilage and the degree of ossification in mammalian embryos. Johnson's method for methachromatic tissue. With cresyl violet for staining DNA and RNA. With thionin for malignant cells of biopsy specimens
Wright stain	For differentiation of blood corpuscles. Used with brilliant cresyl blue for staining platelets and reticulum of immature red cells. For staining blood and bone marrow films

STAINING PROCEDURES

Staining Equipments

- **Staining dishes:** A variety of these dishes are available. Small jars are used for staining single slides. Coplin jars holds 5–10 slides. Large staining troughs with separate baskets enable up to 20 slides to be stained at the same time (Fig. 9.1).
- **Staining racks:** These racks are often used in biomedical laboratories. Two glass rods, 50 mm apart, are fixed across the sink. The slides are laid across these rods and solutions pored onto the slides, using drop bottles. This method is not recommended for prolonged staining procedures (Fig. 9.2).
- **Staining machines:** These are used for staining large numbers of slides by a routine staining procedure. Machines generally operated either on the conveyor belt or linear principle or by passing batches of slides through baths of stain or reagent. Staining machines for conventional tinctorial stains or immunocytochemical methods are available.
- **A hot plate** for heating stains and hardening mounting media.
- **A microscope** for controlling the degree of staining.

Steps of Standard Staining of Paraffin Sections

Before staining, certain preparatory treatment of sections is necessary and involves the following steps:

- **Removal of paraffin wax:** Because paraffin wax is poorly permeable to stains its removal with a solvent is necessary and xylene is used for this purpose. One or two min. immersion in each of two changes of xylene is usually sufficient for sections up to 1 μm in thickness and removal of wax can be increased by warming the slide before the immersion.
- **Removal of xylene with absolute alcohol:** Xylene is not miscible with aqueous and low grade alcohols and

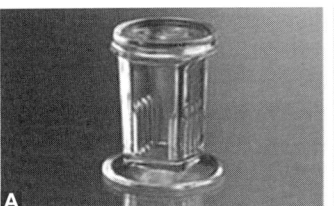
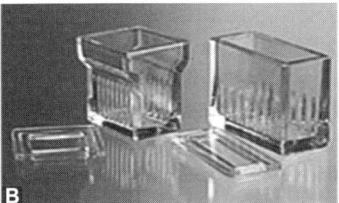
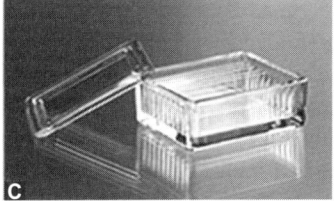

Figs 9.1A to C: (A) Coplin jar; (B) Staining jars; (C) Staining dish

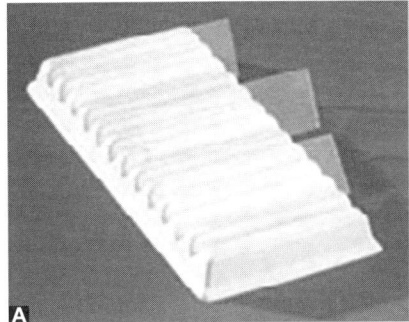
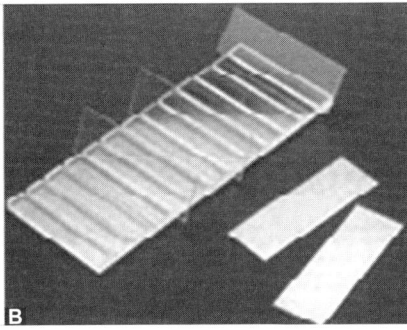
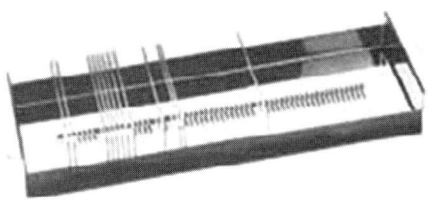

Figs 9.2A to C: (A) Slide holder; (B) Slide racks; (C) Slide tray

it is therefore necessary to remove this with absolute alcohol. One half to one min. in each of two changes of absolute alcohol is adequate for the purpose.
- **Treatment with descending grades of alcohol:** To avoid the possibility of diffusion currents causing damage and detachment of the sections, it is necessary to give absolute alcohol treatment for a minute or two with 90% and sometimes 70% alcohol.
- **Water:** It is desirable to pass sections from a reagent in the sequence which is the same as or similar to solvent of the stain to be used first. This is commonly distilled water.
- **Staining:** This involves the treatment with a single or two or more separate stains, with washing and differentiation between. This requires few minutes or several hours and may include mordant staining.
- **Dehydration:** Mostly paraffin sections are mounted in media miscible with xylene. Hence, the sections should be dehydrated in alcohol before passing to xylene.
- **Clearing:** First the sections are passed through alcohol and xylene mixture (1:1) before treatment with pure xylene. One min. in xylene is sufficient to achieve transparency of the sections and removal of alcohol.
- **Mounting:** A coverslip is applied to protect and preserve the section by using mounting media.

HEMATOXYLIN STAINS

Hematoxylin is the most widely used and versatile dye in histological technique and is used for demonstration of nuclei, myelin, elastic fibers, fibrin, neuroglia, and muscle striations. Hematoxylin is most commonly used as a nuclear stain which is proceeded by staining of cytoplasm, and connective tissues with eosin.

Hematoxylin is extracted from the heart wood (log wood) of the tree hematoxylon campechianum. The hematoxylin is extracted from log wood with hot water, and then precipitated out from the aqueous solution using urea. It is important to know that hematoxylin itself is not a stain, its oxidation product hematin is a natural dye. Hematoxylin can be oxidized by two methods namely natural oxidation and chemical oxidation.
- **Natural oxidation (ripening):** It is done by exposure to light and air. This is a slow process, sometimes taking as long as 3–4 months.
- **Chemical oxidation:** It is done by using sodium iodate or mercuric oxide. The use of chemical oxidizing agents convert the hematoxylin to hematin almost instantaneously, so these hematoxylin solutions are ready for use immediately after preparation, but they have a shorter useful life than the naturally oxidized hematoxylin.

Hematin on its own has poor affinity for tissue and is inadequate as a nuclear stain without the presence of mordant. The most useful mordants for hematoxylin are salts of metals, aluminium, iron and tungsten. Most of the mordants are incorporated into the hematoxylin staining solution, but certain hematoxylin stains require the tissue section to be soaked in the mordant before staining, For example, Heidenhain's iron hematoxylin.

Hematoxylin stains can be classified according to the mordant used in following classes:
- Alum hematoxylins
- Iron hematoxylins
- Tungsten hematoxylins
- Molybdenum hematoxylins
- Lead hematoxylins
- Hematoxylins without mordant

Important hematoxylin stains are discussed below:

Ehrlich's Hematoxylins (1886)

This is probably the most commonly used alum hematoxylins in both normal and morbid histology. It is prepared as follows: Dissolve the hematoxylin in the alcohol before adding the other ingredients. The stain is ripened naturally be allowed to stand in a large flask loosely stoppered with cotton plug, in a warm place and exposed to sunlight. The flask should be shaken frequently and ripening required about 2 months. After ripening the solution is bottled and filtered before use. Hematoxylin can be chemically oxidized by adding 0.3 g sodium iodate in 1 g of hematoxylin. Glycerol acts as a stabilizer and retard evaporation. As the hematoxylin becomes oxidized the color of the solution changes from purplish to deep red. Ehrlich's hematoxylin is generally used as regressive stain. After staining for about 20 min. sections are differentiated in 1% hydrochloric acid in 70% alcohol until nuclei are selectively stained.

Composition of Ehrlich's hematoxylins
Hematoxylin	- 2 g
Absolute alcohol	- 100 mL
Glycerol	- 100 mL
Distilled water	- 100 mL
Glacial acetic acid	- 10 mL
Aluminium potassium sulfate	- 15 gm

Mayer's Hematoxylin (1903)

It is an aluminium hematoxylin which is chemically ripened with sodium iodate. It can be used as a regressive stain as well as a progressive stain. It is used as a nuclear counter stain in the demonstration of glycogen, in various histochemical techniques. It is more vigorous in action than Ehrlich's hematoxylin and require only 5–10 min. for staining. It is prepared as follows: The hematoxylin, potassium aluminium and sodium iodate are dissolved in the distilled water by warming and stirring or by allowing to stand at room temperature overnight. The chloral hydrate and citric acid are added, and the mixture is boiled for 5 minutes. then cooled and filtered. The stain is ready for use immediately. Chloral hydrate acts as a preservative and citric acid sharpens nuclear stain.

Composition of Mayer's hematoxylins
Hematoxylin	- 1 g
Sodium iodate	- 0.2 g
Chloral hydrate	- 50 g
Distilled water	- 1000 mL
Citric acid	- 1 gm
Ammonium/potassium Aluminium	- 50 g

Harri's Hematoxylin

This is an alum hematoxylin which is chemically ripened with mercuric oxide. It is a useful general purpose hematoxylin and gives clear nuclear staining hence used in diagnostic exfoliative cytology. It is used as a regressive stain, but in exfoliative cytology, it can be used as progressive stain. It is prepared as follows: The hematoxylin is dissolved in the absolute alcohol, and is then added to the alum, which has previously been dissolved in the warm distilled water. The mixture is rapidly brought to the boil and the mercuric oxide is then added. The stain is rapidly cooled by plunging the flask in cold water. When the solution is cold the acetic acid is added, and the stain is ready for immediate use.

Composition of Harri's hematoxylins
Hematoxylin	- 2.5 g
Absolute alcohol	- 25 mL
Distilled water	- 500 mL
Potassium aluminium	- 50 g
Mercuric oxide	- 1.25 g
Glacial acetic acid	- 20 mL

Cole's Hematoxylin (1943)

This is an aluminium hematoxylin, artificially ripened with an alcoholic iodine solution. The stain is prepared as follows: The hematoxylin is dissolved in warm distilled water and mixed with the iodine solution. The aluminium is added, and the mixture is bought to the boil and then cooled quickly and filtered. The solution is ready for immediate use. It require 10 minutes for staining.

Composition of cole's hematoxylins	
Hematoxylin	- 1.5 g
Distilled water	- 250 mL
Sat. aq. Potassium aluminium	- 700 mL
1% Iodine in 95% alcohol	- 50 mL

■ Weigert's Iron Hematoxylin (1943)

This is an iron hematoxylin in which ferric chloride is used as the mordant/oxidant. The main use of Weigert's hematoxylin is as a nuclear stain in techniques where acid stain is used as counter stain (e.g. Van Gieson stain). Staining time of 15–30 min. is required. It is useful for CNS tissue. It is prepared as follows: Solution A and B are stored separately and mixed immediately before use. The prepared stain is stable only for few hours. The color of the mixture should be a deep purplish black. If it is muddy brown, discard it. It give brownish black to black color to nuclei.

Composition of Weigert's iron haematoxylins	
Solution (A)	
Hematoxylin	- 1 g
Absolute alcohol	- 100 mL
This allows to ripen naturally for four weeks	
Solution (B)	
30% aq. Ferric chloride	- 4 mL
Concentrate hydrochloric acid	- 1 mL
Distilled water	- 95 mL

■ Heidenhain's Hematoxylin (1896)

It is an iron hematoxylin stain which is used as a cytological stain. Ferric ammonium sulfate is used as an oxidant/mordant. It is used to demonstrate many structures according to the degree of differentiation, like chromatin, chromosomes, nucleoli, centrosomes, mitochondria, yolk, muscle striations and myelin. It is prepared as follows: This allows to ripen naturally for four weeks. Dissolve hematoxylin in the alcohol and then add water. Allow to ripen for four weeks and store in stoppered bottle. For staining first the sections are treated with the mordant solution and then over stained with hematoxylin stain. Then it is differentiated by the same mordant solution. It impart gray—black color to the structures.

Composition of Heidenhain's iron hematoxylins	
Iron aluminium solution:	
Ferric ammonium sulfate	- 5 g
Distilled water	- 100 mL
Hematoxylin solution:	
Hematoxylin	- 0.5 g
Absolute alcohol	- 10 mL
Distilled water	- 90 mL

COUNTER STAINS

The term is used to denote the application of a different color to provide contrast and background to the staining of the component or structure that the technique is designed to demonstrate. They may therefore be nuclear or cytoplasmic, single or multiple and of several colors. They may give a flat, general background color or a degree of tissue differentiation. It is important that the purpose of counter stains is supplementary. In some cases, the judicious selection of a counter stain can result in significant additional information. To be effective, a counter stain should be of a contrasting, subtle color which does not intrude on the major stain. They should be used discretly, never dominating, obscuring or causing a change of color of the primary stain, as may occur if too heavily applied.

Following is a list of some of the most important dyes that may be used as counter stains, some of them are also used as primary stains (Table 9.5).

■ Eosin

Originally, eosin was used alone to color tissues, but its role has now been exclusively in double and multiple staining procedures. It is most suitable stain to combine with an aluminium hematoxylin to demonstrate general histological structures of a tissue. Its particular value is its ability, with proper differentiation, to distinguish between cytoplasm of different types of cells, and between the different types of connective tissue fibers and matrices by staining them with different shades of red and pink. The eosins are xanthene dyes and are of different types viz Eosin Y (eosin yellow, eosin water soluble), Ethyl eosin (eosin S, eosin – alcohol soluble), and Eosin B (eosin bluish, erythrosin B). Out of these eosin Y is much widely used as cytoplasmic stain as 0.5 or 1.0% solution in distilled water. A few crystals of thymol are added to inhibit growth of fungi.

Table 9.5: Counter stains

Cytoplasmic stains		
Red	**Yellow**	**Green**
• Eosin Y • Eosin B • Erythrosin B • Phloxine B • Biebrich Scarlet • Rose Bengal	• Picric acid • Tartrazine • Metanil yellow • Orange G	• Light green SF • Fast green FCF • Lissamine green
Nuclear stains		
Red	**Blue**	
• Neutral Red • Safranin O • Carmine	• Methylene blue • Toluidine blue • Celestine blue • Hematoxylin	

The addition of 0.5 mL of acetic acid in 1000 mL of stain sharpens the staining.

STANDARD HEMATOXYLIN AND EOSIN STAINING METHOD FOR PARAFFIN SECTIONS

■ Deparaffinization

Flame the slide on a burner and then place it in xylene for 3-4 minutes. Repeat xylene treatment with agitation.

■ Hydration

Hydrate the section by passing it through decreasing concentration of alcohol baths and water. The alcohol solutions used are 100%, 90%, 80%, and 70%. Place the section for 30-60 seconds. In each of these alcohol solutions. Wash in tap water and rinse in distilled water. Drain the section well before staining.

■ Staining

- Stain the section with hematoxylin solution for 3-5 minutes. and wash in running tap water.
- Quickly dip the slide in and out of 0.5% (v/v) hydrochloric acid.
- Check the differentiation by using a microscope.
- The nuclei should appear dark purple and the rest of the tissue should appear pale.
- Quickly rinse the slide in tap water for 30-60 seconds.
- Dip the slide several times in dilute ammonia water (the section should appear blue colored).
- Wash in tap water and then rinse in 95% alcohol.
- Agitate the slide in eosin solution for 10-60 seconds. Drain the staining solution.

■ Dehydration

Place the slide in 70%, 95% and absolute alcohol for 30-60 seconds in each. Give two changes in absolute alcohol.

■ Clearing

Place the slide twice in xylene for 30-60 seconds in each.

■ Mounting

Drain the excess xylene and mount in DPX or Canada balsam with a coverslip.

SPECIAL STAINING METHODS

■ Weigert–Van Gieson Staining for Connective Tissues

Procedures for the differential staining of connective tissue fibers and muscle are a very important part of histological technique and their use is often helpful in the diagnosis of pathological changes in tissues.

Principle

In the routine staining method, collagen, elastic fibers and smooth muscles appear pink or reddish in color. In Weigert – van Gieson stain, collagen and most reticulin stain selectively with acid aniline dyes (acid fuchsin). Picric acid acts as counter stain for muscle and cytoplasm and also form complexes with the dyes. This complex has special affinity for collagen. The main disadvantage of this method is its inability to stain young fibrils the deep red. The advantage of this method is that van Gieson's stain gives good results after a wide range of fixative and can be used for paraffin, frozen or cellulose nitrate sections.

Reagents	Weigert – iron – hematoxylin solution: (as described earlier) Van Gieson's solution: Saturated solution of picric acid : 10 mL 1% (w/v) acid fuchsin : 1.5 mL It should be freshly prepared. Acid—alcohol: 1%
Procedure	• Deparaffinize with xylene • Hydrate the sections up to water • Stain with Weigert's iron hematoxylin for 20–40 minutes • Wash in tap water • Differentiate in acid—alcohol 1%, controlling the degree of differentiation microscopically, until the nuclei are just overstained. • Wash in tap water • Counter stain in Van – Gieson's stain for 5 minutes • Blot lightly, do not wash in water • Dehydrate rapidly with 90% and absolute alcohol • Clear in xylene (two changes) • Mount in DPX or Canada balsam mounting medium
Results	Cell nuclei – Black Collagen – Red Muscle fibers, cell cytoplasm and red cells – Yellow

■ Verhoeff's Elastic Fiber Stain

Principle

Histological study of the connective tissue involves the study of elastic fibers, which are present in the skin, ligaments, lungs, and in the elastic laminae of blood vessels. In the presence of ferric salts, the Verhoeff's reagent stains, the elastic fibers and the nuclei with hematoxylin.

Reagents	Verhoeff's stain: Solution A: 5% solution of hematoxylin in absolute alcohol dissolved by heating, cool and filter Solution B: 10% ferric chloride in distilled water Solution C: Dissolve 2 g iodine and 4 g potassium iodide in 100 mL distilled water Mix 20 mL of solution A, 8 mL of solution B and 8 mL of solution C, filter and store in amber colored dropping bottle Ferric chloride solution: 2% (w/v) ferric chloride solution Van Gieson's stain: As described earlier
Procedure	• Dewax the sections • Take the sections to water • Stain in Verhoeff's solution for 15–60 minutes • Wash in distilled water • Differentiate with ferric chloride solution for a few min. controlling the degree of differentiation microscopically • Transfer in 95% alcohol • Wash in water for 5 minutes • Counter stain with Van Gieson's stain for 1–2 minutes • Dehydrate, clear, and mount
Results	Elastic fibers - Blue–black to black Nucleus - Gray to black Collagen - Red Muscle fibers and RBC - Yellow

SPAS Staining for Carbohydrates

Principle

The Periodic-acid Schiff (PAS) reaction is widely used in histopathology and is particularly valuable for demonstrating glycogen, fungi, and mucin. The reaction is due to the oxidation of carbohydrates containing 1,2–glycol groups to aldehydes by oxidation with periodic acid and red color development using Schiff's reagent.

Reagents	0.5% (w/v) periodic acid solution **Schiff' Reagent:** Basic fuchsin : 1 g Distilled water : 200 mL 1 M HCl : 20 mL Sodium bisulfate(anhy) : 1 g Activated charcoal : 0.5 g Dissolve basic fuchsin in 500 mL boiling water, cool and filter. Add HCl. Cool to 25°C, add sodium bisulfate. Store in the dark for 24–48 hours. During storage solution becomes straw colored. Now shake up with charcoal filter immediately, transfer to a brown colored bottle and label and refrigerate it. **Sulfurous acid solution:** 10% aqueous Sodium metabisulfite : 6 mL 1 M HCl : 5 mL Distilled water : 100 mL Harri's alum hematoxylin: As described earlier
Procedure	• Dewax and hydrate • Place in periodic acid solution for 5 to 10 minutes • Rinse in tap water for 2 minutes • Rinse in distilled water • Place in Schiff's reagent for 5 to 10 minutes • Place in sulfurous acid solution for 2 minutes (3 changes) • Rinse in tap water • Stain with Harri alum hematoxylin for 30 seconds • Blue in tap water • Dehydrate, clear and mount
Results	Nuclei : Blue Mucin and glycogen : Purple Basement membrane : Reddish-purple

Sudan Black B in Propylene Glycol Staining for Lipids

Principle

The most common stains used to demonstrate fats are oil soluble dyes. This group of dyes is more soluble in the fat than in alcohol. They are used in saturated form so that their uptake by the fats is made easy. This group of dyes includes the orange red dye Sudan II, Sudan IV, oil red O and Sudan black B. Sudan black B is most sensitive of them.

Reagents	**Sudan black B solution:** Dissolve 0.78 g of Sudan black B in 100 mL of propylene glycol. Add small amount at a time with constant stirring. Heat to 100°C for a few minutes, stirring constantly. Filter through Whatman No. 2 filter paper. Cool to room temperature and then filter again. Store at room temperature and then filter again. Store at 60°C in the oven. The stain will keep for years **Propylene glycol:** (85%) Nuclear fast red: Dissolve 0.1 g of nuclear fast red in 5% aqueous solution of aluminium sulfate with the aid of heat. Cool, filter and add a grain of thymol as a preservative. **Kaiser's glycerine:** Gelatin : 10 g Distilled water(warm) : 52.5 mL Glycerol : 62.5 mL Phenol : 1.25 mL After mixing place small aliquots in brown bottles, melt as needed for use
Procedure	• Dehydrate section in absolute propylene glycol for 10–15 minutes. • Stain in Sudan black B for 10 minutes. • Differentiate in 85% propylene glycol • Wash in distilled water • Counter stains in nuclear fast red for 1 minute. • Wash thoroughly in several changes of distilled water • Mount in glycerol gelatin.
Results	Fats : Blue-black Background : Red

Silver Nitrate Staining for Reticulin (Gordan and Sweet's Stain)

Principle

In the connective tissue, reticulin appears as a fibrillary extracellular framework. The fibrils of reticulin stain black on impregnation with silver nitrate. This type of staining is used to identify a tumor of uncertain origins. Mild degrees of fibrosis in organs can also be recognized by the reticulin stain.

Reagents	Potassium permanganate solution 0.5% aqueous potassium permanganate : 95 mL 3% aqueous sulfuric acid : 5 mL 1% aqueous oxalic acid solution 2.5% iron alum solution Ammonical silver nitrate solution 10% aqueous silver nitrate : 5 mL 3% aqueous sodium hydroxide : 5 mL Ammonia : as required Mix silver nitrate solution with sodium hydroxide solution. The solution will appear turbid. Add ammonia drop by drop with constant shaking until the turbidity disappears. Make final volume to 50 mL by adding glass distilled water 10% aqueous formalin solution 0.2% aqueous gold chloride 5% aqueous sodium thiosulfate 0.5% aqueous safranine

Procedure	• Dewax and bring sections to water • Oxidize in potassium permanganate solution for 1–5 minutes • Wash in water • Bleach in oxalic acid solution for 3–5 minutes • Wash thoroughly in tap water and several changes in distilled water • Mordant in iron alum solution for 10 minutes to 2 hours • Wash in several changes of distilled water	• Impregnate with ammonical silver nitrate solution for 30 seconds • Wash in several changes of distilled water • Reduce in formalin solution for 1 minutes • Wash in tap water and then distilled water • Tone in gold chloride solution for 10–15 minutes • Rinse in distilled water • Fix in sodium thiosulfate solution for 5 minutes • Wash in water for 1–2 minutes • Counter stain nuclei with safranine for 2 minutes • Dehydrate, clear and mount
Results	Reticular fibers : Black Nuclei : Black Other elements : Pink	

Staining of Pigments

Pigments are substances found in living matter. They absorb visible light. They differ in their origin, composition and significance. Pigments are classified into (i) Artefacts, (ii) Endogenous pigments, and (iii) Exogenous pigments.

- **Artefacts:** These are the pigments that result from the methods used during processing of the tissues.
- **Formalin pigment:** This is a dark brown pigment formed by the action of acidic formaldehyde on blood.
- **Mercuric pigments:** These are gray, black granular deposits resulting from the use of mercury containing fixatives.
- **Chrome deposits:** These are brownish black granular deposits result when tissues fixed in chrome fixatives are treated with alcohol.
- **Stains precipitates:** These are highly colored, amorphous and granular precipitates seen in stained sections.
- **Endogenous pigments:** Endogenous pigments are substances often colored, opaque or crystalline found inside the tissues. Examples are hemoglobin, hemosiderin, inorganic iron, bile pigments, melanin, etc.
- **Exogenous pigments:** These are those extraneous substances, often colored, opaque or crystalline, found in tissues. Examples are carbon, iron ore pigments, copper, asbestos, calcium, etc.

Staining of Hemoglobin by Dunn Thompson Method

Hemoglobin is the most widely encountered hematogenous pigment in the tissue. Despite its presence in large amounts in all tissues, it is difficult to stain. It is a poorly preserved in fixatives like Susa fixative. It is well-stained by acid dyes after fixation in formalin. Dunn Thompson staining is a modified Van Gieson staining method.

Procedure	• Bring section to water • Stain in matured aqueous solution of alum hematoxylin for 15 minutes • Wash in tap water • Mordant for 1 minutes in aqueous solution of 4% ferric ammonium sulfate (iron alum) • Stain in the aqueous alum hematoxylin solution of 10 minutes • Rinse rapidly in tap water • Stain in van Gieson solution • Transfer directly to 95% alcohol and differentiate for 1–3 minutes. • Dehydrate, clear and mount
Results	Red blood corpuscles : Green–black Hemoglobin casts or ingested hemoglobin : Light shades of green

Gmelin's Method for Bile Pigments

Bile pigments are iron free and appear days after hemosiderin appeared. The usual method of staining the bile pigment is by Gmelin's reaction. This staining method is based on the progressive oxidation of bilirubin into various colored compounds. Negative reactions should be repeated two or three times before being reported as negative.

Procedure	• Bring section to tap water • Mount a section in water under a coverslip and find the pigment • Leave the slide on the microscope under the high power objective • Apply a drop of strong nitric acid to one side of the coverslip with a Pasteur pipette • Put a small piece of dry filter on the opposite side of the coverslip so as to draw the nitric acid through the section • Immediately watch the pigment through a microscope for a change of color
Results	In a few seconds, the yellowish–brown pigment will change to green, then a blue and purple

Masson–Fontana Ammonical Silver Reaction for Melanin

Melanin is a granular black or yellowish-brown pigment that is normally present in the skin, hair, eye (choroids and iris), meninges and substantial nigra of the brain. It is formed from tyrosine. In pathological conditions such as benign and malignant melanomas, melanin is found in varying amounts, and its demonstration in tissues, may be very decisive. Identification of a pigment as melanin may depend on a negative Prussian blue reaction, a positive argentiaffin (silver) reaction and positive melanin bleach, while of course bearing in mind the situation of the pigment.

Masson–Fontana ammonical silver reaction for melanin is based on the ability of tyrosine derivatives to reduce silver solutions to metallic silver.

Procedure	• Bring sections to water • Treat with Gram's iodine solution for 10 minutes • Wash well in several changes of distilled water • Place the section in the silver solution in the dark for 18–24 hours • Rinse in three changes of distilled water • Tone in 0.1% Gold chloride for 3–5 minutes • Rinse in distilled water • Fix in 5% sodium thiosulfate for 2 minutes • Rinse in running tap water for 2 minutes • Counter stains with 0.54% Safranin or 1% neutral red for 1–2 minutes • Rinse in water, and rapidly in 70% alcohol • Dehydrate, clear and mount
Results	Melanin : Black Argentaffin cell granules : Black

Staining solution

Add strong (28%) ammonia water drop by drop to 20 mL of 10% aqueous silver nitrate until the dark brown precipitate that forms is almost redissolved. Add 20 mL distilled water and leave to stand for 18–24 hours. Place the supernatant in a dark brown bottle and it will keep for weeks. Filter before use.

Perl's Prussian Blue Method for Hemosiderin

Principle
Hemosiderin is a brown granular pigment occurring at the site of previous hemorrhage. It is a product of the breakdown of hemoglobin. In iron deficiency, the hemosiderin iron stores become depleted and insufficient hemoglobin is produced

leading to anemia. It can be demonstrated by the absence of stainable iron in the bone marrow. In case of excess of iron, the excessive iron gets deposited in the organs like spleen, bone marrow, liver, etc. causing hemosiderosis. This can be demonstrated by excessive staining of iron in these organs. The ferric iron of hemosiderin combines with potassium ferrocyanide to form the insoluble prussian blue precipitate.

Reagents	Acidified potassium ferrocyanide solution:
	    Solution A 10% aqueons HCl
	    Solution B 10% aqueons Potassium ferrocyanide solution
	    Mix equal parts of solution A and solution B and keep for 20 minutes
	Nuclear fast red (Neutral red): Dissolve 5.0 g of aluminium sulfate in hot distilled water and add 0.1 g of nuclear fast red. Mix well and filter. Add a crystal of thymol as a preservative

Procedure	• Deparaffinize the section and bring to water • Keep the sections in acidified potassium ferrocyanide solution for 5–20 minutes • Wash thoroughly with distilled water • Stain with nuclear fast red for 5 minutes • Rinse with distilled water • Dehydrate, clear and mount
Results	Hemosiderin : Bright or Prussian blue Nuclei : Red Cytoplasm : Pink

Staining of Enzymes

Histochemical methods for enzymes have played a great role in the identification and evaluation of enzyme activity. The tissues must be prepared in such a way as to preserve and retain the enzymes as much as possible in their original sites. Enzymes should not deteriorate or diffuse during fixation and the final color reaction should be sharp and precise.

Azo-dye Coupling Method of Staining for Alkaline Phosphatase

The alkaline phosphatase together with acid phosphatase make up the group of enzymes that are now called phosphomonoesterases. There are several methods for demonstration of alkaline phosphatase of which azo-dye coupling is mostly use.

Principle
The substrate used is a solution of alpha naphthyl phosphate. The alpha naphthol moiety is released by the enzyme and is coupled with the diazonium salt to form a insoluble colored final reaction product. Fresh frozen cryostat sections are preferably used, but fixed tissues can also be used.

Reagents	**Substrate in buffer:** Dissolve 10–20 mg of sodium alpha-naphthyl phosphate in 20 mL of tris buffer at pH 9.1. Add 20 mg of fast-red TR or fast Black B and stir well. This should be freshly prepared.
	Tris (tris[hydroxymethyl] aminomethane) buffer, pH 9.1:
	    0.2M Tris (24.2 g/L) : 25 mL
	    0.1N HCl (8.5 mL Conc. HCl/L) : 5 mL
	Distilled water : 70 mL
	Mayer's hemalum : as described earlier

Procedure	• Filter the freshly prepared substrate diazonium salt on the slides. Leave for 15–60 minutes (paraffin sections may require up to 12 hours with Fast–Red TR) • Wash in running water for 2–3 minutes • Counter stain in the Mayer's hemalum for 1–2 minutes • Wash and blue nuclei in running water for 20–30 minutes • Mount in glycerin jelly
Results	The site of enzyme activity: Brown with fast–red or Black with fast black B

Azo-dye Coupling Method of Staining for Acid Phosphatase

Principle
The enzyme hydrolyzed the substrate, alpha naphthyl phosphate, to liberate alpha naphthol which couples with a diazonium salt to form an insoluble colored azo-dye. This marks the site of enzyme activity. Fresh or fixed cryostat sections cut at 10–15 µm can be used.

Reagents	**Solution:** Dissolve 10–20 mg of sodium alpha naphthyl phosphate in 20 mL of 0.1 M hydrochloric acid-Veronal buffer mixture at pH 5.0. Add 1.5 g polyvinyl pyrrolidone and leave to dissolve. Add approximately 20 mg of fast garnet GBC salt or fast red ITR.
	Veronal acetate solution:
	    Sodium acetate crystals : 19.4 g
	    Sodium diethyl barbiturate (Veronal) : 29.4 g
	Distilled water : 1000 mL
	To prepare buffer at pH 5.0, mix 25 mL of the veronal acetate solution, 36 mL of 0.1 N HCl and 44 mL of distilled water

Procedure	• Filter the incubating medium onto the sections at 37°C for 30–60 minutes • Wash in running water for 2 minutes • Counter stain, if desired, in Mayer's hemalum for 1–2 minutes • Wash thoroughly in running water for 30 minutes • Mount in glycerin jelly
Results	Site of acid phosphatase activity : Reddish-brown Nuclei : Blue

Benzidine Method for Peroxidases

Principle
Peroxidases catalyze the removal of oxygen from hydrogen peroxide to a suitable acceptor and release free oxygen. Benzidine a colorless compound in the staining solution, is oxidized to blue dye by the free oxygen. Benzidine is carcinogenic and should be handled with care. Fresh unfixed cryostat sections are used.

Reagents	1% ammonium molybdate solution in 0.9% sodium chloride Saturated solution of benzidine in 0.9% Sodium chloride Picric acid in 95% alcohol
Procedure	• Place sections in the 1% ammonium molybdate solution in 0.9% sodium chloride for 4–5 minutes • Transfer sections to a saturated solution of benzidine containing a few drops of 20 volume hydrogen peroxide and leave for about 3 minutes • Transfer to a saturated solution of picric acid in 98.5% alcohol, leave for 5 minutes • Wash in tap water, dehydrate, clear and mount in a synthetic resin medium
Results	Peroxidase granules : Dark blue Cytoplasm : Yellow

Staining for Oxidases

Principle
This method is based on the so called 'Nadi' reaction. Cytochrome oxidase catalyses the oxidative reaction between alpha-naphthol and dimethyl-para-phenylenediamine to form idophenol blue. Use unfixed fresh cryostat sections.

Reagents	• 0.1% solution of alpha naphthol in 1% sodium chloride and M/15 phosphate buffer (9.465 gm Na_2HPO_4 dissolved in distilled water and made up to 1 liter) at pH 5.8 • 0.1% solution of dimethyl-para-phenylenediamine hydrochloride in 1% sodium chloride and M/15 phosphate buffer at pH 5.8 • 'Nadi' reagent: Mix equal parts of the above solutions immediately before use
Procedure	• Incubate the sections in the freshly prepared 'Nadi' reagent at 37°C for at least 5 minutes or maximum 1 hour • Wash in 0.9% sodium chloride in distilled water • If desired, counter stain nuclei in carmalum or any other red nuclear stain • Mount in 5% potassium acetate in water • Ring the coverslip with paraffin wax
Results	Sites of cytochrome enzyme activity : Bluish violet Nuclei : Red

Demonstration of Dehydrogenase

Principle
Succinate dehydrogenase is an anaerobic dehydrogenase, which catalyses the reversible oxidation of succinic acid to fumaric acid. In the presence of a tetrazolium salt, the transfer of hydrogen reduces the tetrazolium salt to water-insoluble colored formazan which marks the site of enzyme activity. Fresh, frozen, unfixed tissue should be used for cryostat sections.

Reagents	• 0.2M Phosphate buffer (pH 7.6) • 0.2M Monobasic sodium phosphate (27.8 g/L) : 13 mL • 0.2M Dibasic sodium phosphate (53.65 g/L) : 87 mL • 0.2M Sodium Succinate: Dissolve 5.4 g of sodium succinate in 100 mL of distilled water • Nitro blue tetrazolium (nitro BT or NBT) solution: 1 mg/mL • 0.85% saline • Formalin-saline (0.85 g of sodium chloride per 100 mL of 10% formalin) • 15% ethanol
Procedure	• Prepare incubation medium as follows: • 0.2 M Phosphate buffer : 5 mL • 0.2 M Sodium succinate : 5 mL • NBT solution : 10 mL • Incubate sections in the above medium at 37°C for 30 minutes • Wash sections in saline • Post fix in formalin-saline solution for 10 minutes • Rinse sections in 15% ethanol for 5 minutes • Rinse in distilled water • Counter stain, if desired, with 0.5% Safranin O for ½ min • Rinse well in distilled water • Mount in glycerine jelly, or dehydrate in alcohol, clear in xylene and mount in a synthetic resin medium
Results	Sites of enzyme activity: Blue purple deposits of formazan pigment

Demonstration of Mast Cell

Mast cells are normally present in small numbers in the connective tissue of all organs, but particularly in the dermal layer of skin (around blood vessels and nerves), and are identified by their cytoplasmic granules. Mast cells have been considered the tissue equivalent of the circulating basophils but, while there is evidence that they arise from a common precursor cell in the bone marrow. There is no evidence that mature basophils are able to differentiate into mast cells. The two cell types are readily distinguished by their morphology in light microscopy and the presence of chloroacetate esterase activity in mast cells.

Mast cells play an important role in immunity, with specific involvement in type I (anaphylactic) hypersensitivity reactions. When IgE antibodies are raised against a particular allergen, they can bind to the mast cell surface Fe receptors. Subsequent exposure to the allergen triggers mast cell degranulation and the release of chemical mediators, such as histamine and heparin, into the surrounding tissues. Mast cells are also involved in delayed hypersensitivity, cytotoxicity, immunoregulation and inflammation. The increased number of mast cells are found in many pathological conditions like hyperplasia in the skin, multiple cutaneous lesions of utricaria pigmentosa, ulcerative colitis, Crohn's disease and in parasitic infections.

Acidified Toluidine Blue Method for Mast Cells

Fixation must be carried out rapidly to avoid cytoplasmic degranulation and deterioration of granule contents. Neutral buffered formalin (10%) is mostly used. Paraffin sections of 3–5 µm thickness are cut from tissue and tissue known to contain mast cells is used as a control.

Reagents	• 0.5% aqueous potassium permanganate • 2% aqueous potassium metabisulfite • Acidified toluidine blue solution (pH 3.2): Prepared by dissolving 0.25 mL glacial acetic acid and 0.02 g toluidine blue in 99.75 mL distilled water
Procedure	• Dewax and rehydrate the sections • Transfer sections to potassium permanganate solution for 2 minutes • Rinse in distilled water • Transfer sections to potassium metabisulfite solution for 1 minute • Wash in tap water for 3 minutes • Rinse in distilled water • Place in acidified toluidine blue solution for 5 minutes • Rinse in distilled water • Dehydrate rapidly, clear and mount.
Results	Mast cell granules and other strongly sulphated acid mucopolysaccharides—purple Nuclei—blue.

Staining of Microorganisms

The detection and identification of microorganisms in histological sections can be of diagnostic importance. This is particularly important in the diagnosis of tuberculosis where the organisms are few in number and when there is confusion between tuberculosis and sarcoidosis and Crohn's disease.

Gram's Stain for Bacteria

Principle
This is the classical method which divides the bacteria into two groups. Gram-positive bacteria retain the stain after decolorization, while Gram-negative bacteria are decolorized. This method is based upon the differential solubility of the Gram stain in alcohol or acetone when the stain is absorbed by different bacteria. Adding of mordant iodine after primary staining precipitates the stain in the protoplasm of gram positive bacteria, which cannot get removed even after treatment with alcohol. Where as Gram-negative bacteria undergo decolorization by treatment with alcohol and hence take up the counter stain.

Reagents	**Crystal violet stain**		
	Crystal violet	:	0.2 g
	Ethyl alcohol	:	2 mL
	Distilled water	:	18 mL
	1% aqueous ammonium oxalate	:	80 mL
	Gram's iodine		
	Potassium iodate	:	2 g
	Iodine	:	1 g
	Distilled water	:	100 mL
	Decolorizer		
	Ethyl alcohol	:	95%
	Counter stain		
	1% Neutral red	:	15 parts
	Carbol fuchsin	:	1 part
Procedure	<ul><li>Dewax and hydrate</li><li>Apply crystal violet stain for 1 minute</li><li>Rinse with water</li><li>Apply Gram's iodine for 1 minute</li><li>Rinse with water</li><li>Apply several changes of 95% ethyl alcohol until no more color appears to flow from slide</li><li>Wash with water</li><li>Apply counter stain for 10 seconds</li><li>Dehydrate, clear and mount</li></ul>		
Results	Gram-positive bacteria	:	Bluish-black
	Gram-negative bacteria	:	Red/pink

Ziehl- Neelsen's or Acid Fast Staining for Acid Fast Bacteria

Principle

Mycobacterium tuberculosis and *Mycobacterium leprae* are the bacteria which are relatively resistant to staining. When stained by a strong stain they resist decolorization by acid. These acid fast bacteria belong to the Genus *Mycobacterium*, like *Mycobacterium tuberculosis, Mycobacterium leprae,* and other atypical mycobacteria. Certain species of *Nocardia*, a fungus like bacterium (*Nocardia asteroids* and *Nocardia brasiliensis*) are also acid fast.

Reagents	**Carbol fuchsin**		
	Basic fuchsin	:	1 g
	Absolute ethyl alcohol	:	10 mL
	5% aqneous Phenol solution	:	100 mL
	Dissolve basic fuchsin in ethyl alcohol. Combine with phenol solution and label		
	1% acid alcohol solution		
	0.2% aqneous methylene blue solution		
Procedure	<ul><li>Dewax and hydrate</li><li>Flood slide with carbol fuchsin and heat until steam rises, reheat at intervals. Stain for 10–15 minutes</li><li>Wash with running tap water</li><li>Differentiate with acid alcohol until only red cells retain the stain on microscopy</li><li>Wash with running tap water for a minimum 10 minutes</li><li>Counter stain with methylene blue for 2 minutes</li><li>Dehydrate rapidly, clear and mount in DPX</li></ul>		
Results	Acid fast bacilli	:	Red
	Cell nuclei	:	Blue
	Red blood cells	:	Pink

Methenamine Silver Nitrate Method for Fungi

Ordinary routine hematoxylin and eosin stain most of the fungi sufficiently enough for them to be recognized. They can also be demonstrated by Gram's stain or its modifications, and most of them are Gram-positive. A few of the fungi are acid fast. The periodic acid Schiff reaction is valuable in the demonstration of mycelia and rounded fungi in tissues.

Principle
This method depends upon the reduction of the silver by the aldehyde produced after oxidation of fungal wall components with chromic acid. It is the best method for the detection of fungi in tissue sections, particularly when they are present in small numbers. The black staining fungi stand out prominently against the light green background.

Reagents	Stock methenamine silver nitrate solution
	5% aqneous Silver nitrate : 5 mL
	3% aqneous Hexamine : 100 mL
	5% aqneous Chromic acid solution
	1% aqneous Sodium bisulfate solution
	Incubating solution
	5% aqneous borax : 2 mL
	Distilled water : 25 mL
	Dissolve borax in the distilled water, add stock solution 25 mL mix well
	0.1% aqneous gold choride yellow
	Counter stain
	0.2% aqneous light green : 10 mL
	Distilled water : 50 mL
	Glacial acetic acid : 0.1 mL
Procedure	• Bring sectios and a control slide to water
	• Oxidize in chromic acid solution for 60 minutes
	• Wash in running tap water
	• Transfer to sodium bisulfate solution for 1 minute
	• Wash in tap water for 5–10 minutes
	• Rinse in several changes of distilled water
	• Impregnate with incubating solution for 30–60 minutes at 58°C. Examine for adequate impregnation
	• Rinse in several changes of distilled water
	• Tone in gold chloride solution for 2–5 minutes
	• Rinse in distilled water
	• Fix in sodium thiosulfate solution for 2–5 minutes
	• Wash thoroughly in tap water
	• Stain with counter stain for 30–45 seconds
	• Dehydrate, clear and mount
Results	Fungi outline : Black
	Inner parts of hyphae and mycelia : Reddish
	Background : Pale green

Hage-Fontana Silver Method for Spirochetes

Spirochetes are most often looked for in smears of blood and exudates. Some of them such as *Borrelia recurrentis* which causes relapsing fever, can be seen by high power objective with direct illumination. Many others are stained by Leishman's and Giemsa's stains. The best method of detecting spirochetes in films and to some extent in section, is the dark ground illumination. Most of the methods in histopathology for demonstrating spirochetes are based on silver impregnation techniques.

    Hage-Fontana silver method is very good for the detection of spirochetes in smears. A thin smear of the suspected material is prepared and allow to dry in air and fixed in Ruge's fluid.

Reagents	Ruge's fluid:
	    Formaldehyde (40%) : 20 mL
	    Glacial acetic acid : 1 mL
	    Distilled water : 100 mL
	    Fixation time is 1 minute
	Mordant:
	    Phenol : 1 g
	    Tannic acid : 5 g
	    Distilled water : 100 mL

Procedure	• Remove smear from the fixative • Wash briefly in running tap water for 10 seconds • Flood slides with mordant and warm over a flame until steam just rises, leave for 20–30 seconds • Wash in running tap water for about 30 seconds • Rinse in distilled water • Flood slide with 0.25% aqueous silver nitrate and add 1 drop of concentrated ammonia • Warm over a flame for 20–30 seconds. A brownish-green color should form • Rinse well in distilled water • Blot and examine dry
Result	Spirochetes : Black Background : Yellow

Staining Methods for Protozoa and Other Parasites

Staining methods for films and smears of materials suspected to contain protozoa and other parasites are by far superior to any sectional techniques. A matter of choice, therefore in the study of pathogenic protozoa is the examination of blood, films and fecal specimens, even though some of these microorganisms are found in tissues. Besides fresh preparation, some smears give better morphological details than sections which usually have some artifacts due to fixation and paraffin embedding.

Reagents	**Schauddin's fixative (stock solution):** Mercuric chloride : 35 g Ehanol 95% : 250 mL Distilled water : 500 mL	Add the distilled water to the mercuric chloride in a heat resistant flask. Place the flask in a boiling water bath to completely dissolve the solute. Allow to cool at room temperature. The excess salt will crystallize out. Pour the superatant fluid into another flask and note the volume. Mix 1 part of 95% ethanol with 2 parts of the saturated mercuric chloride solution. This reagent keeps for years
	Working solution: Add 5 mL of glacial acetic acid to 95 mL of the stock Schauddinn's fixative just before use. **Ethanol-iodine solution** Absolute ethanol : 70 mL Distilled water : 30 mL. Add Iodine crystals sufficient to give brown color **Acidified ethanol solution** Absolute ethanol : 90 mL Distilled water : 10 mL Acetic acid : 0.45 mL **Trichrome stain:** Chromotrope 2R : 0.6 g Fast grebe FCF : 0.3 g Phosphotungstic acid : 0.6 g Glacial acetic acid : 1.0 mL Distilled water : 100 mL	
Procedure	• Make a thin smear on a clean slide • Fix in solution 1 while still wet for 5 minutes • Fix smears from preserved feces for ½ to 1 hour • Place smear in 70% alcohol for 2–5 minutes • Treat with trichrome stain for 10 minutes • Rinse rapidly in acidified ethanol for 3 seconds • Dehydrate in absolute alcohol, clear and mount	**Results:** Cytoplasm of amoebic trophozoites: Blue green with purple tinge. Nuclear chromatin : Purple to red Chromatoid bodies : Purple to red Ingested red cells : Purple to red Background : Pale green

Giemsa or Leishman's staining methods are useful for demonstrating malaria parasites, *Typanosoma*, *Leishmania*, *Toxoplasma* and *Pneumocystis*. *Pneumocystis carinii* can also be demonstrated by Grocott's silver methanamine method.

Amoebae (the most important intestinal protozoa) in tissue sections may be demonstrated, due to glycogen content, with best carmine or PAS method. Phosphotungstic acid-hematoxylin will stain nuclei, chromatoid bars, and fibrils.

STAINING OF FROZEN SECTIONS

There are various methods of staining frozen sections, but two methods which are most widely used are Haematoxylin—Eosin staining and Polychrome—Methylene blue staining.

■ Hematoxylin — Eosin Staining

- Fix the air dried section in pure acetone for 15–20 seconds or in formal alcohol for 30–60 seconds.
- Place in water until no longer 'greasy' or cloudy.'
- Place in Harry's hematoxylin stain for 1–2 minutes.
- Wash in running water for 5–10 seconds.
- Dip in 0.5% sodium borate until blue.
- Place in 70% ethanol for 5 seconds.
- Counter stain in 1% alcoholic eosin, 1 to 2 quick dips.
- Wash well in running water.
- Dehydrate through graded alcohol (80%, 90%, 100%).
- Clear in three changes of xylol.
- Mount in appropriate medium (Canada balsam).

Rapid Hematoxylin and Eosin (H and E) Procedure

- Slide mounted frozen sections (fresh or appropriately fixed) are washed briefly in water.
- Stain in haematoxylin solution (Harris,' Gill's, Mayer's or Carazzi's) for 30 seconds to 2 minutes.
- Rinse in water.
- If necessary, differentiate in 1% acid alcohol.
- Wash in water.
- Wash and blue the section in alkaline tap water (or equivalent) for 30 seconds.
- Counterstain in 1% eosin for 5–30 seconds.
- Rinse in water.
- Dehydrate and mount in synthetic mounting medium.

Results

Nuclei—blue to blue/black
Cytoplasm, collagen—shades of pink

■ Toluidine Blue and Thionine

These closely related dyes offer a good and extremely rapid staining reaction for diagnostic work. The staining pattern is particularly useful for the lymph node and brain evaluation due to the metachromatic qualities of the staining solutions.

Reagents required		Method	Results
• Toluidine blue or Thionine	: 0.5 g	• Use fixed or air dried sections	Nuclei—blue
• Ethanol	: 20 mL	• Apply stain to the section for 20 seconds	Cytoplasm, muscle and connective tissue — pink to purple
• Distilled water	: 80 mL	• Rinse in water	
• Phenol	: 0.5 g	• Mount in water or an aqueous mounting medium. (For permanent mount, dehydrate in acetone, clear in acetone-xylene, then in xylene and mount)	

■ Polychrome Methylene Blue

This is a rapid metachromatic stain which is also of value in the diagnosis of frozen sections. The stain, however, requires considerable time to mature before it is ready for use.

Reagents required	Method	Results
12% Aqueous potassium carbonate: 8.0 mL 1% Aqueous methylene blue: 100 mL Mix together and boil gently for 60 minutes Cool to room temperature, then add 10% Aqueous citric acid 4.0 mL Store in loosely stoppered bottle and allow to oxidize for 12 months before use	• Use a fixed or air dried section • Apply staining solution for 30 seconds • Rinse in water • Mount in water or aqueous mounting medium	Nuclei — Blue Cytoplasm, muscle, connective tissue — pink to purple

■ Alcoholic Pinacyanide

This metachromatic stain is particularly recommended for staining thyroid sections.

Reagents required	Method	Results
Pinacyanole: 0.5 g 70% ethyl or methyl alcohol: 100 mL	• Use fixed or air dried section • Apply stain to the section for 5–15 seconds • Rinse in water • Mount in water or aqueous mounting medium	Nuclei — blue Cytoplasm, collagen — pink Muscle and elastic tissue — violet Plasma cells — red Haemosiderin — orange Thyroid and pituitary colloid and amyloid — bright red

■ Phloxine — Methylene Blue — Azure B

This method gives a permanent stain with a similar appearance to H and E. It is recommended particularly for unfixed tissue where it gives good nuclear definition and clear staining.

Reagents required	Method	Results
Solution A Phloxine : 0.5 g Acetic acid : 0.2 mL Distilled water : 100 mL **Solution B** Methylene Blue: 0.25 g Azure B : 0.25 g Borax : 0.25 g Distilled water : 100 mL 30.2% acetic acid	• Rinse section briefly in water and drain • Apply staining solution A for 1 minute • Wash in water for 10 seconds and drain • Apply staining solution B for 30 seconds • Remove excess stain in 0.2% acetic acid in distilled water Agitate the slide gently until stain ceases to flow from the section (about 20–30 seconds) • Differentiate in three washes of 95% ethanol • Dehydrate in two changes of absolute ethanol, clear in two changes of xylene and mount in synthetic mounting medium	Nuclei and bacteria—blue Collagen and muscle—bright rose to red Erythrocytes—scarlet

■ Methyl Violet for Amyloid

This stain demonstrates amyloid deposits in frozen sections. Use unfixed sections or sections fixed in 70% methanol

Reagents required	Method	Results
Methyl violet: 0.5 g Distilled water: 100 mL 1% acetic acid	Apply stain to section for 1 minute Wash in two changes of distilled water for 30 second each Apply 1% acetic acid for 10–30 seconds Wash in tap water for 1–5 minutes Blot off excess water but do not allow to dry Mount in glycerin	Amyloid—red purple

PRECAUTIONS TAKEN DURING STAINING

- Stains and solutions should be kept covered when not in use.
- The slides should be cooled after removing from the oven and before keeping in the xylene.
- Stains must be filtered before using it.
- After deparaffinization of slides with the xylene they should not be allowed to dry out. Similarly, at the time of mounting care must be taken not to allow xylene to evaporate hence mounting should be done immediately.
- The level of staining solutions should be maintain sufficient to cover the whole slide.
- The slides should be properly drained and blot on the filter paper before putting into the next solution so that one solution should not contaminate other solution.
- Alkali used for bluing should be washed out properly otherwise, it may lead to disagreeable hazy blue color of the nuclei.

CAUSES OF POOR STAINING

- The fixation of the tissue is poor and inadequate.
- Hematoxylin used is overused or over worked out.
- Hematoxylin used is either over ripened or under ripened.
- Improper differentiation of hematoxylin.
- Insufficient bluing and differentiation.
- Insufficient washing of bluing agent and counter staining with eosin.
- Improper differentiation of eosin during washing or dehydration.
- Insufficient dehydration and clearing of sections.
- Contamination of stains.

Table 9.6 shows various staining methods used in histopathology laboratory.

Table 9.6: Various staining methods used in histopathology laboratory

Tissue to be stained	Staining method	Stain used	Counter stain used	Result of staining
Connective tissue	Weigert's-Van Gieson staining	Weigert's-iron Hematoxylin solution	Van Gieson's solution	Cell nuclei—black Collage—red Muscle fibers, cytoplasm, RBC—yellow
Elastic fibers	Verhoeff's staining	Verhoeff's stain	Van Gieson's solution	Elastic fibers—blue black/black Nuclei—grey to black Muscle fibers and RBC—yellow
Carbohydrates	PAS staining	Schiff's reagent	Harri's alum hematoxylin	Nuclei—blue Mucin/glycogen—purple Basement membrane—reddish-purple
Lipids	Sudan black B staining	Sudan black B solution	Nuclear fast red	Fat—blue black Background—red
Reticulin	Silver nitrate staining	Ammonical silver nitrate	Safranine	Reticular fibers—black Nuclei—black Other elements—pink
Hemoglobin	Dunn Thompson staining	Alum hematoxylin	Van Gieson's solution	Rbc—green-black Hemoglobin casts—light shades of green
Bile pigments	Gmelin's method	Nitric acid	-	Bile pigments-yellowish to brown to green to blue to purple
Melanin pigments	Masson-Fontana Ammonical silver reaction	Silver nitrate	Safranine	Melanin—black Argentaffin cell granules—black
Hemosiderin pigments	Perl's prussian blue method	Acidified potassium Ferro-cyanide solution	Nuclear fast red	Haemosiderin—bright prussian blue Nuclei—red Cytoplasm—pink
Alkaline phosphatase	Azo-dye coupling method	Tris buffer	Mayer's hemalum	Site of enzyme activity—brown with fast red or black with fast black B

Contd...

Contd...

Acid phosphatase	Azo-dye coupling method	Veronal acetate solution	Mayer's hemalum	Site of enzyme activity—reddish brown Nuclei—blue
Peroxidases	Benzidine method	Benzidine	Picric acid	Peroxidase granules—dark blue Cytoplasm—yellow
Oxidases	Nadi reaction	Nadi reagent	Carmalum/red nuclear stain	Site of enzyme activity—bluish violet nuclei—red
Dehydrogenase	Tetrazolium salt method	Nitroblue tetrazolium (NBT)	Safranine	Site of enzyme activity—blue purple deposits of formazan pigment
Bacteria	Gram's staining	Crystal violet	Neutral red	Gram-positive bacteria—bluish black Gram-negative bacteria—red/pink
Acid fast bacteria	Ziehl–Neelsen's staining	Carbol fuchsin	Methylene blue	Acid fast bacilli—red Cell nuclei—blue Rbc—pink
Fungi	Methenamine silver nitrate method	Methenamine silver nitrate solution	Light green	Fungi outline—black Inner parts of hyphae and mycelia—reddish Background—pale green
Spirochetes	Hage-Fontana silver method	Aqueous silver nitrate		Spirochetes—black Background—yellow
Parasites	Gomori trichrome staining	Trichrome stain		Cytoplasm of amoeba—blue red with purple ting Nuclear chromatin—purple to red Chromatoid bodies—purple to red Ingested red cells—purple to red Background—pale green

EXERCISE

1. What is the purpose of staining? Why do any tissue components stain? Why are the stains not taken up into every part of the tissue?
2. Classify dyes or stains with suitable example.
3. Enlist various types of dyes or stains with their major uses.
4. What is staining? Describe in short different staining processes used in histological laboratory.
5. What is mordant staining? Explain with example.
6. Describe various steps of staining.
7. Explain equipments, materials and methodology of staining.
8. Describe different types of staining dyes and their properties. What are the common special stains used in histopathology.
9. Describe important hematoxylin stains used in histopathological laboratory.
10. Describe briefly technique of hematoxylin and eosin staining.
11. Write composition of Mayer's hematoxylin, Harri's hematoxylin, Weigert's iron hematoxylin and Heidenhain's hematoxylin.
12. What are counter stains? Describe important counter stains used in histopathology laboratory.
13. Write a note on:
    i. PAS stain
    ii. Coplin Jar
    iii. Reticulin stain
    iv. Stains for bile pigments and melanin
    v. Hematoxylin and Eosin stains
14. What is deparaffinization of tissues?
15. What is dehydration and rehydration of tissue sections.
16. What is hematoxylin? How is hematoxylin stain prepared? Write its uses.
17. How is routine hematoxylin stain prepared? Mention the steps in staining procedure. What are the limitations of this stain in the study of histological sections?
18. Describe PAS staining and bile pigment staining techniques.
19. Describe the theory of staining of tissues.
20. Write down stains used for demonstration of reticulin fibrin, fat, carbohydrate and amyloid.
21. Describe in details stains for carbohydrate, nucleic acid, hemosiderin and *Candida*.
22. Describe Sudan Black stains for lipids and acid-fast stain for bacteria.

23. Describe in detail Z and E staining procedure.
24. Write short notes on following:
    i. Staining of connective tissues
    ii. Staining of hemosiderin
    iii. Staining of alkaline phosphatase
    iv. Gram staining
25. What are pigments? Give types of pigments present in cell?
26. Write note on staining of enzymes.
27. Give an account of staining of microorganisms.
28. Describe staining technique for fungi, spirochetes and protozoa.
29. Write compositions and results obtained by the following stains:
    i. Ehrlich's hematoxylin stain
    ii. Verhoeff's elastic fiber stain
    iii. PAS stain
    iv. Sudan black stain
    v. Silver nitrate stain
    vi. Mason-Fontana ammonical silver reaction stain
    vii. Perl's Prussian blue staining
    viii. Ziehl-Neelson stain
30. What are various causes of failure of staining? What are the precautions to be taken during staining?

OBJECTIVE QUESTIONS

1. _____ is the method by which different tissue components can be easily distinguished from each other.
    a. Clearing   b. Infiltration
    c. Dehydration   d. Staining

2. Nucleic acids carry _____ charge.
    a. Positive   b. Negative
    c. Both   d. None

3. Cytoplamic components usually have _____ charge.
    a. Positive   b. Negative
    c. Both   d. None

4. _____ is an example of natural dye.
    a. Hematoxylin   b. Eosin
    c. Methylene blue   d. Carbol fuschin

5. Nitro group is _____ group.
    a. Chromophore   b. Auxochrome
    c. Metachrome   d. None

6. _____ is an example of auxochrome.
    a. NO_2 b. -N=N
    c. Quinoid   d. -OH

7. _____ impart color to a compound due to presence of specific groups.
    a. Chromophore   b. Auxochrome
    c. Metachrome   d. None

8. Auxochrome is an ionizing group which _____ the color of the dye.
    a. Intensify   b. Fad
    c. Do not change   d. None

9. Acid fuschin is an _____ stain.
    a. Basic   b. Amphoteric
    c. Neutral   d. Acidic

10. _____ is not an acidic component of cell.
    a. DNA   b. RNA
    c. Cartilage   d. RBC

11. Cytoplasm and muscle are _____ in nature.
    a. Acidic   b. Basic
    c. Amphoteric   d. Neutral

12. _____ is not an basic component of cell.
    a. RBC   b. WBC
    c. Cartilage   d. Collagen

13. In vital staining the tissue or the cells which are stained are in _____ condition.
    a. Living   b. Dead
    c. Degraded   d. Fixed

14. The cells which have capacity of reducing ammonical silver (in metallic impregnation) are called _____.
    a. Argentaffin cells   b. Argyrophil cells
    c. Argentiferous cells   d. Argyro ferrous cells

15. A substance that can alter the color of a metachromatic dye is a _____ .
    a. Chromophore   b. Auxochrome
    c. Chromotrope   d. All

16. The dye which combine with certain tissue components to form a color different from the color of the dye.
    a. Vital dye   b. Fluorescent dye
    c. Direct dye   d. Metachromatic dye

17. Staining in which the tissue is first over-stained and then de-stained to remove excessive stain is called as _____ staining.
    a. Progressive   b. Regressive
    c. Direct   d. Mordant

18. Fluorochromes are _____ dyes.
    a. Nitro   b. Thiazine
    c. Azo   d. Quinoid

19. Hematoxylin is a natural _____.
    a. Dehydrant   b. Dye
    c. Clearing agent d. Fixative

20. In Ehrlich's hematoxylin _____ is used as mordant.
    a. Aluminium alum b. Potassium alum
    c. Ferric alum sulfate d. Ammonium alum

21. Eosin is a _____ stain.
    a. Nuclear   b. Cytoplasmic
    c. Counter   d. All

22. Weigert Van Geison staining is used for _____.
    a. Elastic fiber   b. Connective tissues
    c. Carbohydrates   d. Lipids

23. Verhoff's stain is used for _____.
    a. Elastic fiber   b. Connective tissues
    c. Carbohydrates   d. Lipids

24. PAS staining is used for _____.
    a. Elastic fiber   b. Connective tissues
    c. Carbohydrates   d. Lipids

25. Sudan black B in propylene glycol staining is used for _____.
    a. Elastic fiber   b. Connective tissues
    c. Carbohydrates   d. Lipids

26. Stain used for reticulin is _____.
    a. Silver nitrate b. Sudan black B
    c. PAS   d. Verhoff's stain

27. Perl's Prussian blue method is used for staining of _____.
    a. Melanin   b. Bile pigments
    c. Hemosiderin   d. Hemoglobin

28. Bile pigment is stained by _____.
    a. Gmelin's method
    b. Dunn Thompson method
    c. Masson-Fontana method
    d. Gram staining method

29. Benzidine method is used for staining of _____.
    a. Oxidases
    b. Peroxidases
    c. Acid phosphatases
    d. Alkaline phosphatases

30. In staining of mast cells by acidified toluidine blue method, mast cell stained as _____.
    a. Purple   b. Red
    c. Pink   d. Green

31. _____ is used to divide bacteria in two groups.
    a. Gram's stain   b. Z-N stain
    c. PAS stain   d. None

32. Mycobacteria are stained by _____.
    a. Gram's stain   b. Z-N stain
    c. PAS stain   d. None

33. Gomori trichrome staining method is used for demonstration of _____.
    a. Bacteria   b. Spirochetes
    c. Fungi   d. Parasites

ANSWERS

1-d, 2-b, 3-a, 4-a, 5-a, 6-d, 7-a, 8-a, 9-d, 10-d, 11-c, 12-c, 13-a, 14-a, 15-c, 16-d, 17-b, 18-d, 19-b, 20-a, 21-c, 22-b, 23-a, 24-c, 25-d, 26-a, 27-c, 28-a, 29-b, 30-a, 31-a, 32-b, 33-d.

CHAPTER

10

Mounting of Sections

INTRODUCTION

The final stage in the preparation of tissues for microscopy is mounting. Occasionally tissue samples are examined dry (as occurs with sections for electron microscopy and in some procedures for displaying specimens in a museum) but in almost every other situation a liquid medium or 'mountant' is applied.

Mountants with a refractive index (RI) as close as possible to that of the tissue (usually taken as the RI of fixed protein, between 1.53 and 1.54) will effectively render a section transparent. With such specimens the only features visible will be those colored by the staining method used. A medium with a much lower or higher RI than that of the tissue will increase visibility but is beneficial only if an overview of the specimen is required as the resolution can be poor (evident in the extreme if sections are cleared and examined dry; the mountant in this case, air, has a RI of 1.000). In some forms of microscopy (such as phase contrast) the use of a mountant with an RI only slightly different from that of tissue is recommended to supplement contrast enhancement.

CHARACTERISTICS OF MOUNTANT

To be effective, a mountant should possess certain characteristics. These include the following:
- It should be colorless and transparent.
- It should be able to completely permeate and fill tissue interstices.
- It should have no adverse effect on tissue components.
- It should be resistant to contamination.
- It should protect the section from physical damage and chemical activity (oxidation and changes in pH).
- It should be completely miscible with dehydrant or clearing agent.
- It should set without crystallizing, cracking or shrinking (or otherwise deform the material being mounted)

and not react with, leach or induce fading in stains and reaction products (including those from enzyme histochemical, hybridization and immunohistochemical procedures).
- Finally, once set, the mountant should remain stable.

Mounted sections are often stored for many years and the use of an appropriate mountant is critical to avoid deterioration in the specimen.

TYPES OF MOUNTANT

Mounting media are either hydrophobic or hydrophilic. Methods using the former generally call for sections to be dehydrated and cleared before the mounting medium is applied. Sections are mounted in hydrophilic media directly from water.

Within each group, mountants can also be classed as adhesives or non-adhesives. In general, adhesives harden through solvent evaporation and thereby fix the accompanying coverslip to the slide. During this process, the RI of the medium alters, moving away from that of the solvent and towards that of the dry mountant. The exact RI of the applied medium cannot therefore be known. Nevertheless as the RI of hydrophobic (adhesive) mountants usually approximates that of tissue proteins (fixed), they provide firm adhesion of the coverslip, these mountants are the type most frequently used.

Hydrophilic media, although of relatively low RI, are essential for procedures in which dehydrants and hydrocarbon type clearants must be avoided. This will mostly relate to methods for demonstrating lipid, enzyme identification and immunohistochemistry. Disadvantages of hydrophilic mountants are that they may induce stains to leach from the section and many, being non-adhesive, remain soft such that the edge of the coverslip must be sealed to prevent drying out. Suitable agents (ringing media) for this purpose are nail varnish, resinous mountants or paraffin wax.

Hydrophobic Mounts

Canada Balsam (RI = 1.52)

This is an oleoresin obtained from the bark of the fir *Abies balsamea* (of the family Pinaceae), native to North America. The dried resin is freely soluble in xylene and other organic solvents. Originally introduced in about 1832 and widely used until only recently, Canada balsam has a number of disadvantages: it yellows with age; is very slow to harden and; as it becomes increasingly acidic over time, cationic dyes are poorly preserved and the Prussian blue product of Perls' reaction is bleached.

Reagents Required
Canada balsam 55–65 g and xylene 100 mL.

Method
Prepare using the quantities indicated (greater amounts of resin will result in more viscous solutions). RI (solution) 1.523. When dissolved, the solution is filtered through soft filter paper and the desired consistency is obtained by the controlled evaporation of solvent. It should be kept in a dark glass bottle. A few crystals of calcium carbonate in the stock bottle will help to maintain neutral reaction.

Distrene, Plasticizer, Xylene (DPX)

One of the most commonly used mountants, DPX is a colorless, neutral medium in which most standard stains are well preserved. It is prepared by dissolving the common plastic, polystyrene, in a suitable hydrocarbon solvent (usually xylene). A major disadvantage of polystyrene media, however, is that they set quickly and in doing so often retract from the edge of the coverslip. This can be prevented by adding a plasticizer which is thought to resist the effect by forming a mesh with the polymerized plastic.

Reagents Required
Polystyrene (Distrene 80) 18 g, dibutyl phthalate 7.5 mL and xylene 52.5 mL.

Method
Prepare using the quantities indicated. RI (solution) 1.523. Combine the dibutyl phthalate with xylene, mix and dissolve polystyrene. Label and store. It is more advantageous than Canada balsam because slides can be cleaned by excess mountant by stripping it off after cutting around the edge of the coverslip.

Euparal

Euparal is a mixture of eucalyptol, sandarac (a resin from the tree, Tetraclinis articulata grown in North West Africa), paraldehyde and camsal (camphor and phenyl salicylate). Its has relatively low RI (which is usually 1.483 but ranges from 1.478 at 20°C to 1.535 when solid) which makes it useful for mounting unstained sections. Another advantage is that slides may be transferred directly from 95% alcohol, eliminating the need for complete dehydration and clearing. Some fading may occur in hematoxylin stained sections; in this situation the green (or 'vert') copper-containing form of Euparal is advocated.

Resin-Embedded Tissue

Sections of tissue embedded in plastic compounds (such as epoxy resins) can be successfully mounted in a liquid resin of the same type. Sections should be completely dry before applying mountant, which is best set using the same conditions prescribed for tissue blocks.

Photosensitive Resins

Light polymerizing resins have the advantage of very short setting times, requiring in the order of 10–30 seconds exposure to UV light to harden completely. Once cured, however, the mountant cannot be dissolved nor the coverslip removed (as might be necessary for restraining). Acrylic based light sensitive resins are also suitable for fluorescence microscopy.

Hydrophilic (Aqueous) Mounts

Water

Although of low RI (1.333), water serves as a convenient temporary mountant for some whole specimens for examining certain microorganisms live (saline mount) and particularly when checking sections during staining procedures.

Glycerol

Glycerol is also a useful temporary mountant, but with a higher RI (1.460) and longer drying time than water. Ringing the coverslip with a hydrophobic seal will extend the life of mounted sections, although cationic dyes will diffuse into the medium over time. Phosphate buffered glycerol (RI 1.47) is commonly used to mount sections for immunofluorescence. Glycerol may be added to other agents to retard drying and cracking.

Mounting of Sections

Reagents Required

0.2 mol/L phosphate buffer-1 part and glycerol-9 parts.

Method

Prepare using the quantities indicated. The addition of gum arabic (derived from species of Acacia) to a solution of glycerol will result in an adhesive mountant (Farrants medium) with a RI of 1.436. The preparation is acidic but rendered neutral through the inclusion of potassium acetate, which also retards dye extraction from methyl violet stained sections of amyloid.

Glycerin (Glycerol) Jelly

This commonly utilized aqueous mountant is a mixture of glycerol and gelatin and has a RI of 1.47. It should set quite hard but for long-term preservation sections are best ringed and sealed. Various formulations are in use.

Apathy's Medium

Sucrose added to gum arabic preparations increases the RI and prevents overdrying. The inclusion of potassium acetate will prevent leaching of metachromatic dyes.

Reagents Required

Gum arabic 20 g, cane sugar 20 g, potassium acetate 20 g, distilled water 40 mL and thymol 0.02 g.

Method

Dissolve components in warm distilled water. Store in air tight containers.

Polyvinyl Alcohol

Polyvinyl alcohol, often used as a mountant in immunofluorescence microscopy, has been recommended as an alternative for glycerin jelly. Adding paraphenylenediamine to the preparation is effective in retarding photo fading.

Karo Corn Syrup (RI = 1.47)

Karo corn syrup	:	1 volume
Distilled water	:	2 volume
Thymol (preservative)	:	1 crystal

Dilute corn syrup with distilled water and add thymol, mix, label and store at 4°C.

Levulose (Fructose) Syrup (RI = 1.47)

Levulose (fructose)	:	70 g
Distilled water	:	20 mL

Dissolve the levulose in the distilled water by heating at 37°C for 24 hours. Mix well and store.

Farrant's Medium (RI = 1.43)

Gum Arabic	:	50 g
Distilled water	:	50 mL
Glycerol		50 mL
AsO_3 (preservative)	:	1 g

Dissolve gum Arabic in the distilled water with the aid of gentle heat, add glycerol and AsO_3 mix well and label but thymol (100 mg), merthiolate (15 mg) or cresol (0.1 mL) are effective substitutes.

Kaiser's Glycerin Jelly (RI = 1.47)

Gelatin	:	10 g
Glycerol	:	70 mL
Distilled water	:	60 mL
Phenol crystals (preservative)	:	0.25 g

Add gelatin in distilled water and incubate in water bath at 60°C till the gelatin gets dissolved. Add glycerol and crystals of phenol. Mix well, label and store at 4°C.

■ Temporary Mountant

A mixture of equal parts of pure glycerol and distilled water may be used as a temporary mountant with fresh or watery preparations while thick cedar wood oil (RI = 1.52) is suitable with dehydrated specimens.

■ Methods of Mounting Sections (Cover Slipping)

First a clean coverslip of the appropriate size and wipe off the excess of xylene from the side with a dust free cloth. If xylene remain on the section then it will mix with the mounting medium and form air bubbles which become trapped beneath the coverslip. There are four methods of mounting stained sections which are as follows:

Method 1: Place mounting medium on a coverslip Invert glass slide with stained section on the coverslip.

Method 2: Place the mounting medium on a coverslip. Place the coverslip on the stained section on the slide.

Method 3: Place the mounting medium on the stained section. Place coverslip over it.

Method 4: Stained section is placed on the coverslip. Glass slide with mounting medium is placed over the coverslip (Fig. 10.1).

Method 1

- Select the appropriately sized coverslip and place on a white paper sheet.
- Place a drop of mountant in the center of the coverslip.
- Remove surplus clearant from the back of the slide and around the section, leaving a margin of approximately 3 mm. The section should not be allowed to dry out.
- Invert the slide (section face down) over the coverslip and with one end resting on the paper sheet, gradually lower the other end until the mountant touches the section. Mountant will spread quickly over the section, between slide and coverslip. The slide, with coverslip attached, is then turned upright. Any trapped air is gently squeezed out whilst aligning the coverslip.
- The mountant is allowed to set. The time required will depend upon the particular agent used but in some cases warming the slides (37°-60°C) will hasten the process. If the result is inadequate, slides are returned to the solvent (appropriate to the mountant) to have the coverslip removed and the process repeated.

Method 2

- Select the appropriate sized coverslip.
- Remove surplus clearant from the back of the slide and around the section and place the slide on a level surface.
- Place a drop of mountant in the center of the coverslip.
- Invent the coverslip so that drop face the downward.
- Now keep the coverslip over the slide with one end resting on the paper sheet, and gradually lower the other end until mountant touches the section.
- Remove the trapped air by gentle squeezing.

Method 3

- Remove excess clearant from the back of the slide and around the section.
- Place the slide on a level surface and apply a drop of the mountant.
- Hold the coverslip at 45° angle to the surface of the slide, and allow the bottom edge to touch the drop of mountant. When the drop spread along the edge of the coverslip, let go of the coverslip and allow the mountant to spread slowly.
- Remove excess of mountant while wet with a tissue paper or with a razor blade after mountant dried sufficiently in 30 minutes.

Method 4

- Select an appropriate size coverslip, place stained section on it and place it on a leveled surface.
- On a cleaned glass slide, add a drop of mountant in the center.
- Invent the slide and slowly lower the slide on the coverslip until the mountant touches the section.
- Mountant spread quickly over the section.

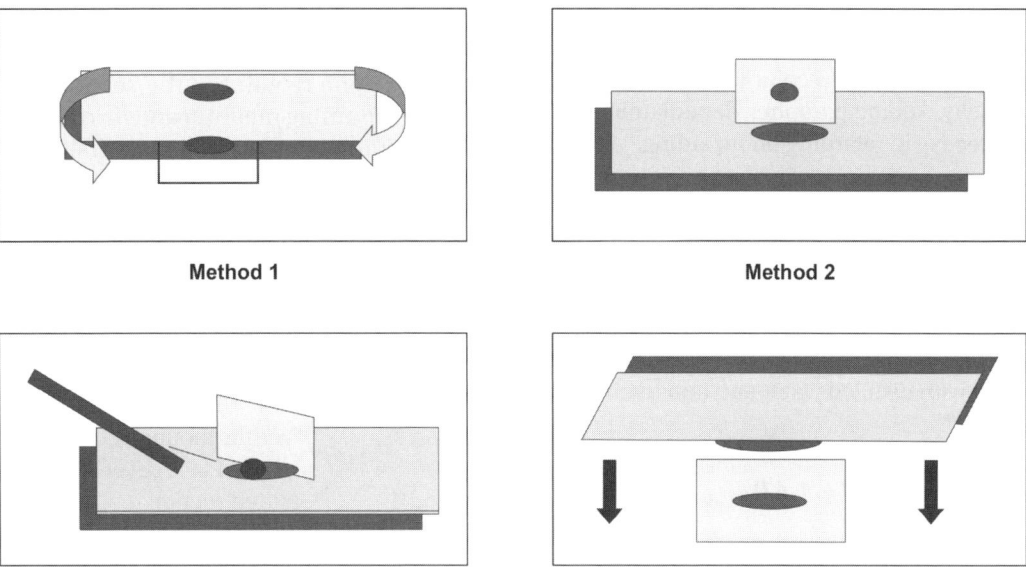

Fig 10.1: Techniques of mounting

- Now, turn the slide upside down.
- Remove the air trapped by gently squeezing.
- Remove excess mountant.

RESTAINING

In some instances, it becomes necessary to gain access to a section previously set in mountant to restain specimens that has faded appreciably, remove the original stain and apply a new technique or to superimpose an additional stain. Mounted tissue may also need to be retrieved for additional assessment such as by electron microscopy or X-ray analysis. In this case, coverslips can be removed by soaking in the solvent appropriate to the mountant. This may require one to two days after which the coverslip is gently removed and sections are rehydrated and treated as required. Alternatively, slides can be left at –20°C for up to one hour then a sharp blade used to carefully prize off the coverslip.

LABELING AND STORAGE OF SLIDES

Slide mounted sections are identified during preparation by inscribing the slide with the tissue accession number or suitable code using a diamond marker or pencil (frosted slides). Care should be exercised when using characters such as A, I, O, T, V and the like as these appear the same when viewed from either side of the slide; incorrectly identifying the side upon which the section is mounted may lead to poor staining or section damage. After staining and mounting it is common practice to affix to the slide a paper label upon which the laboratory number, staining method and date are usually written. This may be supplemented with a bar code or other symbol which can be recognized by a computer supported image scanner. It is important when attaching identifying labels to be aware of the slide storage system to be utilized. Standard 7.5 × 2.5 (3″ × 1″) slides are usually stored, standing on their short side, in metal or plastic drawers. Labels need to be fixed to the opposite end and orientated so the details can be read with the slide in this upright position (Fig. 10.2).

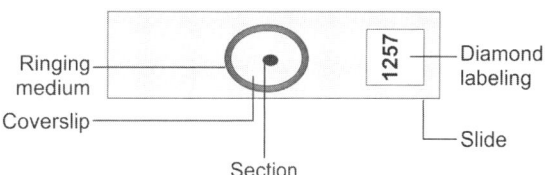

Fig. 10.2: Labeling of slide

COVERSLIPS

Coverslips are made up of borosilicate or silicate glass and it holds the samples in place and protect them from inadvertent movement and contamination. To be compatible with the standard slide, coverslips are 22 mm or 24 mm wide, but vary in length to suit the size of the section. In general a selection of 22 mm, 30 mm, 50 mm and possibly 60 mm (if preparing cell smears) will accommodate most purposes. Round coverslips of different diameters are also available. The coverslips are manufactured to a specified thickness to complement the optical specifications of microscope objectives lenses (the recommended thickness is indicated on the barrel of the lens and is normally 0.17 mm). Various thicknesses are available (with some variation between manufacturers) and are designated No. 1 (0.13–0.17 mm), No. 1½ (0.16–0.19 mm) and No. 2 (0.19–0.25 mm).

RINGING MEDIA

Fluid and semi fluid mountants, including which fail to set completely hard should be sealed at the margin of the coverslip to prevent evaporation of mountant, to immobilize the coverslip, and to prevent shrinkage or sticking of slides on storage. Ringing media may be solid, being melted for use and applied with a bent wire, or fluid being applied with a fine brush, the medium hardening by evaporation. For a solid medium, paraffin wax may be used or Kronig's cement which is composed of 2 parts wax and 7 part powdered colophonium resin. Several liquids ringing media are available commercially such as nail varnish, durofix, etc.

EXERCISE

1. What are mountants? Classify with suitable example.
2. Enlist various characteristics of mountants.
3. Write short note on following:
   i. Canada balsam
   ii. DPX
   iii. Glycerol
4. Give composition of following mounting media:
   i. Karo Corn syrup
   ii. Levulose (fructose) syrup
   iii. Farrant's medium
   iv. Kaiser's glycerin jelly
5. Describe methods of mounting sections with the help of figure.
6. What is restaining? How restaining can be done?
7. Describe method of labeling and storage of slides.
8. Write a note on coveslips and method of coverslipping.
9. What do you mean by ringing media?

OBJECTIVE QUESTIONS

1. The mountants which are used in histology should have refractive index (RI) of _____.
   a. 1.54   b. 2.54
   c. 0.54   d. 3.54

2. A good mounting medium should be _____.
   a. Colorless and transparent
   b. Colored and transparent
   c. Colorless and opaque
   d. Colored and opaque

3. A good mounting media should not set with _____.
   a. Crystallization   b. Cracking
   c. All   d. Shrinking

4. A medium with much lower or higher RI than tissue provides _____.
   a. Good resolution   b. Poor resolution
   c. Average resolution d. No resolution

5. _____ is not an example of hydrophobic mounting media.
   a. Canada balsam   b. DPX
   c. Eupharal   d. Glycerol

6. _____ is not an example of hydrophilic mounting media.
   a. Canada balsam   b. Polyvinyl alcohol
   c. Apathy's medium   d. Glycerol

7. DPX is an _____ mounting media.
   a. Hydrophilic   b. Hydrophobic
   c. Amphoteric   d. None

8. Glycerol is an example of _____ mounting media.
   a. Hydrophilic   b. Hydrophobic
   c. Amphoteric   d. None

9. Canada balsam is an _____ mounting media.
   a. Natural   b. Synthetic
   c. Artificial   d. None

10. _____ is an resinous mounting media.
    a. Eupharal   b. Glycerol
    c. Polyvinyl alcohol d. None

10. DPX is a mixture of _____.
    a. Distyrene, phenol, xylene
    b. Dibutyl, phenol, xylene
    c. Diphenyl amine, phenol, xylene
    d. Distyrene, plasticizer, xylene

ANSWERS

1-a, 2-a, 3-c, 4-b, 5-d, 6-a, 7-b, 8-a, 9-a, 10-a, 11-d.

CHAPTER 11

Cytopathology

Cytopathology is that branch of diagnostic medicine which deals with the study of individual cells and or tissue fragments spread on a slide and stained properly.

Exfoliative cytology deals with the microscopical examination of cells, which are shed (exfoliate) spontaneously from epithelial surfaces of the body, or which may be removed from such surfaces or membranes by physical means. It deals with the examination of cells denuded from a neoplasm (or other type of lesion), recovered from the sediment of the exudate, secretions, or washings from the tissue (e.g. sputum, vaginal secretion, gastric washings, abdominal fluid, prostatic secretion, urine). Exfoliative cytology is a quick and simple procedure and is an important alternative to biopsy in certain situations. This technique is useful only for the examination of surface cells and often requires additional cytological analysis to confirm the results.

TYPES OF EXFOLIATION

Spontaneous or Natural Exfoliation

It is characteristic of normal epithelial surfaces which continuously shed cells from their superficial layers as they are replaced by new cells. Malignant tumor cells exfoliate more readily than those from normal tissue, even though the lesion may be so small for clinical detection.
For example:
- Vaginocervical cells in posterior vaginal fornix.
- Mesothelial cells in effusion of pleural and abdominal cavities.

Artificial Exfoliation

Artificial exfoliation of viable cells from the lesion takes place when the surface of mucosa is scraped by spatula or aspirated using a fine needle.

Exfoliated cells can be found in smears taken directly from epithelial membranes or body cavities, like vagina, buccal mucosa, or from a variety of body fluids and effusions including sputum, urine, pleural fluid and gastric juice.

Applications

- Cytology is used for the diagnosis of malignancy in various organs, particularly those of the respiratory, urinary and female genital tracts. The collection of material for vaginal cytology is readily available with minimal discomfort to the patient, hence it is a relatively simple method for screening for detection of asymptomatic cancer in women.
- Study of vaginal smears to assess the hormonal activity in females is of value in some cases of sterility and certain endocrine disorders.
- Cytology also provides a method for determining genetic sex.
- Cytology also helps in the identification of vaginal infections.
- Cytological examination of the sputum is of value in the diagnosis of malignant disease of the lower respiratory tract, pulmonary asbestosis, and pulmonary fungal infections.
- Cytology of urine is important in the detection of urothelial neoplasia in urinary tract, and tumors of the prostate gland and renal parenchyma.
- Cytological examination of amniotic fluid is useful in the assessment of fetal maturity.

GENERAL CYTOLOGICAL CHANGES IN CELLS DURING MALIGNANCY

Unlike histopathology, in which diagnosis of malignancy is done often on the general behavior and arrangement of the cell aggregates, cytological diagnosis is based on the appearances of individual cells or small groups of cells. Most of the information is obtained from the study of nuclei, whereas the cytoplasm may assist to identify the cell type.

Nuclear Changes in Cancer

- Malignant cells show nuclear enlargement, generally at the expense of the cytoplasmic mass, causing a rise in the nuclear/cytoplasmic ratio.
- There is a variation in shape, many angular forms being present. The nuclear membrane can lose its smooth, even appearance, to be replaced by an irregular contour, sometimes with lobulation.
- Irregular clumping of the nuclear chromatin gives a rough, irregular appearance, in contrast to the smooth granular distribution in benign cells.
- Hyperchromasia is a frequent finding. Increased chromatin material produces an increase in staining intensity.
- Abnormalities in size, shape or number of nucleoli may be seen.
- Multinucleate forms may arise due to abnormal cell division (Fig. 11.1).

Cytoplasmic Changes in Cancer

- Changes in the cytoplasm help in identification of tumor type, but are not reliable for the diagnosis of malignancy.
- Variation can occur in the staining reaction, producing an organophilic or eosinophilic opaque appearance.
- Bizarre variations in size and shape. Tadpole cells and fiber cells are frequently seen.
- Phagocytosis occur in malignant cells, the ingested material appears as cytoplasmic inclusions.
- Vacuolation can occur in both malignant and benign cells.

Nuclear: Cytoplasmic Ratio in Cancer

Normal cells show a fairly constant ratio between the size of the nucleus and that of the cytoplasm. In malignant cells, there are varying degrees of disturbance of the nuclear: cytoplasmic ratio. The nucleus will usually comprise one-third or more of the total cell diameter. In malignancy, the nucleus enlarges too much leaving only a rim of cytoplasm.

CYTOLOGY OF NORMAL GENITAL TRACT

The vaginal and ectocervix (portiovaginalis) are normally covered by non-keratinized stratified squamous epithelium. The mucosa terminates at the external OS of the cervix (opening cervix) where it is replaced by simple columnar epithelium (Fig. 11.2). The location of squamo-columnar junction varies with age.

Squamous Cells of the Ectocervix

The vaginocervical squamous epithelium is composed of basal cell layer, parabasal cell layer, intermediate cell layer and superficial cell layer (Fig. 11.3).

- **Germinal/basal cells:** This is a single celled layer upon basement membrane. Basal cells are not normally exfoliated and are rarely seen in smear. They are almost always traumatically exfoliated. These cells are the smallest (10–12 μm in diameter) cells of squamous epithelium and are round or oval. Cytoplasm is scanty stain dark to deep blue with papanicolaou stain. The

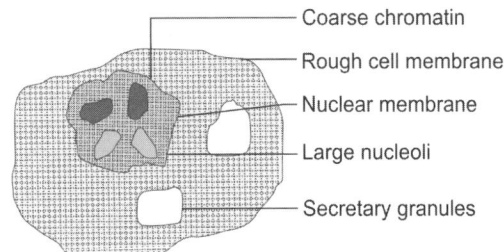

Fig. 11.1: Cellular abnormalities in carcinoma

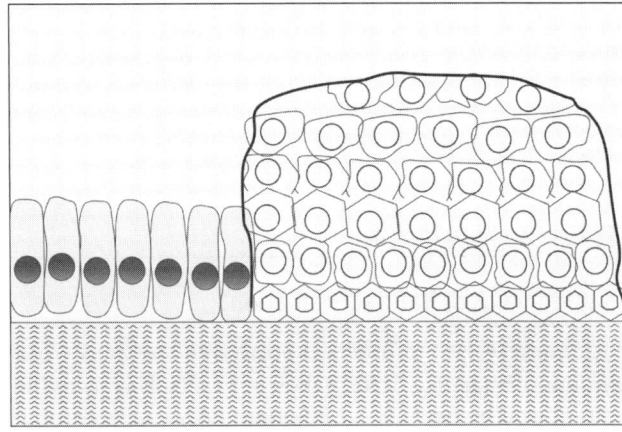

Fig. 11.2: Squamocolumnar junction of uterine cervix

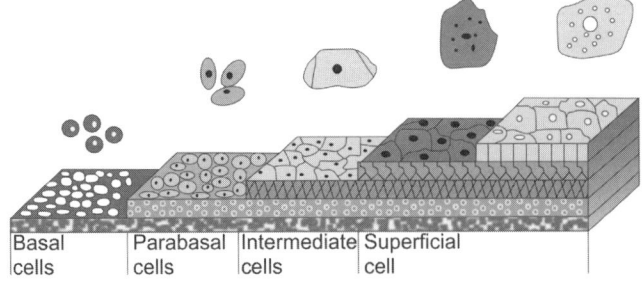

Fig. 11.3: Cells of normal genital track

nucleus is large, round and oval, and hyperchromatic with fine granular chromatic pattern.
- **Parabasal cells:** Superficial to the basal cell layer lies a zone of several rows of polyhedral cells called parabasal cells. When detached, these cells loose their intercellular bridges and appear round or oval. They are 15-25 μm in diameter and are larger than basal cells and uniform in shape. Cytoplasm stains blue and contain vesicular nucleus. Nucleus:cytoplasmic ratio is about 1:3. They are either traumatically exfoliated in sheets or singly from atrophic epithelium (prepuberty, lactation, postmenopausal mucosa or in estrogen deficiency).
- **Intermediate cells:** They originate from parabasal cells and composed of several rows of slightly larger cells. They have cell diameter from 30-60 μm depending upon degree of maturity; those from the lower rows are smaller in size and stain bluish-green; whereas those nearer the surface are larger and may take up the eosinophilic stain. They have a smaller nuclei and larger amount of cytoplasm than the parabasal cells. Nuclear to cytoplasmic ratio is about 1:100.
- **Superficial cells:** They originate from uppermost layer of the intermediate cell layer; and are usually exfoliated physiologically. They have cell diameter of 40-46 μm with pyknotic nuclei and are found in the vaginal smear at preovulatory time, after estrogen therapy or in ovarian tumor. They usually occur singly, polyhedral in shape, with the translucent acidophilic cytoplasm.

■ Columnar Cells of Endocervix

There are three types of endocervical cells, namely secretory, ciliated and nonciliated cells. They are not usually found in vaginal smear and are seen only in endocervical aspirations and endocervical scrapings. Their presence in a vaginal pool indicate inflammatory condition of endocervix.
- **Secretory cells (15-60 μm):** These are tall columnar epithelia with basally located, oval nucleus. They stain irregularly and cytoplasm contains secretory vacuoles.
- **Ciliated columnar cells:** They are smaller (10-25 μm) and appear cylindrical/pyramidal in shape in smear. Cilia are present on luminal surface. They stain darker than the mucus secreting cells.
- **Non ciliated endometrial cells:** They are non secretory endocervical cells (20-30 μm) which are compressed by the surrounding cells.

■ Columnar Endometrial Cells

Endometrial cells may be found normally only during menstrual flow and the following few days, early in pregnancy and during abortion and postpartum period. Their presence at other times or after menopause indicates abnormal endometruim, e.g. polyp, endometritis, submucus fibroid, endometrial hyperplasia and adenocarcinoma. However, endometrial cells can be obtained by endometrial aspiration or scraping, their shape and size depends on the phase of menstrual cycle. The cytoplasm stains green to pink and is scanty and nucleus stain dark blue and round and hyperchromatic.

■ Endometrial Stromal Cells

The superficial stromal cells are found cells with round/spindle-shaped nucleus.

METHODS OF SPECIMEN COLLECTION AND SUBMISSION

Technicians are rarely involved in the collection of specimens. They should, however, be aware of the method of specimen collection and the sources of error. Some of the specimens are collected by the patient or attending nurse. These include urine, sputum, and gastrointestinal specimens. The majority of specimens for the cytological investigations are collected by the attending physician during physical examination. These include vaginal and cervical smears, breast secretions, urine and sputum. Uterine cancer is diagnosed from the study of vaginal secretions. Cancer of the urinary tract is diagnosed by the study of urine and breast cancer from breast secretions through nipple. Malignant cells in any of the body cavity fluids indicates involvement of the serous membrane of that particular cavity, e.g. pleura, peritoneum. Prostatic carcinoma can be diagnosed by examining the secretions from the prostate by massage.

It is the most important step in cytopathology. At least one half to two thirds of false negatives are the result of patient conditions present at the time of sample collection and submission and the skill and knowledge of the individual who obtains the specimen. Thus, trained personnel are required for sample collection and submission.

Samples collected for cytological examination can be divided into two parts: Gynecological samples and non-gynecological samples. Various steps of cytological technique includes the following steps:
- Gynecological sample collection
- Non-gynecological sample collection
- Preservation of sample
- Smear preparation
- Fixation
- Staining
- Mounting.

GYNECOLOGICAL SAMPLE COLLECTION

It includes the following steps:

■ Patient Preparation

Proper patient preparation is the beginning of good cervical cytology. The patient should be instructed before coming for smear collection:
- Patient should not douche the vagina for at least a day before the examination.
- No intravaginal drugs or preparations (tampons, birth control prams, jellies, vaginal creams) should be used for at least one week before the examination.
- Patient should abstain from coitus for one day before the examination.
- Sample should be collected two weeks (10–18 days) after the first day of her last menstrual period.

■ Test Requisition

Under the supervision and guidance of the physician, a laboratory requisition must be legibly and accurately filled out before obtaining the cellular sample. The requisition should request the following information:
- Patient's name
- Age and or date of birth
- Menstrual status (LMP, hysterectomy, pregnant, post-partum, hormone therapy)
- Previous abnormal cervical cytology result, previous treatment, biopsy or surgical procedure
- Patient's risk status for developing cervical cancer
- Source of specimen, e.g. cervical, vaginal
- Clinical history- hormone/contraceptive used
- Relevant clinical findings (abnormal bleeding, grossly visible lesion, etc.).

■ Labeling of Sample

The glass slide or specimen vial must be labeled with a unique identifier, usually the patient's first and last names, at the time of sample collection of the cellular sample. Individual laboratories may require a section identifier such as date of birth, medical record number, social security number, or collection date. The laboratory must have a written procedure that specifies the requirements for proper specimen identification. For glass slides, the required information is written in solvent resistant pen or pencil on the frosted end of the slide. For liquid based samples, the required information must be fixed to the vial.

■ Visualization of Cervix for Collection of an Adequate Sample

Collection of a cervical cytology specimen is usually performed with the patient in the dorsolithotomy position. A sterile, or single-use bivalve speculum of appropriate size is inserted into the vaginal without lubrication. Warm water may be used to facilitate insertion of speculum. The position of the speculum should allow for complete visualization of the OS and ectocervix.

A cervical cytological sample is considered satisfactory for cytological diagnosis when their composition reflects the mucosal lining of the cervix, encompassing ectocervical, squamous metaplastic cells and endocervical columnar cells in fair numbers. It is found that majority of epithelial abnormalities that lead to an invasive cancer originate in the squamocolumnar junction (transformation zone TZ). As stated by the British Society for Clinical Cytology (BSCC) a cervical smear if properly taken should contain cells from the whole TZ. The sample should contain a sufficient quantity of epithelial cells, and both metaplastic and columnar cells should be present. Lubricant should not be used while examining, as it can obscure the cells during smear preparation.

The TZ may be easily visualized or may be high in the endocervical canal. The location varies not only from patient to patient, but in an individual over time. Factors producing variation in the location of TZ includes the changes in vaginal pH, hormonal changes, including pregnancy, childbirth, and menopausal status, and hormonal therapy. Thus, the location and visualization of TZ require more extensive clinical procedures.

■ Collection Devices

There are variety of collection devices available for sampling the endocervix, TZ, and ectocervix. They include endocervical brushes, wooden and plastic spatulas, plastic "broom type" sampler, cytobrush, etc. The choice of a particular device dependent on variation in the size and shape of the cervix and the clinical situation.
- **Wooden Ayre's and plastic spatulas:** With a visible TZ, a single sample obtained with wooden spatula is adequate in women. When spatula is used for sample collection, it should be applied with some degree of firmness and rotated around the full circumferences of the cervix. Wooden spatula is preferable to plastic spatula, because it has mildly rough surface that can collect more material. It has the disadvantages that the method may occasionally be traumatic to the patient and the tip of the spatula which do not fit to the external OS

may fail to remove some of the valuable material from the TZ. Hence, plastic spatula is used (Fig. 11.4).
- **Endocervical brush:** It is a small bottle brush like device with one end having fine bristles made up of nylons. This device is strictly for taking materials from endocervix. The brush is gently inserted in the endocervix and rotated one turn pressing on the upper and lower wall (Fig. 11.5).
- **Cervex brush device:** It is a flexible plastic brush which follows the shape of the endocervix, TZ and ectocervix and is suitable for every cervix shape (Fig. 11.6).
- **Cytobrush:** It is similar to that of endocervical brush except that the projected tip is without bristles. This can be used for obtaining cells from the whole cervix. (Fig. 11.7).

Use of cotton swab for collection of cervical smear is discouraged, in view of the drying artefacts and loss of cells, which are caused by this method. A combination of two devices, usually spatula and endocervical brush, give better results. Triple smear or the vaginal-cervical–endocervical (VCE) technique provides the best results. However, feasibility and cost factor need to be taken into consideration.

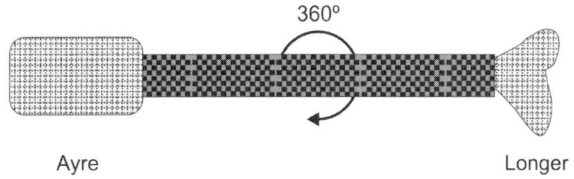

Fig. 11.4: Ayre's spatula

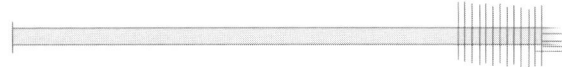

Fig. 11.5: Endocervical brush

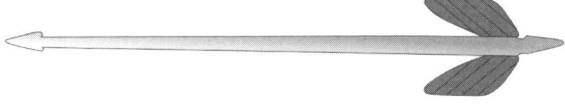

Fig. 11.6: Cervex brush

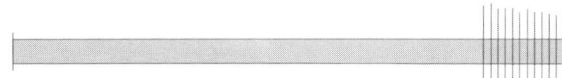

Fig. 11.7: Cytobrush

Technique of Sample Collection

Collection of Cervical/Vaginal Smear

i. **Using spatula and endocervical brush:** The viginal fornix and ectocervix should be sampled before the endocervix/TZ. First, a sample of the ectocervix is taken using a plastic or wooden spatula. The notched end of the spatula is rotated 360° around the circumference of the cervical OS, retaining the sample on the upper surface of the spatula. Grossly visible lesions, including irregular, discolored or friable areas should be directly sampled and can be placed on a separate slide, especially if the lesion is distant from other collection areas.

   Sampling of endocervix requires insertion of the endocervical brush into the endocervical canal until only the bristles closest to the hand are visible. The brush is rotated 45–90° and removed. At this time the sample on the spatula is spread evenly and thinly lengthwise down one-half of the labeled slide surface, using a single uniform motion. The endocervical brush is then rolled along the remaining half of the labeled slide surface by turning the brush handle and slightly bending the bristles with gentle pressure. The brush should not be smeared with force or in multiple directions The entire slide is then rapidly fixed by immersion or spray and the collection devices are discarded.

   For liquid based preparation the ectocervix should be sampled using the same procedures for conventional smears. However, the spatula with cellular material is rinsed in the specimen vial and then discarded. The endocervical specimen is collected using the same technique as mentioned above, however, the endocervical brush is rinsed in the vial and then discarded.

ii. **Using "broom like device":** The ectocervix and endocervix are collected simultaneously with "broom like device". The central bristles of the broom are inserted into the endocervical canal until the lateral bristles bend fully against the ectocervix. The sampling device is rotated 360° in the same direction five times while maintaining gentle pressure. The broom is removed with a single paint stroke motions and the cellular sample is transferred down the long axis of the labeled surface of the slide. The broom is turned over and the paint stroke motion is repeated over the same area. The slide is rapidly fixed either by immersion or spray and the device is then discarded.

For liquid based preparation, the ectocervical and endocervical specimens are collected with the broom like device simultaneously by the same procedure as above. The broom is rinsed in the specimen vial and then the device is discarded.

Collection of Vaginal Pool Smear

In this the sample is collected from the posterior fornix pool using a plastic pipette (Fig. 11.8) with suction bulb. The pipette is gently introduced into the vagina until resistance is encountered. Compress the suction bulb during the introduction of the pipette to avoid collection of cellular material of the lower vaginal origin. The cellular material is spread on a glass slide and fixed immediately. This technique has the advantage of a higher detection rate of endometrial carcinoma and upper vaginal carcinoma. But the disadvantage is that there is more opportunity for epithelial degradative changes as material may have been present in the fornix for a day or more.

Sample Collection by Endometrial Aspiration

It is an uncommon method due to risk of infection. After preliminary visualization and cleaning of cervix a sterile cannula is introduced into the uterine cavity and aspiration is then carried out with a syringe. The specimen is squirted on a clean glass slide, gently spread and rapidly fixed. The method provides rapid diagnosis of endometrial carcinoma.

NON-GYNECOLOGICAL SAMPLE COLLECTION

The various non-gynecological samples includes sputum, urine, body fluids, endoscopy specimens, cerebrospinal fluid, fine needle aspirates, joint fluids, amniotic fluids and seminal fluid.

Sputum

Sputum is examined in the cytology laboratory for the detection of malignant cells, pulmonary asbestosis, and organism like *Pneumocystis carinii*. Ideally three consecutive early morning specimens should be sent from the patient. To avoid the contamination by food particles, the sputum should be coughed up by the patient before the teeth are brushed or before breakfast is eaten. If more than one specimen is received on the same day they should be combined to make the smears. The specimen is poured into a petridish unless the container is of wide enough for inspection. Its appearance is recorded and if food material is present or the specimen seems to consist only of saliva further specimen should be requested. These specimens should not be rejected without examination because there may be possibility of malignant cells in them.

The smear should be made from any white areas in the specimen which are likely to come from the tumor and from any streaks of blood. If there is not white or blood stained areas are seen then the smears should be made from different parts of the specimen. The material can be picked up from the petridish using orange sticks or forceps and spread carefully on at least two slides. The slides are immersed immediately in 95% alcohol for 20 minutes. Smears from each specimen should be fixed in separate containers so as to avoid the possibility of cells floating from one specimen to another (Fig. 11.9).

Urine

Cytological examination of urine is useful in the diagnosis of malignancy in the urothelium or in the kidney. Preparations for cytology should be made from freshly voided urine, within two hours. of its production. Midstream specimen, i.e. urine passed after the bladder has been emptied in the morning should be requested as they may contain freshly shed cells. If the urine cannot be processed within two hours. or have to reach the laboratory through post, should be

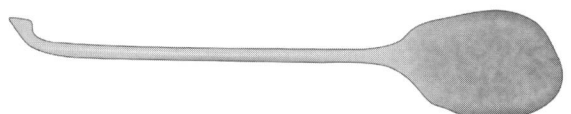

Fig. 11.8: Disposable plastic pipette

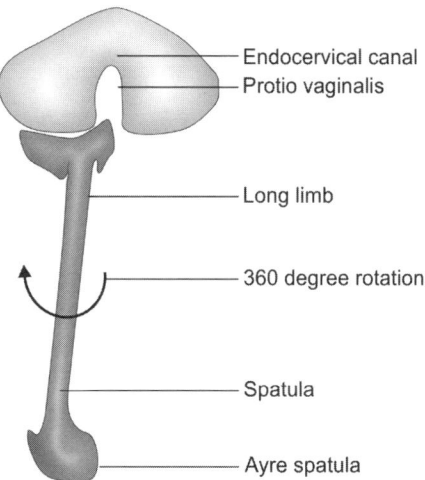

Fig. 11.9: Method of obtaining cervical material for fast smear

prefixed with an equal quantity of a mixture of ethyl alcohol and glacial acetic acid. Mostly urine specimens contains scanty cell content, hence it is necessary to cytocentrifuge the specimen to concentrate the cells. After centrifugation the preparations are fixed immediately with an aerosol spray fixative.

■ Serous Effusions

The term serous effusion refers to the fluid-accumulated in the three serous cavities namely pleural, pericardial and peritoneal. It forms an important source of useful diagnostic information in cytology. It helps in the diagnosis of certain benign processes like florid tuberculosis or rheumatoid pleurisy and recognition of malignant cells.

Pleural, pericardia and peritoneal fluids can be collected in tubes or syringes that may be either plain or contain anticoagulant to prevent coagulation. Various coagulants used are: Sodium citrate, hepain and EDTA.

Sodium citrate (3.8% solution)	:	5–100 mL fluid
Heparin	:	2 mg in 20 mL fluid
EDTA	:	20 mg in 20 mL fluid

Cells in heparinized fluids do not deteriorate rapidly and also get adhered to slides firmly. Freshly tapped specimens are preferred for cytology, the if facilities of immediate processing are available. If immediate processing is not possible, it can be preserved in the refrigerator for a period of 24–48 hours. Preservations of cells by prefixation in 50% ethanol is also possible. For prefixation spray fixatives are recommended when samples have to send to a distant laboratory. 20–30 mL fluid is sufficient to get enough cells for cytological evaluation.

After receiving the specimen in the laboratory, the gross appearance and the amount of fluid received are recorded. The gross appearance includes clear, transparent, straw colored, yellow, brown, red, chylous, purulent, mucoid or haemorrhagic.

10–15 mL of specimen is centrifuged at 2,500 rpm for 5 minutes. If the quantity of fluid is too little for centrifugation then an equal amount of normal saline can be added before centrifugation. If the fibrin clot has already formed, the clot may be smashed against the sides of the tube with an applicator. One to two drops of the sediment is used for preparation of smear.

For clear, sparsely cellular specimen (which do not yield sediment after centrifugation at 2,000 rpm for 10 minutes), cytocentrifugation method is used. Cytocentrifuge concentrates small number of cells suspended in a fluid specimen. Spinning samples at 2,000 rpm for 2 minutes sediments cells directly to slides. The blotter or filter card simultaneously absorbs the fluid medium. This results in a monolayer of well-preserved cells within an area of 6 mm. The major drawback of cytocentrifuge is the possibility of distortion of cellular morphology due to air drying artefacts, this can be avoided by immediate fixation or by use of equal volume of polyethylene glycol.

■ Cerebrospinal Fluid

Cerebrospinal fluid (CSF) specimens should be processed immediately without any delay because the cells quickly become fragile and their morphology deteriorates. The volumes of CSF available for examination is very small, hence centrifugation is necessary for preparation of smears. Approximately 0.5 mL of CSF is pipetted out into two or more cuvettes and cytocentrifuge at 700 rpm for 5 minutes. The sediment is used for preparation of smear. One slide is sprayed with fixative and the second slide is air dried.

■ Joint Fluid

Synovial fluid aspirates are mostly examined for crystals which can be characterized by using a polarizing microscope. Anticoagulant should not be added to the fluid and if clot has formed a part of it should be included with a deep and well-mixed fluid spread on the slide. Crystals are mostly of sodium urate and calcium pyrophosphate dihydrate and both are birefringent. Urate crystals are negative birefringence and calcium pyrophosphate crystals are positive birefringence. If the cell content is scanty and no crystals are seen, a centrifuged deposit of the fluid should be examined.

■ Amniotic Fluid for Estimation of Fetal Maturity

The cytological examination of amniotic fluid is used for assessment of fetal maturity. Fetal maturity can be estimated from the proportions of fat filled fetal squamous found in the amniotic fluid. Two drops of well-mixed amniotic fluid are mixed with one drop of 1% aqneous Nile blue sulfate and mixed with wooden stick on a slide. The mixture is heated gently and covered with coverslip. The percentage of anucleate orange stained cells (orange cells) is determined by counting a total of five hundred cells. The whole slide should be screened properly. Large clumps of orange cells are not possible to count and a rough estimate must be made.

Fat droplets may also be seen. The count of orange cells is interpreted as:

Less than 1%	:	Up to 34 week maturity
1–10%	:	34–38 week maturity
10–50%	:	38–48 week maturity
More than 50%	:	Term

Vaginal secretions suspected of draining from ruptured membranes may be examined for fetal squamous. If orange staining cells are found the fluid will be of amniotic origin.

Seminal Fluid

Analysis of semen specimens is required for the investigation of infertility and follow-up of vasectomy cases. Semen specimens must be examined within two hours of production as one of the essential investigations is that of sperm motility. The smear of seminal fluid is prepared by mixing four drops of it with two drops of sodium bicarbonate diluting fluid and allowing to stand for a few minutes.

Other Specimens

- **Bronchial brushings:** Roll brush over clean, dry slide. Fix immediately with spray fixative or 95% ethyl alcohol. The brush(es) used to prepare bronchial brushing slides may be swished in a container of 70% ethyl alcohol to dislodge remaining specimen. Submit labeled slides and liquid together with the request form to the laboratory.
- **Bronchial washings:** Collect in a clean container, label and send to the laboratory.
- **Oral lesions:** Scrap the oral lesion with a tongue depressor, and spread material on a clean slide and fix immediately.
- **Nasopharynx:** Cotton tipped applicator is used to obtain material for cytological examination.
- **Larynx:** Cotton swab smear of the larynx may be useful adjunct to clinical diagnosis if biopsy is not recommended.
- **Esophagus:** Esophageal washing and brushing are usually recommended for collecting cytological sample from esophagus.
- **Stomach:** Cytology specimen can be collected from the surface of the lesion by scraping (abrasion) under direct vision of a flexible endoscope. The cells collected can be directly smeared on a glass slide, gastric lavage can also be used for cytological investigations.
- **Breast cyst aspiration:** If aspirate is scanty, fluid is to be smeared one drop at a time on a clean slide and the slide is to be rapidly air dried. If aspirate is abundant, collect in a clean container and send fresh to the cytology department. Indicate the volume aspirated.
- **Breast secretions (Nipple discharge):** Drops of fluid from the nipple are smeared directly on clean glass slides. Submit 3 to 5 slides whenever possible. Half of the smears are to be fixed immediately with spray fixative or immersed in 95% alcohol for 20 minutes. Another half of the smears should be left to air-dry without fixative. Clearly label all slides to indicate whether they are air dried or alcohol fixed.

Endoscopy Specimens

Specimens may be obtained during endoscopy examination of the stomach, esophagus, or bronchus. There are collected under direct vision by brushing the lesions with a nylon brush. The brush is smeared across four labeled slides which are then immediately placed in fixative. Biopsies obtained during endoscopy yield useful information for cytological evaluation.

FINE NEEDLE ASPIRATION CYTOLOGY

Cells from any site of the body can be obtained by fine needle aspiration under negative pressure. Fine needle aspiration cytology (FNAC) of superficial nodule and thyroid lesions have become a routine diagnostic procedure. FNAC is being increasingly used in the recent years in the diagnosis of bone lesions, breast lesions and in lesions of internal organs (pancreas, prostrate, salivary glands, etc.).

Advantages:

- Eliminates the need for more complicated diagnostic tests.
- Less traumatic than usual knife biopsy.
- Rapid and accurate, permits early treatment.
- Investigation of a mass is possible without excision.
- Provides preoperative knowledge of deep seated lesions.

Disadvantages:

- Danger of dissemination of tumor cells in the needle tract or natural cavities.
- It may cause internal bleeding and complications like air emboli, pneumothorax.
- Accuracy of the method has been questioned—the point of the needle may miss the target.

Indications:

- When surgery is not possible:
  - Patient refuses surgery or tolerate anesthesia poorly.
  - Exploratory mass in a poor risk patients.
  - Difficult or dangerous site of location of mass.
- When surgery is contraindicated:
  - Clinically an obvious malignant mass.
  - Clinically, the mass is a cyst or obviously benign.
  - Age of patient and other factors, like pregnancy.

Requirements

- **Needles:** Standard disposable 22–24 gauge 1–1 ½ inch needles are used for plain FNAC. The length and caliber of the needle should fit the size, depth, location and the consistency of the target. For small subcutaneous lesions, one-inch 2–3 gauge needle is ideal while for a deep-seated breast lesion, the longer and larger needle is required. Finer needles are also recommended for children, and for vascular organs like thyroid.
- **Syringes:** Standard disposable plastic syringes of 10 mL are used. The syringe should be of good quality and should produce good negative pressure. 5 mL syringes can be used for vascular organs like thyroid. One important factor is to check the tight fit of the needle on the syringe tip. A loosely fitting needle can render the procedure useless and may injure the patient.
- **Syringe holder:** A syringe piston handle can be used, leaving one hand free to immobilize the lesion. This is not absolutely essential and is a matter of choice of the aspirator.
- **Slides:** A plain glass slide of good quality are used. Slides should be clean, dry, transparent and grease free.
- **Fixative:** About 95% alcohol is generally used which should be kept in Coplin jars.
- **Other supplies:** Test tubes, marking pencils, alcohol, swabs for skin, watch glass, saline, adhesive dressing, gloves, etc. are needed. All materials required are assembled in advance before starting the procedure. This is extremely important as delay fixation can make interpretation of smears difficult (Fig. 11.10).

Aspiration Procedure

Position the Patient

Any comfortable position can be chosen depending on the convenience to palpate the lesion and the comfort of the patient. FNA is usually carried out with the patient lying supine on an examination couch.

Immobilization of the Lesion

The skin is cleaned firmly with an alcohol swab (as used for routine injection). Local anesthetic may not be necessary. Apprehensive patients must be reassured about the procedure. The session is fixed between the thumb and index finger of the left hand, with the skin stretched. Try to avoid significant muscle mass while fixing the lesion because it is not only painful, but also muscle tends to plug the needle tip, preventing further material from entering the needle.

Penetrating the Lesion

Fixing the lesion with one hand, grasp the syringe with the needle attached (with or without syringe holder) by the dominant hand and introduce through the skin into the lesion, carefully and swiftly. The angle and depth of entry vary with the type of lesion. For small lesions, aspiration of central portion is indicated. For larger lesions that may have necrosis, cystic change or hemorrhage in the center, aspiration may be done from the periphery. If pus or necrotic material alone is aspirated from larger lesions, FNA can be repeated immediately from the periphery. With experience, a change in tissue consistency will be felt as the needle enters the lesion. If the needle goes tangentially missing a small slippery lesion or if penetrates beyond the lesion, representative material will not be obtained.

Creation of a Vacuum and Obtaining the Material

Suction is applied after entering the lesion and while maintaining the suction, the needle is moved vigorously back and forth in a sawing or cutting motion, changing the direction a few times, ensuring that the needle is inside the mass throughout; the whole procedure taking only 4–8 seconds. Do not rotate the needle or pump the plunger in the syringe in and out. Purpose of the suction is to pull the tissue against the cutting edge of the needle and to pull the dislodged tissue fragments and cells into the lumen of the needle. The material is procured by cutting motion of the needle and not by suction.

Release of Vacuum and Withdrawal of the Needle

When material is seen in the hub of the needle, the procedure if discontinued. Before withdrawing the needle, suction is

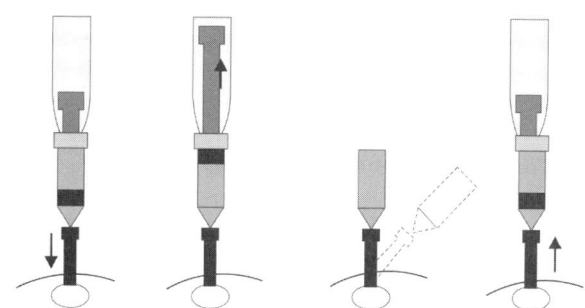

Fig. 11.10: Technique of fine needle aspiration cytology

released and needle pulled straight out. The piston is just allowed to slowly fall back by itself (never push). Failure to release negative pressure within the session will cause the aspirated material to enter the syringe, which is difficult to recover.

Preparation of Smears

Direct Smearing

The aspirate present in the core of the needle is blown on the clean slides. Smears are made immediately by applying a gentle pressure with another dry slide. For Pap staining both slides are immediately placed in a Coplin jar containing fixative. A small amount of saline solution is aspirated to rinse the needle core and syringe. The saline is then passed through a membrane filter and process. The aspirate is referred to as 'dry' if it consists of numerous cells suspended in a small amount of tissue fluid and has a creamy consistency. Such a dry smear represents the perfect sample for most malignant tumor.

Indirect Smearing

A 'wet' aspirate consists of a small number of cells suspended in fluid or blood. The process of centrifugation and preparation of smear from deposit is called indirect smearing. When aspirated cellular material is abundant, then even the paraffin cell block can be prepared. Moreover, material from the aspirate can be utilized for special staining, immunobiochemistry cell marker studies, chromosomal analysis and tumor marker.

Fixation and Staining

Different methods of fixation and staining are used in FNAC. Different stains such as May Grunwald, Giemsa, Leishman, combined Leishman and Giemsa (LG), and alcohol fixation and staining with Pap or H and E. Pathologists who had their basic training in gynecological cytology finds it convenient to employ alcohol fixation and Pap staining, whereas those having a background in hematology prefer air-dried Giemsa stained smears.

Leishman – Giemsa Stain (LG)

Solutions
- Leishman stain: 1.5 g Leishman powder dissolved in 1000 mL of acetone free methanol.
- Giemsa stain: Dissolve 1.0 g of Giemsa powder in 66 mL glycerin and 66 mL methanol to get stock Giemsa stain.

Procedure
- Cover the slide with Leishman stain for 1 minute.
- Add equal volume of Giemsa stain.
- Keep it for 10-15 minutes and wash in running tap water.
- Dry the smear and mount with coverslip.

PRESERVATION OF CYTOLOGICAL SPECIMENS

Preservation of cellular morphology until the sample can be processed is essential for accurate cytological interpretation. Specimens may be sent to the laboratory without preservatives or prefixatives, if facilities for immediate processing are available. The duration between collection and preparation of the sample before cellular damages occur depends on pH, protein content, enzymatic activity and the presence or absence of bacteria. The following are few methods of preservation of specimens.

Specimens with High Mucus Content

These include specimens such as sputum, bronchial aspirates, mucocele fluid, etc. All these specimens can be preserved for 12 to 24 hours if refrigerated. Refrigeration slows down the bacterial growth, which causes cellular damage. Mucus apparently coats the cells, protecting them against rapid degeneration. The cells in specimens diluted with saliva are not as well-protected and may deteriorate more rapidly.

Specimens with High Protein Content

Specimens like pleural, peritoneal or pericardial fluids can be preserved for 24 to 48 hours with refrigeration. The protein-rich fluid in which the cells are bathed acts as a tissue culture medium in preserving cellular morphology.

Specimens with Low Mucus or Protein Content

Specimens such as urine or CSF will be preserved for only 1-2 hours even if refrigerated. The fluid medium in which these cells are bathed contains enzymatic agents capable of causing cell destruction. Refrigeration may inhibit bacterial growth but does not protect the cells.

Specimens with Low pH

Specimens such as gastric material, must be collected on the ice and be processed within minute of collection to prevent cellular destruction by HCL.

PREPARATION OF SMEARS

The successful evaluation of cytological material depends; to a great extent, on the technical quality of the preparations. It is desirable that smears are made and fixed by trained staff in order to obtain uniformly spread smear. The smears are made either directly from the collected specimen or from a concentrated specimen. Concentrated specimens are obtained by centrifugation or by the use of membrane filter. Specimens such as cervical smears, spinal fluid, or breast secretions can be examined unconcentrated by making a direct smear. Watery exudate like urine, gastric contents, serous fluid, pleural fluid, ascitic fluid, and others require concentration of specimen prior to smear preparation because they contain only scanty diagnostic evidence. Irrespective of the type of specimen, the smears must be promptly made and fixed, refrigeration is effective only for a short period.

■ Concentration by Centrifugation

Thick specimen: A specimen having sufficient amount of protein in the form of mucus or albumin require initial fixing with equal amount of 95% alcohol. Then it is centrifuged at 2,500 rpm for 20 minutes. The sediment is mixed with remaining drops of fluid.

Watery specimen: Watery specimens like urine and gastric fluid are low in protein and hence require an additional adhesive like Mayer's albumin or pooled serum or human plasma. The specimen is centrifuged at 2,500 rpm for 20 minutes after mixing with greater amount of human pooled serum or plasma. During centrifugation the collected sediment get coated with a film of adhesive.

■ Smear Preparation

The technical quality of smear greatly determines the accurate evaluation and diagnosis. The skill of making good smears comes through experience. A good smear is thin, spread evenly, and free from lumps. An adhesive agent is either added to the specimen before centrifugation or spread over the surface of the slide. Addition of adhesive agent prevents the cells from "floating away" during processing. The smear can be prepared by three methods depending upon the type of specimen. These are streaking method, spreading method and pull apart method.

Streaking

The specimen is streaked over the slide so as to cover 2/3 of the areas of slide. The streaking should be fast enough and uniform so as not to allow the specimen to dry. The spreading medium should be kept neither too thick nor too thin. This method is used for specimens like mucoid secretions (vaginal secretions), sputum and gastric contents. The smears must be placed immediately into the fixative before any drying occurs (Fig. 11.11).

Spreading

A selected portion of the specimen is transferred to a clean glass slide. Excess material is removed with an applicator stick by 'sawing' out at the sharp glass edge. Mucoid secretion is spread over the slide using teasing process. The film should be moderately thick. The method maintains the cellular inter-relationship which is sometimes disturbed by the streaking technique. This procedure is used for sputum specimen's and bronchial aspirates (Fig. 11.12).

Pull Apart

This method is recommended for mycous secretions like urinary sediment, vaginal pool, breast secretions, serous fluid, etc. It forms the most desirable smear for cytological examination. A drop of the secretion is placed at the center of the slide. An another slide is used to prepare the smear. The spreader slide is placed at an angle of 30–35° and is pull back until it touches the drop of the specimen and then is pushed forward along the slide (Fig. 11.13).
- Keep another slide at 30–35°.
- Pull back the spreader up to drop.
- Push forward evenly.

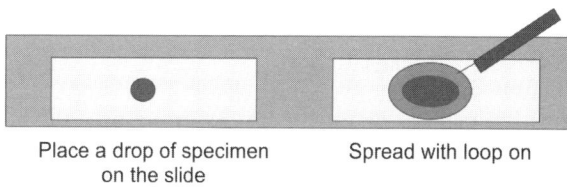

Fig. 11.11: Method of streaking

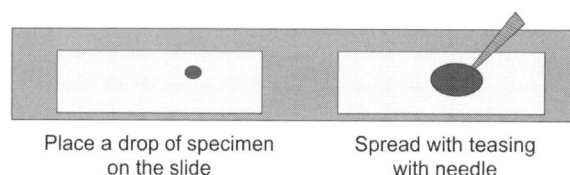

Fig. 11.12: Method of spreading

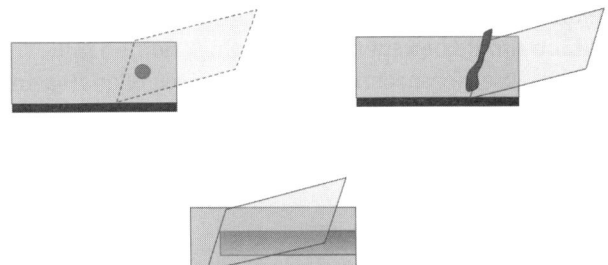

Fig. 11.13: Pull apart

■ Membrane Filters

Cellulose acetate membrane filters of graded pore size are useful for the concentration of cells from most body fluids like urine. They are particularly useful where only a few cells are present. The cells are collected onto a single membrane. A variety of pore sizes are available, the most useful size is 5 μm. The specimen is filtered through a membrane attached to a special funnel type holder using controlled negative pressure.

- After filtration the cells are fixed by placing the membrane in 96% alcohol immediately.
- The membrane is then clipped onto a slide.
- Stain the membrane by Papanicolaou method.
- Dehydrate and clear the membrane.
- After clearing the membrane filter pad is cut into several strips.
- Special mounting medium is required for certain types of membrane filters.
- Fixation of cells in fluid specimens may be carried out by adding an equal volume of formal—saline prior to filtration, but generally the cells adhere to the membrane more readily and securely if fixation follows filtration.

FIXATION AND FIXATIVES

To prevent cellular distortion it is essential that all smear preparations for cytological study be fixed immediately before drying of the material occurs. The fixative should be capable of penetrating rapidly with good preservation of cell morphology.

Air drying of thin smears is used only for specimens which require Romanowsky stains. If transport of sides in liquid is not problem, the most suitable fixative is 95% ethyl alcohol. A useful container and carrier for smear fixatives is the polyethylene screw—capped Coplin jar grooved to take up 10 slides. It is suitable for transportation of smears from wards and clinics to the laboratory, but should not be used for postal transportation because of inflammable nature of the fluid.

Smears which require to be sent by post to a cytology laboratory may be fixed with a protective aerosol spray and placed in suitable wooden, cardboard or plastic slide mailers. These sprays give an effective and convenient form of fixation and are cheap also. They usually consists of polyethylene glycols, methylated spirit or isopropyl alcohol, and propellants. The alcohol fixes the smear and wax sets to form a water soluble protective coating.

Most smears adhere well to the glass slide because they contain a certain amount of mucus and there is little danger of the cells floating off the slides into the fixative. When the specimens are less likely to adhere to the slide a fixative may be dropped onto the slide from a dropper bottle or an aerosol spray fixative may be used.

All the smears should be left to fix for at least for 15 minutes. Fixative solutions may be used more than once but must be filtered so that any free cells are not transferred from one specimen to another. Slides may be left in fixative for up to seven days without deterioration.

■ Routine Fixatives

The process of submerging of freshly prepared smears immediately in a liquid fixative is called wet fixation. This is the ideal method for fixing all gynecological and non-gynecological smears and any of the following alcohols can be used.

- **95% ethyl alcohol:** It is common fixative used now-a-day for safety reasons and satisfactory results. A mixture containing tertiary butyl alcohol and 95% ethyl alcohol in the ratio of 3:1 is also effective. Addition of 3% glacial acetic acid increases the nucleoprotein fixing properties. This is the standard fixative in cytology and give excellent nuclear and cytoplasmic morphology.
- **Ether alcohol mixture:** This fixative was originally recommended by Papanicolaou. It consists of equal parts of ether and 95% ethyl alcohol. It is an excellent fixative, but ether is not used in most of the laboratories because of its safety hazards, odor and hygroscopic nature.
- **100% methanol:** It is an acceptable substitute for 95% ethanol. Methanol produces less shrinkage than ethanol.
- **80% propanol and isopropanol:** Propanol and isopropanol cause slightly more cell shrinkage than ether-ethanol. By using a lower percentage of these alcohols the shrinkage is balanced by the swelling effect of water on cells. However, 80% propanol is a substitute for 95% ethanol.
- **Denatured alcohol:** It is methanol that has been changed by the addition of additives in order to render it unsuitable for human consumption. It contains ethanol as the main ingredient (90%), methanol (5%) and isopropanol (5%).

Coating Fixatives or Spray Fixatives

They are substitutes for alcohol fixatives. They are either aerosols applied by spraying the cellular samples or a liquid base which is dropped onto the slide. They are composed of an alcohol base, which fixes the cells and wax like substances, which forms a thin protective coating over the cells like carbowax, polyethylene glycol, etc. These fixatives have dual action in that they fix the cells and when dry, form a thin protective coating over the smear. These fixatives have practical value in situation where smears have to be mailed to a distant cytology laboratory for evaluation.

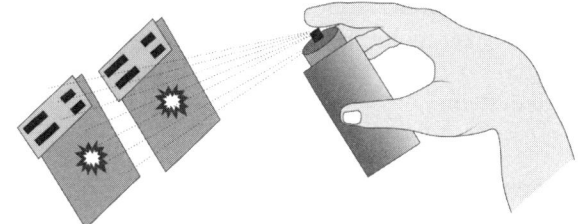

Fig. 11.14: Use of spray fixatives for smear

Precaution Taken During Using Spray Fixative

- The spray must be smooth and steady and the operation of the nozzle must be checked before the smear is obtained.
- The distance between the nozzle of the spray and the smear to be sprayed must be about 10 to 12 inches (25–30 cm) as shown in the Figure 11.14. If the spray is held too close to the smear, several problems may occurs like the cells may be dislodged by the force of the sprays, or the evaporation of the spray vehicle may freeze and irreversibly damage the cells, an artifact may also occur, etc. If the nozzle is too far from the target, insufficient fixative will reach the surface.
- Smear coated with spray fixative are air dried and placed in cardboard slide containers and forwarded to the laboratory.
- It is necessary to protect patients and the medical personnel from the inhalation of the spray by using a face mask or by performing spraying procedure under a protective glass plate or a laboratory hood.

Examples of Spray Fixatives

1. **Polyethylene glycol (Carbowax 1500):**

Absolute alcohol	:	100 mL
Carbowax 1500	:	3 g
Glacial acetic acid (pH 5.8–6.0)	:	0.2 m

   The carbowax is softened in an incubator. Alcohol is added to dissolve the carbowax. Acetic acid is added after cooling and mixed well. Such fixatives containing carbowax provide a covering film for the smear as it dries and are used in dropper bottles or sprays. This fixative is used for smears which required to be transported through the post. The carbowax is removed by alcohol at the beginning of the staining procedure.

2. **Fixative for fine needle washings:** It has composition:

Carbowax	:	10 g
Distilled water	:	100 mL
Absolute ethyl alcohol	:	400 mL

   The carbowax is dissolved in warm water and when cool mixed with the alcohol.

3. **Fixative for urine specimens to travel by post:** It has composition:

Monoethylene glycol	:	350 mL
Diethylene glycol	:	18 mL
Borax pentahydrate	:	3.5 mL
Glacial acetic acid	:	50 mL
Distilled water	:	570 mL

   2.5 mL of this fixative is sufficient for up to 30 mL of urine.

Special Purpose Fixatives

Carnoy's fixative: It has composition

Absolute ethyl alcohol	:	60 mL
Chloroform	:	30 mL
Glacial acetic acid	:	10 mL

Carnoy's fixative is mostly used for heavily blood stained specimens like endometrial aspirates. The red blood cells are lysed by this fixative and this enables the remaining cell population to be seen more clearly. This fixative is commonly used for urgent biopsies but is also recommended for exfoliative cytology. It permits good nuclear staining. The fixation is done in 30 minutes to 3 hours. The fixative is used for fixing small pieces of tissue and for urgent biopsies. The absolute alcohol helps in drying. The tissue is transferred directly to absolute alcohol.

Ethyl alcohol—glacial acetic acid fixative: It has composition:

Ethyl alcohol	:	75 mL
Glacial acetic acid	:	25 mL

The fixative is used for fixing the urine specimen which cannot be processed within two hours. Urine is mixed up with equal volume of this fixative.

Schaudinn's fixative: This is a rapidly penetrating fixative used in diagnostic exfoliative cytology. It preserves smears which are to be stained by hematoxylin and eosin.

Mercuric chloride (saturated solution)	:	6 mL
Absolute alcohol	:	33 mL
Glacial acetic acid	:	1 mL

Fix smears for 2 minutes or more. Wash in distilled water. Remove mercuric chloride pigment by adding a few drops of a saturated solution of alcoholic iodine. Rinse in water and proceed to stain.

CYTOLOGICAL STAINING TECHNIQUES

The most commonly used stain in gynecological cytology is the Papanicolaou stain. This stain is specially suitable for cervical smears. It gives sharp nuclear staining and good differential colouring of acidophilic and basophilic cells. Various staining techniques used in cytology are as follows.

■ Papanicolaou Method (1942, 1954): Modified Method

Papanicolaou stain is the most popular stain for gynecological cytology and was originally developed to demonstrate the cyclic changes taking place in the squamous epithelium of the female genital tract in response to alteration in hormone levels. This staining method is designed to give sharp nuclear staining, transparency of cytoplasm, and good differential coloring of acidophilic and basophilic cells.

The cytoplasm of the parabasal squamous cells stains a deep greenish-blue, intermediate cells a pale greenish-blue and as the cells reach full maturity the cytoplasm stains pink. Orange G in the stain is selective for any keratin that may be present. The stained cytoplasm retains a degree of transparency, which reduces eye fatigue and the nuclei are precisely stained with Harri's hematoxylin. The cytoplasmic staining may be influenced by several factored including changes in pH as a result of infection and also by the thickness and fixation of the smear. However, Papanicolaou stain provides a good differential stain and as a result, is used widely for other routine cytology smears.

The solutions required are Harri's alum hematoxylin, Orange G (OG 6) and a triple dry mixture designated EA 36, or EA 50. All these solutions may be purchased commercially and give consistently good results. The formulae are as follows:

Orange G solution (OG 6):
0.5% Orange G stock solution in 95% Alcohol: 100 mL
Phosphotungstic acid: 0.015 g

Harri's hematoxylin:
Hematoxylin	:	1 g
Absolute alcohol	:	10 mL
Potassium alum	:	20 g
Distilled water	:	200 mL
Mercuric oxide	:	0.5 g

The hematoxylin is dissolved in absolute alcohol and potassium alum in distilled water with the aid of heat. The two solutions are mixed together. The mixture is boiled, removed from the flame and mercuric oxide is added bit by bit. The flask containing the solution is then immersed in cold water bath. After cooling it is filtered and store in a colored bottle.

EA 36 or EA 50 (Eosine Azure):
- Light green SF(yellowish) 0.1% in 95% ethyl alcohol: 45 mL
- Bismarck brown 0.5% solution in 95% ethyl alcohol: 10 mL
- Eosin yellowish 0.5% solution in 95% ethyl alcohol: 45 mL
- Phosphotungstic acid: 0.2 g
- Lithium carbonate (saturated aqneous solution): 1 drop.

Mix well and stored in tightly capped, brown bottles. A variation of the above, known as EA 65 requires 0.25% light green and is recommended for sputum staining.

Procedure for manual Papanicolaou staining:
- Fix the smear in equal parts of 95% alcohol and ether.
- Hydrate the smear in decreasing concentrations of alcohol 80%, 70%, 50%, (6 dips in each).
- Rinse gently in distilled water.
- Stain in diluted Harri's hematoxylin for 6 minutes or for 2–3 minutes in concentrated hematoxylin.
- Gently rinse in distilled water.
- Dip in 0.25% HCl 6 times or in 0.5% HCl 3 times.
- Check the slides under the microscope to see if the nuclei are properly stained. If overstained, decolorize again in acid–alcohol and if understained return to hematoxylin stain. Continue process until the nuclei are distinct and the cytoplasm of the cells is clear and slightly-blue in color.
- Dehydrate the slides by running through distilled water, 50%, 70%, 80%, 95%, (6 dips in each).
- Stain in OG 6 for 2 minutes.
- Rinse in 95% alcohol, 3 changes (6 dips in each).
- Stain in EA 36 or EA 52 for 2 minutes.
- Rinse in 95% alcohol (3 separate changes).
- Dehydrate by passing through absolute alcohol (2 changes).
- Clear by rinsing in a mixture of absolute alcohol and xylene (6 dips) followed by three changes in xylene (6 dips).
- Mount in permount or EPX mounting medium.

Result:
- Nuclei : Blue with clear, sharp details
- Cytoplasm : Varying shades of pink, blue, yellow, green–gray

If the contrast is unsatisfactory, decolorise with acid—alcohol, wash thoroughly in tap water and repeat the staining procedure increasing or decreasing the staining time as deemed properly.

Quick Papanicolaou Staining Technique

Use 50 mL of Coplin jars instead of dishes
- Fix smears in 95% ethyl alcohol : 1–2 minutes
- Hydrate in running tap water : ½–1 minutes
- Stain with Harri's hematoxylin with acetic acid : ½ minute
- Rinse in running tap water : 1 minute
- Dip in weak ammonium hydroxide solution : 5–10 dips until smear appears dark blue
- Rinse in running tap water : 1 minute
- Dip in 95% ethyl alcohol : 25 dips
- Stain with OG 6 (ortho) : ½ minute
- Dip in 95% ethyl alcohol : 10–20 dips
- Stain with EA 50 (ortho) : ½ minute
- Give 2 changes in 95% ethyl alcohol : 10–20 dips each
- Give 2 changes in absolute ethyl alcohol : 10–20 dips each
- Give 2 changes in xylene : 20 dips each

This technique is used for rapid staining of gynecological smears.

Precaution During Staining

- Immediate fixation of smears is essential.
- Smears should never be allowed to dry before placing the coverslip.
- Hematoxylin is filtered everyday before use.
- All solution and other stains are filtered daily after use, to keep them free of sediments.
- Keep stains and solutions covered when not in use.
- Avoid contamination from one smear to another.
- Stains are discarded and replaced as the quality of the stain deteriorates.
- Place the coverslip on the micro-slide slowly without trapping air bubbles.
- Avoid contamination during coverslipping.

Automatic Staining

Automatic stainer can process large numbers of smears with excellent results.

Autostainer

Slides held in rack are automatically rotated around baths containing stains and other reagents. Time schedule for staining can be obtained by calibrating a timing dial. The reagents are renewed weekly. The instrument has the advantage that it can easily be adapted for staining techniques. It uses laboratory prepared reagents and it allows for complete adaptability in staining times. After staining the slides are mounted with DPX.

Papanicolaou Staining Schedule for Automated Stainer

Step no.	Reagent	Time
1.	Water	1 minute
2.	Harri's hematoxylin	3 minutes
3.	Water	1 minute
4.	0.1% HCl in 70% ethanol	15 seconds
5.	Water	15 seconds
6.	1% NH_4OH in 70% ethanol	1 minute
7.	95% ethanol	1 minute
8.	95% ethanol	1 minute
9.	95% ethanol	1 minute
10.	95% ethanol	1 minute
11.	OG modified	2 minutes
12.	95% ethanol	1 minute
13.	95% ethanol	1 minute
14.	EA modified	3 minutes
15.	100% ethanol	1 minute
16.	100% ethanol	1 minute
17.	100% ethanol	1 minute
18.	100% ethanol	1 minute
19.	Xylene	1 minute
20.	Xylene	1 minute

Remove from machine and mount in DPX.
Results: As per manual staining method.

Shorr Staining Technique (1941)

This staining method gives less cytoplasmic transparency and poorer nuclear definition than the papanicolaou stain. But it may be used for hormonal studies (endocrine cytology) as it gives good cytoplasmic differentiation, but it is not a very satisfactory method for detection of malignant cells. This method requires a single differential staining mixture.

Staining Solution

Ethyl alcohol 50%	:	100 mL
Biebrich scarlet (water soluble)	:	0.5 g
Orange G	:	0.25 g
Fast green FCF	:	0.075 g
Phosphotungstic acid	:	0.5 g
Glacial acetic acid	:	1 mL

Procedure

1. Fix smears while moist in equal parts of ether and alcohol. 1-2 minutes is adequate.
2. Stain for 1-2 minutes in Shorr's stain.
3. Rinse in 70% alcohol to remove excess of stain.
4. Transfer to 95% alcohol, followed by absolute alcohol for a few seconds in each.
5. Clear in xylene and mount in synthetic resin mountant.

Results

Nuclei	:	Red
Superficial cornified cells	:	Brilliant orange – red
Non cornified cells	:	Green/blue

■ Methylene Blue Wet film Technique (Philips 1954)

This is a simple and rapid staining method which is useful for the screening of large numbers of specimens, especially fresh sputum for malignant cells. The preparations are not permanent and should be examined immediately.

Staining Solution

Methylene blue	:	1 g
Distilled water	:	100 mL

Procedure

1. Place a small amount of fresh sputum (select purulent or blood flecked particles) or 2-3 drops of centrifuged deposits from the body fluid, on a clean microscope slide.
2. Place about one drop of methylene blue stain beside the specimen.
3. Hold the slide at least 20 cm above the Bunsen flame and gently warm the slide, at the same time mixing the stain and specimen with forceps, until the excess fluid contributed by the stain has evaporated. Do not over heat the slide or allow the smear to dry.
4. Cover the slide with a large coverslip and examine immediately. The stain will fade after about an hour, hence should be recorded photographically if found suspicious.

Results

Nuclei	:	Shades of blue

■ Romanowsky Stains (1891)

This is commonly used stain for cytology specimens which have been rapidly dried after they have been spread.

Staining Solutions

May-Grunwald

May Grunwald stain + Sorensen's phosphate buffer pH 6.8 (equal volume) are mixed and filter into a Coplin jar.

Giemsa Stain

Giemsa stain	:	5 mL
Sorensen's phosphate buffer	:	45 mL

Mix and filter into a Coplin jar.

Procedures

1. Fix the air dried slides in absolute methyl alcohol for 10-20 minutes.
2. Rinse in buffer pH 6.8.
3. Stain in freshly prepared May–Grunwald for 8 minutes.
4. Drain off the excess stain and stain in freshly prepared Giemsa for 10 minutes.
5. Differentiate in buffer pH 6.8.
6. Allow smears to dry if necessary, they can be gently blotted before mounting.

Result

Cytoplasm	:	Mauve
Nuclei	:	Purple

SPECIAL STAINS

■ Stains for Hormonal Assessment

Vaginal cytology is an important tool for the assessment of gynecological endocrine function. Changes in the vaginal smears occurs due to the effect of hormones on the vaginal epithelium from the childhood to the post-menopausal period of a woman's life. The vaginal epithelium is more sensitive to endocrine fluctuations than other tissues, hence any change in vaginal epithelium reflect variation in one or more hormones.

Hormonal activity can be evaluated on the basis of microscopic examination of Papanicolaou stained vaginal smear. The Karyopyknotic index (KPT) and the maturation index (MI) are the two methods used to assess hormone activity.

Smear

Smears should be taken from the lateral walls of the upper third of the vagina. The material should be rapidly, but carefully smeared onto the glass slide and immediately placed into fixative. Care is necessary to preserve clumps of the cells which could have diagnostic significance.

Staining

The staining should provide a good nuclear morphology, with clear cytoplasmic differentiation. The Papanicolaou technique fulfills this dual function well. Similarly, Short staining method I is suitable for hormonal studies of vaginal smears.

Changes in vaginal smear: Hormones affect the vaginal epithelium in three ways: Proliferation, maturation and exfoliation.

These changes are reflected not only in epithelial element of the smears, but also show cyclic variations of the populations of other cells. Above criteria help in ascertaining the degree of estrogenic effect in the smear. Assessment can be made in two ways:
- The proportions of epithelial cell types can be counted.
- A subjective assessment of the epithelial cell types present

Maturation Index

In maturation index (MI) the number of parabasal, intermediate and superficial cells are counted in a total of two hundred cells. The totals of three cell types are expressed as a percentage. The MI is based on cell maturation which is determined by means of the morphology and staining reaction of the non cornified squamous epithelial cells. These are classified as superficial intermediate and parabasal cells. A total of at least 200 squamous cells are counted and each class of cells are expressed as a percentage.

Example: MI is expressed as percentage of parabasal, intermediate and superficial cells MI = 10/20/70 indicates 10% parabasal cells, 20% intermediate cells and 70% superficial cells. High estrogenic activity is indicated by a predominance of superficial intermediate cells while low activity is indicated by the predominance of parabasal cells.

Indications: Assessment of ovarian functions: After hysterectomy, during menstrual disorder and in premature menses (childhood).
- Assessment of abnormal hormonal production: Before, during and after pregnancy (Threatened abortion), fertility study, hormone producing tumors, and various endocrine disorders.
- Assessment and guidance for hormone therapy.

Table 11.1: Cytohormonal averages in different age groups

Age group	Maturation Index	Variation (+)
Newborn	0/90/10	10
Infancy	80/20/00	20
Preovulatory	00/40/60	10
Postovulatory	00/70/30	15
Menopause	00/80/20	20
Postmenopause	50/50/00	45
Estrogen therapy	00/10/90	10
Progesterone therapy	00/90/10	10
Androgen therapy	20/80/00	10

Karyopyknotic Index

Karyopyknotic index (KPI) is a more accurate and dependable method of assessment. It depends upon nuclear morphology, which is more stable than cytoplasmic staining. Superficial cornified squamous epithelial cells show condensed, deeply stained structures (pyknotic) nuclei, with pink to red stained cytoplasm. The calculation of KPI is done by counting a total of 200 squamous cells in a Papanicolaou stained smear. The cornified squamous cells are expressed as a percentage of the total number of squamous cells. More accurate results are obtained by taking vaginal smears at about 3 or 4 days interval through the menstrual cycle.

■ Stains for Sex Chromatin (Barr Bodies)

About 20 to 30% of cells from the female show a mass of chromatin beneath the nuclear membrane which is not found in males. Chromatin bodies are described as a sharply demarcated plano convex chromatin mass attached to the nuclear membrane. Sex chromatin mass represents the inactive X chromosome in the interphase nucleus of the female. In males there is no inactive X and hence, no sex chromatin. Assessment of the sex chromatin is the primary investigation to be required for patient suspected of having a sex chromosome abnormality.

Buccal Smear

After cleaning the mouth the patient with water, the inside of the cheek is scraped firmly with a spatula, the broad end of an Ayres spatula is convenient. The slightly turbid buccal fluid is spread on five glass slides, these are fixed immediately with spray fixative. One of the fixed slides is used for fluorescent staining and other two for permanent preparations using cresyl fast violet or acid thionin. Unfixed slides are stained immediately with lactic acetic-orcein.

Staining by Cresyl Fast Violet Method

Staining solution:

Cresyl fast violet acetate	:	1.0 g
Distilled water	:	100 mL

Procedures:
- Fix smears with spray fixative or 95% alcohol for 30 minutes.
- Transfer to 50% alcohol for few minutes.
- Rinse in distilled water.
- Stain with cresyl fast violet acetate solution for 5 minutes.
- Rinse quickly in tap water.
- Differentiate in 95% alcohol, till the cytoplasm becomes colourless, for about 2–5 minutes.
- Quickly dehydrate in absolute alcohol.
- Clean in two changes of xylene.
- Mount in DPX.

Results:

Nuclei	:	Pale mauve
Sex chromatin	:	Deeply stained
Cytoplasm	:	Almost colorless

Acid Thionin Method

Staining solutions:
Stock thionin solution: 1% thionin in 50% alcohol.
Stock buffer solution:

Sodium acetate	:	9.714 g
Sodium barbiturate	:	14.714 g
Distilled water to make	:	500 mL

Working solution of thionin:

0.1 N HCl	:	32 mL
Stock buffer solution	:	28 mL
Stock thionin solution	:	40 mL

This solution keeps for 6–8 weeks.

Procedures:
- Fix the smear with spray fixative.
- Keep in 0.2% solution of celloidin in ether- alcohol for 2 minutes.
- Wipe the back side, air dry for a few seconds and immerse in 70% alcohol for 5 minutes.
- Wash in two changes of distilled water for 5 minutes.
- Hydrolyze in 1 N HCl for 5 minutes.
- Wash in two changes of distilled water for 5 minutes in each.
- Stain for five minutes in working thionin solution.
- Differentiate and dehydrate in 70%, 95% and absolute alcohol (1 minute in each).
- Clear in xylene and mount in DPX.

Results:

Nuclei	:	Pale mauve
Sex chromatin	:	Deeply stained
Cytoplasm	:	Almost colorless

Lactic Acid Orcein Technique

Staining solutions:
Stock solution:

Synthetic orcein	:	1 g
Glacial acetic acid	:	45 mL, Boil, cool and filter

Working solution : Dilute stock solution with an equal volume of 70% lactic acid and filter.

Procedures:
- Spread the buccal specimen immediately on the slide.
- Add 2 drops of lactic acetic orcein on to the slide.
- Place a coverslip on the slide, thus spreading the stain over the smear.
- Leave for 20 minutes, then blot the coverslip firmly to squash the cells and remove excess stain.
- Examine immediately with a high power objective.

Results:
Cells—faint pink
Nuclei—slightly darker pink
Sex-chromatin—dark red.

Stains for Lipids

Oil Red Method

It is a useful method to indicate two major lipid classes. For detailed morphology oil red O method is used with Mayer's hemalum.

Preparation of Solution

The working solution is prepared an hour in advance by mixing three parts of a stock solution of oil red O (saturated in 99% isopropanol) with two parts of distilled water and filtering just before use.

Procedures:
- Fix the smear in formalin vapour fo 5 minutes.
- Wash in running tap water for 10 minutes.
- Rinse in 60% isopropanol.

- Stain for 15 minutes in Oil red O.
- Differentiate in 60% isopropanol until a delipidized control section appears colorless.
- Wash in water and counter stain nuclei with Mayer's hemalum for 3 minutes.
- Rinse in distilled water and mount in glycerin jelly.

Results:
Unsaturated Hydrophobic lipids and mineral oil-red phospholipids-pink.

Stains for Nucleic Acid

Acridine Orange Fluorescence Method

This method is based on the principle that the fluorochrome dye, acridine orange, which has an affinity for nuclei acids, can emit visible light when excited by an ultraviolet or blue light, usually of 350–400 nm wavelength. At pH 6.0, this dye will demonstrate DNA green or greenish-yellow and RNA orange-red with fluorescence microscopy. Malignant cells have a large amount of RNA in their cytoplasm and so they are readily seen by their orange red fluorescence under low power magnification. This method permits quick scanning of smear preparation. Positive or doubtful cases are usually confirmed by Papanicolaou stain.

Solution:
- Potassium dihydrogen ortho-phosphate (0.067 M): Dissolve 9.072 g of KH_2PO_4 (I) in distilled water.
- Disodium hydrogen ortho-phosphate (0.067 M): Dissolve 9.465 g of Na_2HPO_4 (II) in distilled water.
- Phosphate buffer (pH 6.0): 87.8 mL of solution I is mixed with 12.2 mL of solution II.
- Acridine orange stock solution: Dissolve 0.1 g of acridine orange in 100 mL distilled water and store in a dark bottle at 4°C.
- Acridine orange staining solution: Mix 10 mL of acridine orange stock solution with 90 mL of phosphate buffer (pH 6.0).
- Calcium chloride differentiator (0.1M): Dissolve 11.09 g of calcium chloride in 1,000 mL distilled water.

Procedures:
- Fix smear in ether—alcohol mixture for 15 minutes.
- Pass through descending grades of alcohol (80%, 70%, and 50%) to distilled water.
- Rinse briefly in 1% acetic acid and wash in two changes of distilled water for 1 minute each.
- Stain in acridine orange staining solution for three minutes.
- Wash in phosphates buffer for 1 minute.
- Differentiate with 0.1 M $CaCl_2$ until the nuclei are clearly outlined (about 1 minute).
- Wash thoroughly with phosphate buffer solution.
- Mount with a coverslip using phosphate buffer as the mountant.
- Examine by fluorescence microscopy.

Giemsa Staining For Parasites (Blood Films)

Blood films should be stained as soon as possible as delay may result in stain retention. Romanowsky stains such as Giemsa, Leishman or Field, can be sued for staining of parasites in blood films. Giemsa staining require dilution in buffered water or buffered saline before use.

Giemsa Stain (Stock solution)

Giemsa stain powder	:	0.6 g
Methanol (acetone free)	:	50 mL
Glycerol	:	50 mL

Dissolve the Giemsa stain in methanol in a brown bottle containing a few glass beads. Add glycerol, mix and place the bottle in a water bath at 50–60°C for two hours to dissolved the stain. Shake gently at half hour intervals. The stain should stand at room temperature for three weeks and should be filtered before use. If kept air-tight, the stain is stable for several months.

Working Solution

The commercial stock solution or the solution prepared as above should be diluted 1:10 with buffer for thin films and 1:50 for thick films. Phosphate buffer used for dilution of the stain should be neutral or slightly alkaline pH 7.0–7.2.

Procedures:
- Fix the thin blood film in absolute methanol for 1 minute and air dry the smear.
- Prepare an appropriate dilution of the stock using phosphate buffer.
- Stain with the working Giemsa stain. At the end of the staining period, gently flush the stain off the slide with water. Do not tip off the stain before washing, as this will leave stain deposits over the smear.
- Dip the slide briefly in the buffer or rinse under gently running tap water.
- Wipe the undersurface of the slide to remove excess stain.
- Allow it to air dry in a vertical position.

Results
Malarial parasites

Chromatin of parasite	:	Dark red
Cytoplasm of parasite	:	Blue
Schuffner's dots	:	Red
Maurer's dots	:	Red-mauve

Trypanosomes
    Nucleus : Mauve-red
    Kinetoplast : Dark red
    Cytoplasm : Pale mauve
    Flagellum : Pale mauve

Leishmania
    Nucleus : Mauve-red
    Kinetoplast : Dark mauve-red
    Cytoplasm : Pale mauve

Microfilariae
    Nuclei : Dark purple
    Sheath of Wucheresic bancrofti : Dark pink
    Sheath of Loa loa : Pale gray or unstained

MOUNTING OF SMEAR OF CELL SAMPLES

- Place required amount of mounting media (DPX, permount or Eukitt) on a 24 × 50 mm cover glass (not a slide).
- Remove the slide from the xylene with the help of forcep.
- Hold labeled end of the slide in the left hand with thumb on top and second and third fingers underneath.
- Hold the cover glass in right hand with thumb on the bottom and second and third fingers on top.
- Tilt slide and cover glass so that they meet at the bottom of the slide.
- Gently release cover glass with second and third fingers so that the mounting medium spreads evenly over the smear and the air bubbles escape from the top of the cover glass. If there are any air bubble, press the top of the cover glass with the other end of the forcep and release the air bubbles at the edges of the cover glass.
- Clean slides and back of the slide with tissue paper to remove excess of mountant and xylene.
- Place slide on warming tray 40°C for at least 15 minutes.

EXCERCISE

1. Define cytopathology and exfoliative cytopathology.
2. What is exfoliation? Describe types of exfoliation.
3. Write application of cytopathology.
4. Describe general cytological changes in cells during malignancy.
5. Write role of laboratory technician in collection of specimen for cytological examination.
6. Describe methods of collection of gynecological samples.
7. Write sample collection in non-gynecological cytopathology.
8. Describe collection of sputum and serous effusion.
9. Describe various sample collection devices.
10. Write about preservation and the fixation of samples in cytopathology.
11. How cervix is visualized for collection of sample?
12. Describe method of collection of sputum, urine, and CSF for cytological examination.
13. How is fetal maturity estimated by cytological examination?
14. Describe methods of preparation of smears for evaluation of cytological materials.
15. Write function of membrane filters in cytology.
16. What is the importance of fixation in cytological study?
17. Classify fixatives used in cytopathology.
18. Describe preservation of cytological smears.
19. Describe in detail Papanicolaou method of cytological staining.
20. Write PAP stains.
21. Write principle, reagents and method of PAP staining.
22. Write manual and rapid PAP staining techniques.
23. What is auto stainer? Give schedule of Pap staining by automated stainer.
24. Write precautions to be taken during PAP staining.
25. Write short notes on :
    i. Shorr staining
    ii. Methylene blue wet film
    iii. Romanowsky stain.
26. "Vaginal cytology is an important tool for assessment of gynecological endocrine function" explain the statement.
27. Describe the procedure for evaluation of hormonal activity.
28. Write a note on hormonal assessment in cytology.
29. What are chromatin bodies (Barr bodies)? How they are demonstrated in cytology.
30. Describe oil red method for staining of lipids.
31. Write principle, reagents, procedure and result of nucleic acid staining by acridine orange fluorescence method.
32. How are blood films stained in cytopathology? Give the result of staining.
33. What is FNAC? Write its purpose, advantages and disadvantages.
34. Write indications of FNAC.
35. Describe the technique of FNAC in detail.
36. Write requirements of FNAC.

OBJECTIVE QUESTIONS

1. In malignancy the nucleus _____ too much leaving only a rim of cytoplasm.
   a. Enlarges
   b. Reduce
   c. Degenerate
   d. Appear

2. Malignant cells show nuclear enlargement, generally at the expense of the cytoplasmic mass, causing a rise in _____ ratio.
   a. Mitochondrial : nuclear
   b. Nuclear/cytoplasmic
   c. Cytoplasmic : mitochondiral
   d. Nucleus : nucleolus

3. The squamocolumnar junction is also called as _____.
   a. Tansient zone
   b. Transfer zone
   c. Transformation zone
   d. Temparament zone

4. Ayre's spatula is a _____ spatula.
   a. Metal
   b. Rubber
   c. Plastic
   d. Wooden

5. A small bottle brush like device with one end having fine bristles made up of nylons is called as _____.
   a. Wooden Ayre's
   b. Endocervical brush
   c. Cervex brush device
   d. Cytobrush

6. Syvonial fluid aspirates are mostly examined for crystals which can be characterized by using a _____ microscope.
   a. Polarizing
   b. Bright field
   c. Dark field
   d. Electron

7. The cytological examination of amniotic fluid used for_____.
   a. Hormonal assessment
   b. Malignancy
   c. Assessment of fetal maturity
   d. All

8. The term serous effusion refers to the fluid-accumulated in the _____.
   a. Lungs
   b. Stomach
   c. Brain
   d. Three serous cavities

9. Analysis of semen specimens is required for the investigation of _____ and follow-up of vasectomy case.
   a. Infertility
   b. Tumor
   c. Hormone
   d. Inflammation

10. Sex chromatin mass represents the inactive X chromosome in the _____ nucleus of the female.
    a. Interphase
    b. Prophase
    c. Telophase
    d. Metaphase

ANSWERS

1-a, 2-b, 3-c, 4-d, 5-b, 6-a, 7-c, 8-d, 9-a, 10-a.

CHAPTER 12

Museum Techniques

Every histologist must be able to prepare rare or important specimens for permanent preservation and display. Colored photographs should be taken whilst it is fresh.

FUNCTIONS OF PATHOLOGY MUSEUM

A well, organized pathology museum serves following functions:
- A permanent exhibition of common pathological conditions for undergraduate and postgraduate education.
- A collection of specimens illustrating rare conditions of specimens of histochemical interest.
- A collection of specimens which can be used as the basis of pathology quizzes, tap—slide programs, medical exhibitions, examination vivas, lecture demonstration, etc.
- A permanent sources of histological material for teaching, research, etc.
- A permanent source of photographic material, both gross and histological, for exhibition, publications, etc.

■ Basic Museum Techniques

The museum technique involved following steps: Reception, preparation, fixation, restoration, preservation, and presentation.

Reception of Specimen

Specimens may come from a number of sources like hospitals operation theaters, postmortem room, or research laboratories. It is necessary to make accurate records. This include maintenance of reception book in which all specimens are recorded, including all the relevant details. These consists of diagonis, name of the patient, and donor, i.e. pathologist or surgeon, and hospital and histological section number. After receiving the specimen, it is given an accession number. This is followed by the year of entry example, 1/04; 1/06. The specimen will carry this number until it is given a final catalogue number according to its place in the collection.

The initial number is then written on a tie on type parcel label in indelible ink and the label is firmly tied to the specimen.

Preparation of Specimen

When the specimen is fresh or already in a fixative, gross trimming and dissection is necessary and should be carried out immediately.

If the specimen arrived in an unfixed state, it must not be allowed to dry, as irreversible discoloration occurs. The specimen must never be washed in water otherwise hemolysis will result, causing permanent staining of the final mounting solutions.

In an unfixed state the specimen still retains its natural color, and its photographed after initial trimming. If the specimen is fixed and do not have natural color than photograph should be taken after restoration of color by one of the recommended techniques.

Fixation of the Specimen

There are number of fixatives that can be used in order to preserve a specimen as a permanent museum mount and to restore its original color, but the most acceptable fixatives is formalin.

Usually, specimens removed at operations or at necropsy have already been placed in a formal saline solution before being send to the museum. This is the initial fixative for museum specimens in which the restoration of color is possible.

Most extensively used fixative is Kaiserling's fixative having pH of 7. It has following compositions:

Kaiserling's fixative		
Formalin	:	1000 mL
Potassium acetate	:	85 g
Potassium nitrate	:	45 g
Water	:	Up to 10 liter

Kaiserling's solution I		
Formalin (40%)	:	400 mL
Potassium acetate	:	60 g
Potassium nitrate	:	30 g
Tap water	:	2000 mL

The specimen should be placed in sufficient large container having 3 or 4 times, its volume of fixative. In most cases one fixation is sufficient, but with large specimens it is necessary to give one or two changes. The period for which the specimens should remain in the fixative depends upon its size, shape and consistency for example, small specimen - three days, large specimen — fourteen days.

- **Fixation of hollow viscera:** Cut hollow organs should be padded out with cotton wool, but if uncut they can pressure inflated, e.g. through urethra into the bladder, through ureters into pelvicalyceal system, through trachea into lung, and by direct injection in the cysts.
- **Fixation of solid organs:** Organs such as liver and spleen may be perfused through the main artery, but if this is impossible due to blockage of the artery, it should be immediately sliced in the required plane to allow adequate fixation of the exposed surfaces.
- **Fixation of limbs:** Injection method can be used. If the bisected specimen is to be preserved than the limb is first frozen by solid CO_2 after placing the limb in 95% alcohol. This makes the limbs hard and thus can be bisected with a bandsaw in the required plane. The two halves are then place face down in a container of fixative to thaw and fix.
- **Fixation of heart:** Specimens of heart are usually cut before being sending to the museum. In order to maintain the natural shape all the cavities and major vessels are padded out with cotton wool before fixation. If the heart received fresh and uncut, then it is placed in an adequately large container of fixative and additional fixative is perfused through the coronary ostia with a syringe.
- **Fixation of brain:** As brain is very soft, it is difficult to handle in fresh state. It is necessary to fix brain before cutting. It should be allowed to rest on the base of the container and supported with cotton wool. After a week of fixation the brain become sufficiently hard to bisect or sliced with knife easily.

Restoration of Specimens

After fixation the natural color of the specimen may lost hence it is necessary to restore the specimen to as near its natural color as possible. It is carried out by Kaiserling's method.
- Fix the specimen for at least two weeks in Kaiserling's I solution.
- After fixation wash the specimen gently in running water. Then transfer to Kaiserling's solution II, for restoring the color.

Kaiserling's solution II
80% Industrial alcohol

Watch the specimen carefully during this stage. Remove the specimen from alcohol when maximum color contrast has been obtained. This require about ½–1 hour or upto 4 hours.
- Wash again in running water and place in Kaiserling's solution III.

Kaiserling's solution III		
Formalin (40%)	:	5 mL
Potassium acetate	:	150 g
Glycerol	:	300 g
Distilled water	:	900 mL

Adjust the pH of solution to 8.0 with 1 N NaOH. Specimen may be kept in this until they are ready for mounting in museum jar. If the specimen is left too long in alcohol, the color will become fade and this effect is irreversible.

Preservation of Specimens

The final preserving solution is Kaiserling's solution III in which the specimen remains until it is well-permeated. Initially the specimen floats and covered with soaked lint, then slowly sink to the base of the container.

Presentation of the Specimen

The specimen in the medical museum are mounted in glass jars. These are basically cylindrical-shaped with lid. The specimen is suspended by string. The jar is filled nearly upto the top with preserving solution and a piece of lid covered the top. Over this wet sheep's bladder was stretched, tied around the tip of the jar and when dry, painted.

Nowadays perspex 'jars' are used. These plastic jars have advantage that they can be completely filled with mounting solution, the specimen can be attached to rigid supporting plates within the jar, and they are light and strong. But plastic jars have disadvantages that they are attacked by absolute alcohol and get dissolved in methyl salicylate.

The specimen is attached to the plate either by tying or by impaling it onto Perspex spixes previously fixed to the plate. Nylon thread of 0.01 inch diameter or Japanese thread is used for holding the specimen.

Preserving solution
- Formalin (40%) : 40 mL
- Potassium acetate : 100 g
- Glycerol : 200 mL
- Distilled water : Up to 1000 mL

The pH of the above solution is maintained at 7.0 with disodium hydrogen phosphate. The specimen is left in the above solution for several days and then mounted in a fresh filtered sample of the same composition, to which 3 g sodium dithionite/1,000 g of tissue is added at the time of mounting in the museum jar. The jar is then firmly sealed by self tapping screws or rubber stoppers or polythene rod. The jar is then washed thoroughly in water, dried and reception or accession number is written clearly on the jar in water proof ink. Specimens can be preserved in this way for 25 years and the colors can be well-maintained (Fig. 12.1).

■ Organization of Specimens

It is necessary that the specimens can be easily located and accompanied by relevant information.

Arrangements

Specimen can either be classified by an anatomical system, i.e. all liver conditions together, or heart conditions together, etc. or by disease system, i.e. all tuberculous specimens, all parasites together, etc. Mostly first method us used.

Numbering

After deciding the anatomical division of the collection, a simple prefix letter is given to each example:
- C for Cardiovascular
- R for Respiratory
- S for Skeletal
- B for Breast

This letter should be followed by numbers to indicate the main anatomical breakdown or division of each system. Example:
- C1 for Heart
- C2 for Valves
- C3 for Arteries
- C4 for Veins

This is then followed by a point and then a number indicating the disease process, example:
- C1.1 for Congenitial conditions of heart
- C1.2 for Inflammatory conditions of heart
- C1.3 for Parasites

These numbers are then followed by the appropriate specimens examples: C1.11, C1.12, C1.13 would be examples of congential heart conditions. In this way later additions or amendments do not interfere with the general arrangement.

Another way of numbering is based on the systematized nomenclature of pathology (SNOP) of American College of Pathologist. In this system, the organ or structure is identified by a digit topographical number (T) example: Stomach = T63, fallopian tube = T86, and disease process is represented by a four digit morphological number (M) example: Adenocarcinoma = M 8143, tuberculosis = F9492, etc.

■ Labeling

The specimen jars are labeled either by simple hand painted labels or with machine engrain labels. 'Dymo' tape label can also be used for labeling.

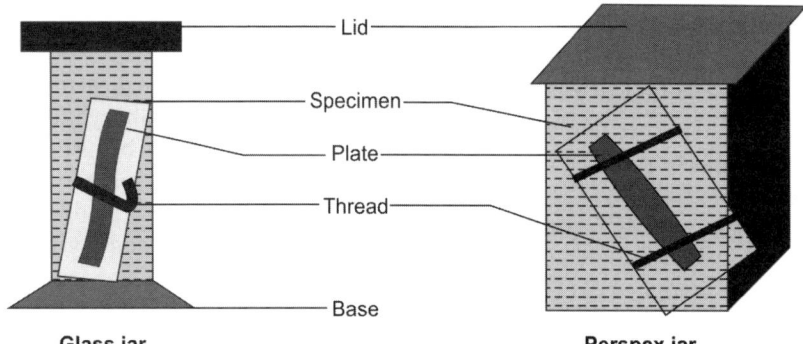

Fig. 12.1: Mounting of specimen

Cataloguing

The simple loose leaf catalogue is sufficient to hold all the necessary information relating to each specimen and, as the collection enlarges, it is helpful if there is a separate catalogue for each anatomical system. If possible, all the information relating to each specimen should be contained on one catalogue sheet. The sheet will have the diagnosis of the conditions at the top and brief description of the specimen and a brief case history at the bottom.

SAFETY IN THE MUSEUM

Always handle museum specimens with care and respect. All specimens consist of generously donated human tissue.
- The specimens are preserved in fixative solutions which contain a variety of toxic compounds.
- For reasons of hygiene, never take food or drink in the museum.
- Never leave a museum specimen on the floor, or in any precarious position.
- If a specimen is leaking, turn it upside down to prevent further leakage, then immediately inform Museum Technical Officer or a member of academic staff.
- If a specimen is broken, do not attempt to wipe up the spillage. Use the kitty litter provided to absorb the fumes, then clear the area and immediately inform academic staff.

EXCERCISE

1. Describe various steps of museum technique.
2. Describe fixation of specimen for museum.
3. What are the various functions of well organized pathology museum ?
4. What is restoration of specimen ? How is it carried out?
5. Give composition of Kaiserling's solutions I, II, and III.
6. Describe organization of specimen in pathology museum.
7. Write about safety in the museum.

OBJECTIVE QUESTIONS

1. An unfixed specimen must not be washed with water because it results in:
   a. Hemolysis   b. Hydrolysis
   c. Oxidation   d. Decolorization
2. The first step of museum technique is
   a. Restoration   b. Reception
   c. Preservation   d. Fixation
3. During reception the number given to a speciman is called
   a. Slide number   b. Tube number
   c. Accession number   d. Catalogue number
4. Kaiserling's fixative is used for fixative during
   a. Decalcification   b. Museum technique
   c. Staining   d. None
5. The process in which the natural colour of specimen is recovered is called as
   a. Fixation   b. Staining
   c. Restoration   d. Clearing
6. Restoration is carried out by using Kaiserling's solution no.
   a. I   b. II
   c. III   d. all
7. In preservation of sepcimen _____ is used.
   a. Kaiserling's solution I
   b. Kaiserling's solution II
   c. Kaiserling's solution III
   d. None.
8. During preservation of specimen the pH 7 is maintained by using
   a. Na_2HPO_4 b. NaH_2PO_4
   c. Na_3PO_4 d. $Na_2S_2O_6$

ANSWERS

1-a, 2-b, 3-c, 4-b, 5-c, 6-d, 7-c, 8-a.

CHAPTER 13

Safety in Histopathology Laboratory

Safety in histopathological laboratory is very important and is concerned with the various people working in it. Following are some of the basic safe working procedures which will ensure safety in histopathology laboratory.
- Staff training
- Basic organization and common sense
  - Infectious hazards
  - Disinfectants
  - Fire dangers
  - Solvent storage
  - Chemical storage
  - Radiation
  - Spillage of reagents
  - Chemical waste disposal
- Equipment hazards
  - Electrical
  - Mechanical
- Practical safety in routine use
  - Fresh tissue
  - Frozen section techniques
  - Paraffin embedding
  - Plastic embedding
  - Microtomy
  - Staining
- First aid action in reagent accidents

STAFF TRAINING

The most important way to avoid accidents in histopathology laboratory is to give correct training to the staff working in it. The training can be given by:
- Providing provision of a safety manual describing various hazards and safe working procedure for the department.
- Arranging lecturers on safety.
- Introduction of safety training programs.
- Regular safety inspections.
- Availability of well-stocked first aid techniques for staff.
- Maintenance of an accident book to record incidents so that lesson can be learned for the future.

BASIC ORGANIZATION AND COMMON SENSE

Safety is promoted by good organization having:
- Clean, tidy laboratory.
- Spacious floor.
- Well-planned safe methods.
- Cool mind, i.e. no stress.
- Introduction to new safety designs of the laboratory protection.
- Personal hygiene (no eating, drinking, and no smoking in laboratory).
- Washing of hands after handling chemicals.
- Use of protective gloves.
- Use of safety fillers for pipetting.
- Transport specimens in a carrier.
- Good quality of glasswares.
- Proper disposal of wastes.

INFECTIOUS HAZARDS

There is a danger of infection from fresh tissues or fluids in histopathology and cytology laboratories.
- Whenever possible all tissues should be fixed before handling otherwise they should be handled in a safe manner.
- Disposable aprons and gloves must be used.
- Do not nick the fingers when cutting unfixed tissues.
- Disinfect instruments after using them.

- In special cares use safety cabinets.
- In cytology avoid formation of aerosols from fluids or sputa.

Disinfectants

Disinfectants are used for sterilization of the equipments. Mostly phenolic types are used for organic and tuberculous material but not for viruses. Hypochlorites and glutaraldehyde is used for viruses. Aldehydes are used in two forms : as formalin vapors for cryostats and safety cabinets and as activated glutaraldehyde, which is useful for shipping surfaces of cryostats and centrifuges.

Fire Hazards

The histopathological laboratories should follow fire regulations, and must have the requisite numbers and types of fire extinguishers and fire blankets. Smoke detectors should be installed and site of fire bells known. The procedures to adopt in the event of fire and the escape route to the assembly point should be made clear to all staff and be clearly signposted for visitors.

Chemical Hazards

There is a great danger in the histopathology laboratory because of the large quantities and varieties of flammable reagents with low flash points. The regular handling of these materials can lead to an attitude of carelessness regarding their fire potential. To reduce this risk, attention must be paid to correct the storage methods. The amount kept in the laboratory should only be large enough to be sufficient for regular use. The stocks of alcohols and solvents required for daily use should be stored in metal fireproof cabinets. Bulk stocks should be maintained in fire resistant rooms with heavy metal fire proof doors. Ideally, there should be a heat triggered automatic carbon dioxide extinguisher system fitter. Because of the dangers of fire, highly corrosive or oxidizing agents such as nitric acid must never be stored with solvents such as acetone, solvents should not be stored at low temperature, but if it is necessary, then they should be stored in domestic type of refrigerator.

Chemical Storage

A chemical store should be well planned to allow sufficient space for avoiding overcrowding of stocks. Chemicals which may interact should not be stored adjacent to one another and stocks should be checked regularly. Any signs of decomposition or deterioration should be disposed off safely. Hazardous, dangerous or poisonous chemicals should be separately locked in a cupboard. Solutions like ammonia should be kept in cool and pressure should be carefully releases at regular intervals. All chemicals should be labeled with proper names.

Spillage of Reagents

An emergency procedure must be ready for use in case of a major spillage. Emergency showers should be provided for cases of personal contamination and eye wash facilities should be available. Supplies of protective clothing such as plastic overalls boots, gloves, safety glasses, and respirators should be stocked. Emergency equipment in the form of mops, brushes, shovels, and buckets must be readily available. In case of inflammable solvent spillage, sources of ignition should be sealed off and ventilation increased. The spillage should be contained by rags or saw dust and a solvent—dispersing agent applied. Acid spills should be treated with soda ash to neutralize them and mopped up with plenty of water. Sodium bicarbonate can be used. All liquids should be mopped up and transferred to buckets of water to increase dilution while solids should be shoveled into buckets for disposal. If there is a spillage of radioactive material, then liquid spills must be mopped up with paper towels and the area washed with cold water and dried.

Chemical Waste Disposal

In dealing with the disposal of large amounts of chemical waste, it may necessary to consult with the local authority or waste disposal firm. When small amounts are to be disposed, flush them into the drainage system, provided there is adequate dilution and the chemicals do not inactivate local sewerage system. But there are some solvents which require specialized treatment for this disposal scheme must be followed:
- Solvents must be returned to the stores in their original containers to which a waste solvent label should be attached.
- Mixtures are appropriately labeled and contaminants noted.
- Radioactive waste must be kept separately and send to RPL.
- Empty solvent containers should not be allowed to accumulate but returned to the chemical company.

RADIATIONS HAZARD

The use of radioactive materials should be strictly controlled. The department, which uses these substances, must follow stringent standards and a senior member of staff should be appointed in this work must undergo a medical examination before starting and are required to wear film badge dosimeters to record the amount of exposure. Regular blood counts are required and if radioactive iodine is used, then a thyroid scar may be needed. Stocks must be kept in locked lead lined boxes marked with symbol for radiation. An accurate form of record keeping is essential, any material removed from stock is recorded, along with the amount used and that returned. Gloves should be worn and benches should be covered with benchkote, all work should be carried out in trays to minimize the risks of spillage. Radioactive solvent waste must be sent to specialized sources such as the regional physics laboratory for disposal.

EQUIPMENT HAZARDS

Electrical

With increasing use of electrical equipments in the laboratory there is an equally increase in the risk of electric shock. The greatest risk is due to improper earthed connections occurring in the plug. To overcome this wiring should be carried out by a skilled electrician.

- Multiples of plugs must not be used at one socket as this can lead to overloading and fire risk.
- Any equipment allowed to run continuously should be inspected frequently.
- All electrical equipments should be regularly checked by a qualified electrician, particular attention being paid to the leads and sockets, especially those subject to movement. Even though all the equipments are assumed to be electrically safe, according to Health and Safety at Work Act, it is essential that they should be checked by an electrician before it is put into service.

Mechanical

- The equipment which may cause mechanical hazard in laboratory is centrifuges. If they are misused the result can be catastrophic.
- Heads, trunnions and carriers must not be interchanged and the balancing of the load should be done carefully.
- The speed should be increased slowly and the rotor must be allowed to stop before opening the lid. The rotor should not be stopped by hand.
- Regular servicing is important. Similarly autoclaves must also be operated correctly, otherwise a pressure build up and explosion would be disastrous. The maximum working pressure should be regularly checked and excess pressure should be released from pressure release valve.
- Similarly, the precaution should be taken for drying ovens and vacuum embedding ovens.

PRACTICAL SAFETY IN ROUTINE USE

Fresh Tissues

- In the histopathology laboratory, the most hazardous material is fresh tissues. The specimen reception room and the cut up area should be properly designed for this purpose.
- The specimen reception bench should have a smooth surface which can be wiped down in case of spillage. The cut up area should have a good system of forced ventilation which can be boosted if required.
- Fresh specimen should be handled carefully. The room should be sterilized with formaldehyde vapors if used for infectious specimens and subsequently washed down with disinfectant.
- Staff who are regularly handling fresh specimen and who are in contact with tuberculous materials should have an annual chest X-ray.
- Only fixed tissues should be transported from the postmortem room. Specimens required for frozen section should be best frozen there and taken to the cryostat.
- Syringes, needles, blades after use should dispose of in a commercially available used sharps box, which can be sterilized if required before incineration.

Fixation

- Most of the chemicals used for fixation are poisonous. The most common is formaldehyde, the pungent fumes of which affect the eyes and the mucous membranes of the nose and throat, hence the laboratory should be well-ventilated.
- During handling tissues fixed in formalin, gloves should always be worn.
- Mercuric chloride is a poison and routine use of fixative mixtures containing this substance should be discouraged.

Cytology

- In cytology, a safety cabinet must be used for known infectious fluid and sputa. The sterilization of bacteriological loop may creat problems of sparking off of infectious material if Bunsen burner is used for flaming. Use of disposable plastic loops overcome this problem.
- The centrifuge should be cleaned daily with glutaraldehyde and if infected material is spun in a centrifuge capped tubes are best used to avoid aerosol formation.

- If the tubes of centrifuge breaks, content of centrifuge should be sterilized by autoclaving.

Decalcification

- The concentrated mineral acids used for decalcification should be handled carefully. Tissues fixed in formalin should be washed before decalcifying in HCl because of the dangers of forming carcinogenic fumes of bis (chloromethyl) ether.
- Increasing use of X-ray cabinet for checking on decalcification may cause health hazard, hence users should be encourage to wear a film badge dosimeter.

Frozen Section Technique

- It require fresh material which may be infectious and create danger to handlers (tumors/tuberculosis).
- It is best to carry out this procedure in a safety cabinet to avoid carrying of the organisms.
- It is better to fix the specimen prior to freezing.
- After using the instrument should be properly sterilized and the cabinet should be sterilized by formalin fumes.
- The use of carbon dioxide gas for freezing avoid the risk of fire caused by solvents, but handling of carbon dioxide cylinders require precaution.

Paraffin Wax Processing

- The processing of tissues involves the use of alcohol, flammable solvents and waxes on automatic tissue processors.
- Most bunsen burner is used readily for embedding which may cause a fire hazard. This can be avoided by storing solvents in separate rooms.
- All electrical plugs and sockets in this room should be made sparkles to lessen the chance of igniting.
- Wax baths should have safety cut outs to prevent overheating.

Microtomy

- Microtome knives are a source of danger hence magnetic knife guards should be used.

Staining Procedures

- Stains used may have less or more dangerous.
- Picric acid is used as fixative and stain and must be stored under water.
- Basic fuschin is carcinogenic and should be handled carefully.
- Ammonical silver solutions used in reticulin staining and neurological staining may form explosive silver compounds if left dry.
- Similarly perchloric acid, sodium azide, etc. should be handled carefully.

First Aid Action in Reagent Accidents

Following procedure should be provided as an emergency first aid treatment:

- If chemical splashed on skin, wash-well with water, remove contaminated clothing.
- If reagent splashed in eye, wash an affected eye with water or use eyewash facilities.
- If the reagent is swallowed, drink sufficient water to dilute poison.

EXERCISE

1. Enlist various basic safe working procedure which will ensure safety in histopathology laboratory.
2. Describe in detail safety in histopathology laboratory.
3. Enlist various precaution to be taken to avoid electrical hazards, chemical hazards and mechanical hazards.
4. Describe various safety precautions to be taken during
    i. Fresh specimen handling
    ii. Fixation
    iii. Decalcification
    iv. Frozen sectioning
    v. Cytology
    vi. Paraffin wax processing
    vii. Staining
5. Give safety precautions during the process of decalcification, paraffin wax processing, staining and cytological preparations.

OBJECTIVE QUESTIONS

1. In chemical splashed on skin wash well with _____
   a. Water
   b. Dilute acid
   c. Dilute alkali
   d. Dilute alcohol

2. If the reagent is sollowed, drink sufficient _____ to dilute it.
   a. Lemon juice
   b. Water
   c. Carbonated drink
   d. None

3. _____ is used to avoid accidents with microtome knife.
   a. Magnetic knife guard
   b. Plastic knife guard
   c. Metal knife guard
   d. Rubber knife guard

4. Histological laboratory should be well _____ to avoid exposure to vapours of poisonous chemicals.
   a. Equipped
   b. Furnised
   c. Fibricated
   d. Ventilated

5. To avoid electrial hazards in histopathology laboratory following steps must be taken:
   a. Avoid use of multiple plugs in one socket
   b. Frequent inspection of equipment
   c. Both
   d. None

6. Highly corrosive/oxidizing agent must never be stored with solvents like:
   a. Acetone
   b. Alcohol
   c. Chloroform
   d. All

7. Basic fuschin is _____ and should be handled carefully.
   a. Carcinogenic
   b. Mutagenic
   c. Teratogenic
   d. Narcotic

ANSWERS

1-a, 2-b, 3-a, 4-d, 5-c, 6-d, 7-a.

CHAPTER
14

Advances in Histopathology and Cytopathology

MICROWAVE IRRADIATION OF PRIMARY TISSUE FIXATION

Microwave (MW) irradiation of tissue fixation was first introduced by Mayers, who reported that direct exposure to MWs generated by a 630 Watt device produce a satisfactory fixation of human postmortem tissues.

The MWs are a form of non-ionizing radiation commonly generated by domestic ovens at a frequency of 2.5 GHz. The heat produced during irradiation of MW is considered to be the primary factor responsible for many of the effects of MWs in tissue fixation, processing and staining.

Domestic MW ovens operating at 2.45 GHz and at 600 Watt output produces satisfactory fixation of most tissues by irradiation in normal saline to a temperature of 50–68°C. When only a small volume of tissue is irradiated then only 120 seconds are required.

Advantages

Microwave fixation does not have any deleterious effect on special stains. Antigens are often better preserved by MW irradiation than routine 10% formalin.

Following procedure can be adopted for large throughput laboratories with the requirement of a high speed of turn-around.

- The specimen is sent to the laboratory in 10% buffered formalin to avoid autolysis during transportation of fresh specimen.
- Following examination and sampling of these specimens 2 mm thick blocks are placed in cassettes, completely immersed in normal saline and irradiated to a temperature of 62°C for 30 seconds.
- After irradiation the tissue blocks are processed through cycles of absolute alcohol, chloroform or xylene and wax in a vacuum-assisted automated processors.
- Cycles of 1 ½ hours is used for endoscopy and small biopsies and 3 ½ hours for all other tissue blocks.

During the interval between MW irradiation and commencement of tissue processing, the tissue blocks can be held in 70% alcohol, Carnoy's solution, 10% buffered formalin or even in normal saline.

ULTRASONIC DECALCIFICATION

The ultrasonic (US) decalcifying bath uses ultrasonic power and temperature control to facilitate significant reductions in the time required to prepare and decalcify bone and tissue samples (Fig. 14.1).

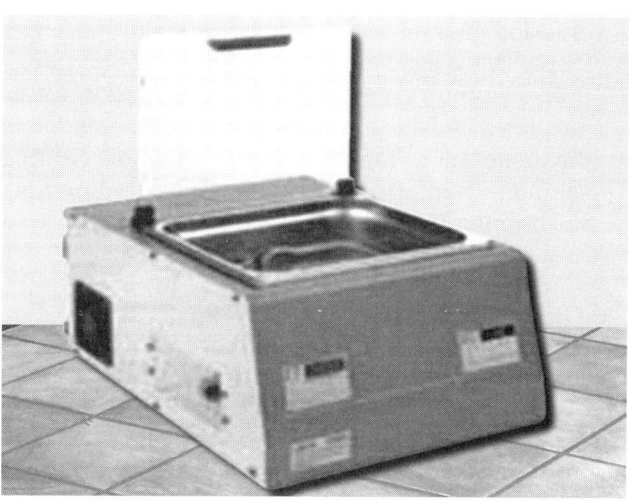

Fig. 14.1: Ultrasonic decalcifier

- The ultrasonic decalcifying bath promotes the rapid destruction of crystalline structures like calcium phosphate, magnesium phosphate and calcium carbonate.
- In combination with appropriate solutions it provides maximum cell or tissue preservation and a significantly accelerated diffusion process.
- In this tissue is maintained at 17°C during the process which prevents the samples from being warmed excessively by the chemical reaction of the decalcifying solution. This guarantees 100% decalcification.

■ Advantages

- Preservation of the morphological structures and the antigenity of the samples.
- No artefacts are generated from shrinking or swelling and all further histological and immunohistochemical methods can be applied to the samples.
- The decalcifying procedure can be carried out with different solutions.
- A quick result can be obtained with strong mineral acids (such as hydrochloric, nitric or formic acid). Their use, however, may result in the loss of morphological and or immunohistochemical information. In this process, these acids work successfully within 15–60 minutes in numerous kinds of specimens.
- Decalcifying times can be reduced by 60–65% compared with conventional procedures. The ultrasonic burst opens the crystal structures containing calcium resulting in faster removal and binding of Ca^{2+} ions in the outer solution.
- The strong integrated cooling protects the tissue from temperature rises caused by the chemical reaction.
- High performance fixation of the specimens can be made in the instrument. The ultrasound accelerates the diffusion speed of the fixation molecules into the target tissue. This is dependent on the molecular structure.
- It also supports clearing and cleaning procedures integrated into the process. Surplus fixation solution in the tissue will be rapidly transferred into the clearing solution. Even primary dehydration procedure time will be optimized.

MICROWAVE-STIMULATED TISSUE PROCESSING

Rapid manual microwave-stimulated paraffin wax processing of small batches of tissues gives excellent results which are comparable to tissues processed by longer automated non-microwave methods. Processing is undertaken in a dedicated microwave oven (Fig. 14.2) which is fitted with precise temperature control and timer, and an interlocked fume extraction system to preclude accidental solvent vapor ignition. Agitation is provided by an air-nitrogen system.

Domestic microwave ovens with a temperature probe and timer accurate to seconds are suitable for tissue processing. A turntable or inbuilt radiation disperser facilitates even reagent heating. Toxic and flammable solvent vapors generated during processing cannot always be adequately vented from these ovens and present an ignition hazard if the electrical system is unprotected. Ovens should therefore be used within a fume cupboard to minimize this problem. Calibration of domestic ovens is essential for optimum results and the accuracy of the temperature probe, duration of cycle time, and net power levels at various settings must be determined before the oven is used to process tissues. Table 14.1 gives schedules for microwave-stimulated processing.

■ Equipment

Tissues are processed in conventional plastic cassettes. Transparent glass or solvent-resistant plastic containers of about 200 mL capacity are ideal for processing batches of up to 14 cassettes per container.

■ Fixation

For rapid processing, tissues are fixed by microwave irradiation, or in 95% ethanol (600 mL), polyethylene glycol PEG 400 (45 mL) from which specimens can be transferred directly to dehydrant. Formaldehyde fixed tissues must be rinsed in running tap water for 5 minutes before microwave processing and an extra dehydration change incorporated in

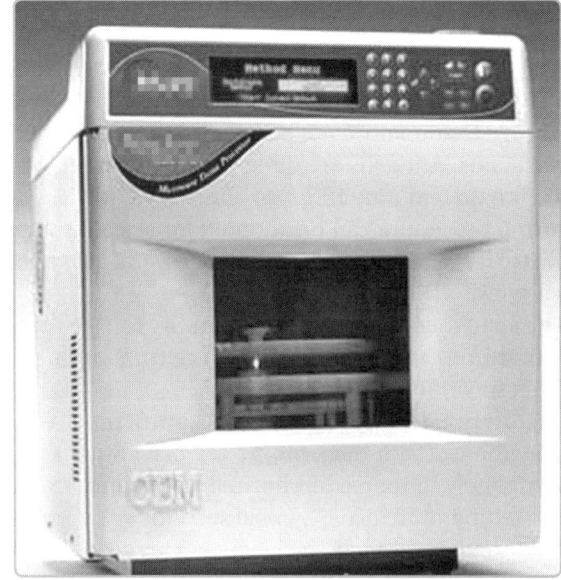

Fig. 14.2: Microwave tissue processor

Table 14.1: Schedules for microwave-stimulated processing. Method of Kok, Visser and Boon

STEP	Temp (°C)	Tissue block thickness		
		<1 mm	1-2 mm	2-5 mm
100% ethanol	67	5 minutes	15 minutes	60 minutes*
100% isopropanol	74	3 minutes	15 minutes	45 minutes
PARAMAT wax	67	2 minutes	15 minutes	30 minutes
	82	5 minutes	20 minutes	60 minutes
Embed				
Total time		15 minutes	65 minutes	195 minutes

*Reduce to 10-15 minutes if tissues do not contain fat. Both volumes 200 mL, power level 450 watt

the schedule. Processing times for formaldehyde fixed tissues need to be increased above those provided for coagulant fixed tissues. Picric acid fixed tissues should not be microwave processed as there is an explosion risk even in well-washed tissues.

■ Hints for Microwave Tissue Processing

Tissue blocks should be as thin as possible. Length and width are not as important.
- Process blocks of similar thickness together.
- Reagent volumes should be at least 50 times that of specimen volume.
- The temperature probe should be placed centrally in processing baths.
- Use a dummy load to check heat generation.
- Reagents boil on minimum settings — an equal volume of reagent irradiated together with the primary load effectively halves the energy received by the primary load.
- Preheat paraffin wax baths in a conventional oven.
- An increase in the number of cassettes or fluid volumes will require a concomitant increase in power and or time to achieve the correct processing temperature.

ULTRASOUND-STIMULATED TISSUE PROCESSING

Ultrasonics are used in histopathology to accelerate fixation, tissue processing for electron microscopy, the decalcification of bone, tissue softening in post-embedding adjuvants, improving the sensitivity of immunohistochemical reactions, conventional staining and for accelerated tissue processing. Unfixed tissue blocks 1-2 mm thick can be fixed and processed to paraffin wax using ultrasonic-stimulation in 1 hour 45 minutes. The ultrasound gives best effect at frequencies of 100 kHz-1 MHz. At lower frequencies cavitation phenomena and attendant heat, pressure and streaming effects may damage tissues and care must be exercised.

Processing is performed in reagent containers suspended in a detergent solution within the transducer tank of an ultrasonic cleaner operated at 50 watts. An immersion heater is used to elevate bath temperatures for paraffin wax infiltration. Tissues are placed in metal or plastic cassettes for processing.

Coagulant fixatives provide optimal stabilization for ultrasonic-stimulated processing. Tissues are dehydrated in ethanol and cleared in toluene, or preferably methyl benzoate or methyl salicylate. Cells and organelles such as cilia, microvilli and desmosomes are all well-preserved. Old and friable specimens sometimes exhibit marginal distortion and erosion.

Table 14.2 gives schedules for ultrasonic-stimulated tissue processing.

Table 14.2: Schedule for ultrasonic-stimulated tissue processing. Method of Gagnon and Katyk

Step	Rapid method	Routine method
	Tissues 1-2 mm	Tissues 5 mm
Fixation	20 minutes	60 minutes
100% ethanol	1.5 minutes	1.15 minutes
	2.10 minutes	2.30 minutes
	3.25 minutes	3.90 minutes
Methyl benzoate	5 minutes	30 minutes
Toluene or substitute	1.5 minutes	1.15 minutes
	2.5 minutes	2.15 minutes
Paraffin wax	1.10 minutes	1.30 minutes
	2.10 minutes	2.30 minutes
	3.10 minutes	3.30 minutes
Total time	1 hour 45 minutes	5 hours 30 minutes

AUTOMATIC KNIFE SHARPNERS

Nowadays automatic knife sharpening machine is extensively used due to:
- Tremendous saving of time and labor
- Production of well-sharpened knife with uniform bevel
- More efficient.

But they are undoubtedly expensive. The commonly used knife shapers are Shandon and Temtool automatic knife sharpeners. Out of which Shandon machine is used extensively (Fig. 14.3).

In this the knife is held in a holder attached to the main spindle, in such a way that the cutting edge is in contact with a glass/metal plate. A mechanism is provided for adjusting the height of the glass plate at agree with the bevel of the knife. There is a combined oscillatory and rotary motion which spread the abrasive evenly over the surface of the plate. There is a damping device which automatically turns the knife over at suitable intervals to ensure that the each facet is sharpened equally. There is a speed control for regulating the speed of the sharpening. For badly nicked knife, slow speed is recommended.

Cleaning: It is important that the knife should be thoroughly cleaned after honing or stropping. If any traces of metal dust remain on the knife edge that it may get transferred to the sections during cuttings and subsequently give a false positive Prussian blue reaction for ferric iron.

ULTRAMICROTOMY

In principle, it is the offspring of the standard microtome, in that it also is a mechanical device that involves a stationary knife (glass/diamond) and a moving specimen. The specimen or block, is a plastic embedded tissue that advances in nanometers rather than microns.

Operationally, the only difference is that smaller samples are handled which in turn require a binocular dissecting microscope mounted over the blade. The tissue sections are too thin to see their thickness with the naked eye, one usually estimate thickness by the color of the diffraction pattern of the section as it floats off the knife onto the surface of a water bath. The sections are too thin to be handled directly, they are therefore transferred with wire loops, or picked-off the water directly onto an EM grid. This process requires a good light source mounted to cast the light at just the correct angle to see the color pattern (Fig. 14.4).

Since, the plastics are hard enough to break steel knives, freshly prepared glass knives or commercially available diamond knives are used. Mostly glass knives are used, whereas diamond knives are used only in research laboratories by trained technicians. Diamond knives have the advantages of a consistent knife edge (unlike glass which varies with each use) and can last for years if treated properly. They are usually resharpened several times before discarding. But the disadvantage of diamond knife is that they are very expensive. Ultramicrotome are cast in heavy metal to minimize vibrations (which lead to uneven sections) and are mounted on shock absorbent tables, and preferably, kept in draft free environments of relatively constant temperature. To further minimize vibrations, the block's mechanical advance mechanism is replaced with a thermal bar, which advances the tissue by heating a metal rod. This can exquisitely precise and is the ultimate in thin sectioning. Of course, with this advancement comes increased cost and maintenance and decreased ability to withstand rough treatment. Mechanically advanced ultramicrotome remains as the workhorse of the cell biology laboratory.

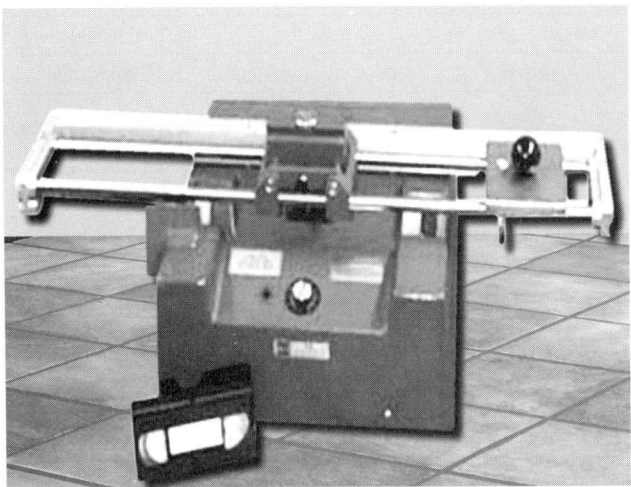

Fig. 14.3: Automatic knife sharpner

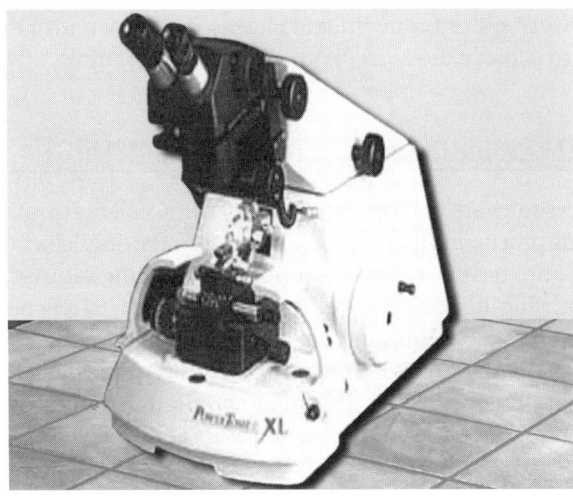

Fig. 14.4: Ultramicrotome

AUTOMATIC STAINING METHOD

Manual slide staining procedure occupies a considerable amount of technician's time. To accelerate the process slide staining machine was designed on modern principles for carrying out practically all slide staining techniques of cytology and histology (Fig. 14.5). Automatic slide staining machine, is compact and rugged equipment designed with the latest technology for automatic staining of slides in different reagents according to preprogrammed chronological user selectable cycles. Throughout the process the slides are shaken (Switch selectable) for effective staining in a slide carrier. The capacity of stainer is usually of 16 slides. The last trough, i.e. 12th station is provided with an inlet and outlet to enable washing of the residual chemicals. The unit is supplied with 11 glass staining troughs, 1 trough with inlet and outlet, 1 slide carrier, 5 timing discs for chronological programming calibrated for 60 minutes and 1 notch cutting plier.

The schedule of automatic staining is as follows:

- Xylene I — 3 minutes
- Xylene II — 3 minutes
- Absolute alcohol I — 3 minutes
- Absolute alcohol II — 2 minutes
- 70% alcohol — 3 minutes
- Distilled water — 3 minutes
- Cole's hematoxylin — 10 minutes
- Tap water — 5 minutes
- 0.25% HCl in 75% alcohol — 1 minute
- 2% sodium hydrogen carbonate — 2 minutes
- Tap water — 5 minutes
- 0.5% eosin — 5 minutes
- Tap water — 90 seconds
- Absolute alcohol III — 2 minutes
- Absolute alcohol IV — 2 minutes
- Absolute alcohol—xylene — 2 minutes
- Xylene III — 3 minutes

Transfer sections to a final bath of xylene prior to mounting.

Results

Nuclei	– Blue to blue black
Nucleoli	– Red or purple or blue
Cartilage	– Pink or light blue
Cement line of bone	– Blue
Calcium and calcified bone	– Purplish-blue
Basophilic cytoplasm	– Purplish

ENDOSCOPY

Endoscopy allows physicians to peer through the body's passage ways. Endoscopy is the examination and inspection of the interior of body organs, joints or cavities through an endoscope. An endoscope is a device using fiber optics and powerful lens systems to provide lighting and visualization of the interior of a joint.

An endoscope uses two fiber optic lines. A "light fiber" carries light into the body cavity and an "image fiber" carries the image of the body cavity back to the physician's viewing lens. There is also a separate port to allow for administration of drugs, suction, and irrigation. This port may also be used to introduce small folding instruments such as forceps, scissors, brushes, snares and baskets for tissue excision (removal), sampling, or other diagnostic and therapeutic work. Endoscopes may be used in conjunction with a camera or video recorder to document images of the inside of the joint or chronicle an endoscopic procedure. New endoscopes have digital capabilities for manipulating and enhancing the video images.

This Figure 14.6 shows a rigid endoscope used for arthroscopy. The "image fiber" leads from the ocular (eye piece) to the inserted end of the scope. The "light fiber" is below and leads from the light source to the working end of the endoscope.

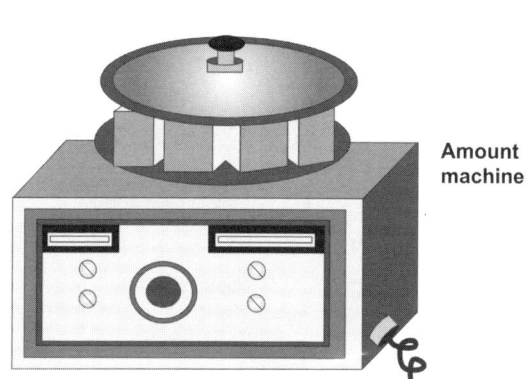

Fig. 14.5: Automatic stainer

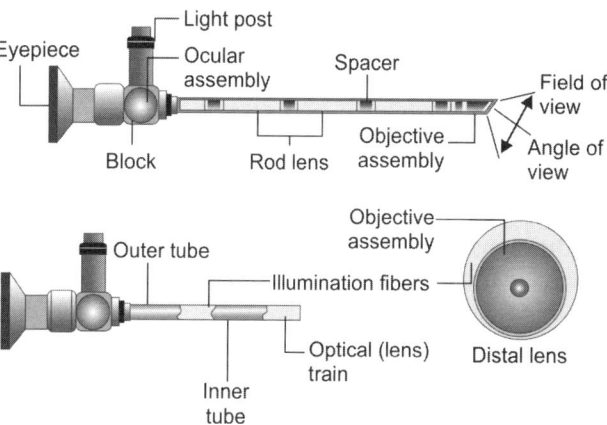

Fig. 14.6: Endoscope

Purpose of Endoscopy

Endoscopy can be used to diagnose various conditions by close examination of internal organ and body structures. Endoscopy can also guide therapy and repair, such as the removal of torn cartilage from the bearing surfaces of a joint. Biopsy (tissue sampling for pathologic testing) may also be performed under endoscopic guidance. Local or general anesthetic may be used during endoscopy, depending upon the type of procedure being performed. Endoscopy is a minimally invasive procedure and carries with it certain minor risks. However, these risks are typically far outweighed by the diagnostic and therapeutic potential of the procedure.

Types of Endoscopy

Fiber optic endoscopes now have widespread use in the medicine and guide a myriad of diagnostic and therapeutic procedures including:

- **Arthroscopy** is an examination of joints for diagnosis and treatment (arthroscopic surgery).
- **Bronchoscopy** is an examination of the trachea and lung's bronchial trees to reveal abscesses, bronchitis, carcinoma, tumors, tuberculosis, alveolitis, infection, inflammation.
- **Colonoscopy** is an examination of the inside of the colon and large intestine to detect polyps, tumors, ulceration, inflammation, colitis diverticula, Crohn's disease, and discovery and removal of foreign bodies.
- **Colposcopy** is direct visualization of the vagina and cervix to detect cancer, inflammation, and other conditions.
- **Cystoscopy** is a examination of the bladder, urethra, urinary tract, uteral orifices, and prostate (men) with insertion of the endoscope through the urethra.
- **Endoscopic biopsy** is the removal of tissue specimens for pathologic examination and analysis.
- **Gastroscopy** is an examination of the lining of the esophagus, stomach, and duodenum. Gastroscopy is often used to diagnose ulcers and other sources of bleeding and to guide biopsy of suspect GI cancers.
- **Laparoscopy** is visualization of the stomach, liver and other abdominal organs, including the female reproductive organs, for example, the fallopian tubes.
- **Laryngoscopy** is a examination of the larynx (voice box).
- **Proctoscopy**, sigmoidoscopy, proctosigmoidoscopy is an examination of the rectum and sigmoid colon.
- **Thoracoscopy** is an examination of the pleura (sac that covers the lungs), pleural spaces, mediastinum, and pericardium.

COLPOSCOPY

It is a diagnostic procedure used in the prevention of cervical cancer and involves the use of a magnifying device called a colposcope to examine an illuminated, magnified view of the cervix, the tissue of the vagina, and vulva. The enlarged view provided by the colposcope allows the colposcopist to visually distinguish normal from abnormal appearance of tissue and to take direct biopsies for further histology.

Purpose of Colposcopy

The purpose of colposcopy is the prevention of cervical cancer through the early detection and treatment of precancerous lesions (CIN). The German physician, Dr Hans Hinselmann in 1925, developed the procedure. Women who receive abnormal smear results can be referred for colposcopy which is used to identify and grade the abnormality.

- **Colposcope:** It is the most important piece of equipment used during a colposcopy. It functions as a ligh binocular microscope, which magnifies the view of the cervix, vagina and vulvar surface and enables the colposcopist to identify areas on the surface that show abnormalities. Two chemicals, acetic acid and iodine solutions are used in colposcopy to improve the visualization of the abnormal area (Fig. 14.7).

The patient is asked to lie with her bottom close to the lower edge of a purpose-built table. The valva is then examined for any suspicious lesions and then a speculum is gently placed in the vagina. The transformation zone (the area on the cervix where many precancerous and cancerous lesions develop), is swabbed lightly with acetic acid to remove the mucus that covers the surface, and to highlight abnormal areas.

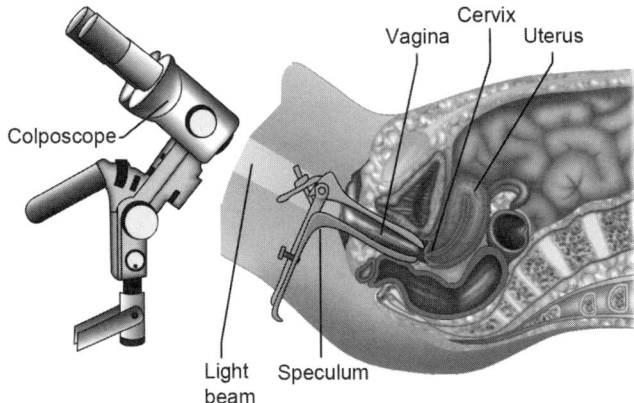

Fig. 14.7: Colposcopy

The colposcope is then positioned at the opening of the vagina and the area is thoroughly examined. Area of the cervix, which turn white after the application of acetic acid or have an abnormal pattern are often considered for biopsy. If no lesion is visible an iodine solution may be applied (The Schiller test) to the cervix to help highlight area of abnormality. Mature, normal cells will stain a dark-brown color whereas abnormal cells will not stain and biopsies may be taken from these non-staining areas. After a complete examination, the colposcopist determines the area with the highest degree of visible abnormality and a small sample of the tissue will be removed (biopsy) using small biopsy forceps. Many samples may be taken, depending on the size of the area. Thus, a combination of acetic acid and iodine tests are used by most colposcopists to determine if an abnormality is likely to be precancerous or not.

A diagnosis will be made by:
- How white the tissue goes after using acetic acid?
- How quickly the tissue turns white?
- How smooth or irregular the surface is?
- The different patterns of the blood vessels under the surface of the cervix.

All biopsies taken are sent to a laboratory for histology.

AUTORADIOGRAPHY

Radiography is the visualization of the pattern of distribution of radiation. In general, the radiation consists of X-rays, gamma (γ) or beta (β) rays, and the recording medium is a photographic film. For classical X-rays, the specimen to be examined is placed between the source of radiation and the film, and the absorption and scattering of radiation by the specimen produces its image on the film. In contrast, in autoradiography the specimen itself is the source of the radiation, which originates from radioactive material incorporated into it. The recording medium, which makes visible the resultant image, is usually photographic emulsion.

An autoradiograph is an image on an X-ray film or nuclear emulsion produced by the pattern of decay emissions (e.g. beta particles, gamma rays) from a distribution of a radioactive substance. Alternatively, the autoradiograph can also be available as a digital image (digital autoradiography), due to the recent development of scintillation gas detectors or rare earth phosphorimaging systems. In biology, this technique may be used to determine the tissue localization of a radioactive substance, either introduced into a metabolic pathway, bound to a receptor or enzyme, or hybridized to a nucleic acid. The film or emulsion is opposed to the labeled tissue section to obtain the autoradiograph (also called an autoradiogram). The auto- prefix indicates that the radioactive substance is within the sample, as distinguished from the case of historadiography or microradiography, in which the sample is X-rayed using an external source.

The use of radio labeled ligands to determine the tissue distributions of receptors is termed either in vivo or in vitro receptor autoradiography if the ligand is administered into the circulation (with subsequent tissue removal and sectioning) or applied to the tissue sections, respectively. The ligands are generally labeled with H^3 (tritium) or I^{125}. The distribution of RNA transcripts in tissue sections by the use of radiolabeled, complementary oligonucleotides or ribonucleic acids ("riboprobes") is called in situ hybridization histochemistry.

■ Autoradiography Method

- Living cells are briefly exposed to a 'pulse' of a specific radioactive compound.
- The tissue is left for a variable time.
- Samples are taken, fixed, and processed for light or electron microscopy.
- Sections are cut and overlaid with a thin film of photographic emulsion.
- Left in the dark for days or weeks (while the radioisotope decays). This exposure time depends on the activity of the isotope, the temperature and the background radiation (this will produce with time a contaminating increase in 'background' silver grains in the film).
- The photographic emulsion is developed (as in conventional photography).
- Counterstaining, e.g. with toluidine blue, shows the histological details of the tissue. The staining must be able to penetrate, but not have an adverse affect on the emulsion.
- Alternatively, pre-staining of the entire block of tissue can be done, (e.g. with osmium on plastic sections coated with stripping film or dipping emulsion. This avoids the need for individually (post-) staining each slide.
- It is not necessary to coverslip these slides.
- The position of the silver grains in the sample is observed by light or electron microscopy
- **Note:** The grains are in a different plane of focus in the emulsion overlying the tissue section. Often oil with a 100X objective is used for detailed observation with the light microscope.
- These autoradiographs provide a permanent record.
- Full details of the batch of emulsion used, dates, exposure time and conditions should be kept for each experiment (Fig. 14.8).

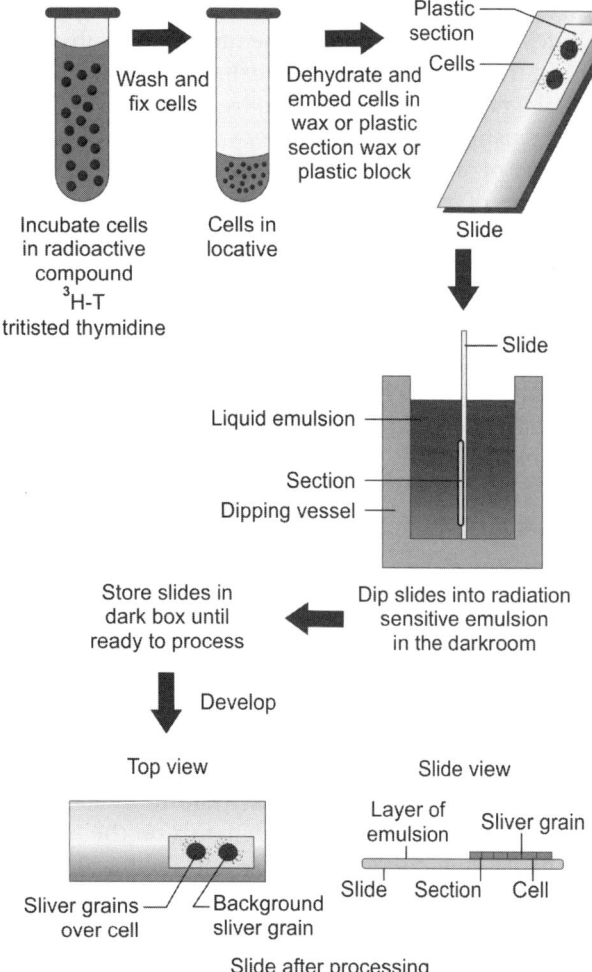

Fig. 14.8: Steps of autoradiography

IMMUNOHISTOCHEMISTRY

"Immuno" refers to antibodies and "histo" means tissue, thus immunohistochemistry or IHC means the process of localizing proteins in cells of a tissue section using the principle of antibodies binding specifically to antigens in biological tissues.

■ Applications of Immunohistochemistry

- It is widely used in the diagnosis of abnormal cells, such as hose found in cancerous tumors.
- IHC is widely used in basic research to understand the distribution and localization of biomarkers and differentially expressed proteins in different parts of a biological tissue.
- It is an effective way to examine the tissues.
- It is widely used technique in the neurosciences enabling researchers to examine protein expression within specific brain structures.

Antibody

The antibody used for immunohistochemistry can be polyclonal or monoclonal. Monoclonal antibodies are generally considered to exhibit greater specificity. Polyclonal antibodies are made by injecting animals with peptide Ag, and then after a secondary immune response is stimulated, isolating antibodies from whole serum. Thus polyclonal antibodies are a heterogeneous mixture of antibodies that recognize several epitopes. Antibodies are also called primary or secondary reagents. Primary antibodies are raised against an antigen of interest and are typically unconjugated (unlabelled). Secondary antibodies recognize immunoglobulins of a particular species and are conjugated to either biotin or a reporter enzyme such as alkaline phosphatase or peroxidase. Some secondary antibodies are conjugated to fluorescent agents.

■ Methods of Immunohistochemistry

Immunohistochemical detection of antigens in tissue can be carried out by two methods viz. direct method and indirect method.

- **Direct method:** In the direct method labeled antibody (conjugated antiserum) react directly with the antigen in tissue sections and is a one-step staining method.
- **Indirect method:** In the indirect method staining uses one antibody against the antigen being probed for, and a second, labeled, antibody against the first. In this an unlabeled primary antibody (first layer) reacts with tissue antigen and a labeled secondary antibody (second layer) react with the primary antibody. The second layer antibody can be labeled with a fluorescent dye or an enzyme.

■ Immunohistochemical Protocol For Formalin Fixed, Paraffin Embedded Tissues

- **Fixation:** Place tissue in 10% formalin (pH 7.4) for up to 24 hours.
- **Processing and embedding:** Process tissue through to paraffin using standard histological methods and embedded in paraffin and allow to cool.
- **Sectioning and mounting:**
  - Cut tissue sections at 3–5 μ. Mount on slides treated to enhance tissue adherence.
  - Dry slides at 60–70°C for 1–2 hours or dry slides overnight at 37°C.
  - Cool to room temperature if slides are to be stored.
- **Deparaffinization or rehydration:**
  - Dewax slides in xylene for 3 to 5 minutes.
  - Hydrate slides in 100%, 95%, 80% ethanol for 3 minutes each, then immerse slides in tap water for 5 minutes.

- **Endogenous peroxide quenching:**
  - Immerse slides in 3% hydrogen peroxide solution for 10 minutes, then wash slides in phosphate buffer solution (PBS) 2 times for 3 minutes each.
- **Pretreatment/antigen retrieval:**
  - Heat induced epitope retrieval is used:
    - Place racked slides in citrate, EDTA, or Tris HCl buffer
    - Heat samples near boiling for 10–20 minutes.
    - Rinse in PBS at lest 3 × 1 minute before proceeding For enzyme pretreatment:
      » Add enzyme (pepsin, trypsin, proteinase K) to cover tissue, put in moisture chamber, and incubate at 37°C for 10 minutes.
      » Rinse off enzyme using PBS squirt bottle. Rinse in PBS at least 3 × 1 minute before staining.
- **Primary antibody:**
  - Dilute the primary antibody if necessary.
  - Place the slides in a humidity chamber to decrease reagent evaporation.
  - Incubate according to the recommended time and temperature, then wash slides in PBS for 3 × 3 minutes.
  - Instructions are specific to Lab Vision's UltraVision Detection Kit: TP-015-HA. Follow manufacturer's recommendations.
- **Secondary antibody (link):**
  - Cover tissue with 4–5 drops of UltraVision biotinyulated goat anti-polyvalent secondary antibody.
  - Incubate at room temperature of 10 minutes, then wash in PBS for 3 × 3 minutes.
- **Streptavidin/peroxidase (label):**
  - Add drops of steptavidin peroxidase to cover sec-tion, incubate at room temperature for 10 minutes, then wash in PBS for 3 × 3 minutes.
- **Substrate/chromogen:**
  - Mix AEC buffer and AEC chromogen according to UltraVision instructions 20 minutes before application (20 μl AEC chromogen per 1 mL AEC buffer).
  - Cover section by adding drops.
  - Incubate at room temperature for 10 minutes, then wash slides in PBS for 3 minutes.
- **Counter staining:**
  - Place slide rack in hematoxylin bath for 1–4 minutes. (adjust accordingly).
  - Wash in water bath 7–8 times, PBS for 1 minute, then tap water for 3 minutes.
- **Coverslipping:**
  - For permanent mounting, dehydrate through 100% alcohol and in xylene for 3 × 1 minute.
  - Mount coverslip with permanent mounting media.

Disadvantages

The major disadvantage of immunohistochemistry is that, unlike immunoblotting techniques where staining is checked against a molecular weight ladder, it is impossible to show in IHC that the staining corresponds with the protein of interest. An antigen-antibody interaction can be accomplished in a number of ways. In most common method an antibody is conjugated to an enzyme, such as peroxidase, that can catalyse a color-producing reaction. Alternatively, the antibody can also be gagged to a fluorophore, like fluorescein, rhodamine, etc.

TISSUE MICROARRAYS

Tissue microarrays (TMAs) are used to analyze the expression of genes simultaneously in multiple individual tissue samples on one slide. TMAs are composed of small 0.6–3.0 mm cores of tissue from donor tissue paraffin blocks which are arrayed at a high density on a slide. Tissue microarrays have allowed tissue traditional analysis of conventional histologic paraffin blocks to become miniturized and high-throughput. Histochemical and molecular detection techniques can be used on the TMA slides, and thus allow TMAs to be powerful tools to examine gene expression profiling in disease states across a variety of patients and disease conditions.

Characteristics of Tissue Microarrays

- 50–500 tissues or more can be analyzed per slide block
- High throughput
- Relatively low cost
- Can be stained with a variety of stains such as H and E stained
- Slides can be analyzed with a wide-variety of techniques
- Automated analysis and data collection with many techniques.

Tissue Microarray Synthesis

Tissue microarrays are produced using a microtome which sections tissue into 4–5 micrometer sections. These core tissue biopsy sections are taken from specific areas of interest from paraffin-embedded tissue blocks. These cylindrical cores of tissue are re-embedded into an arrayed blank recipient blocks. Using this method, more than 500 tissue cores can be arrayed on a single slide (Fig. 14.9).

Techniques in Histopathology and Cytopathology

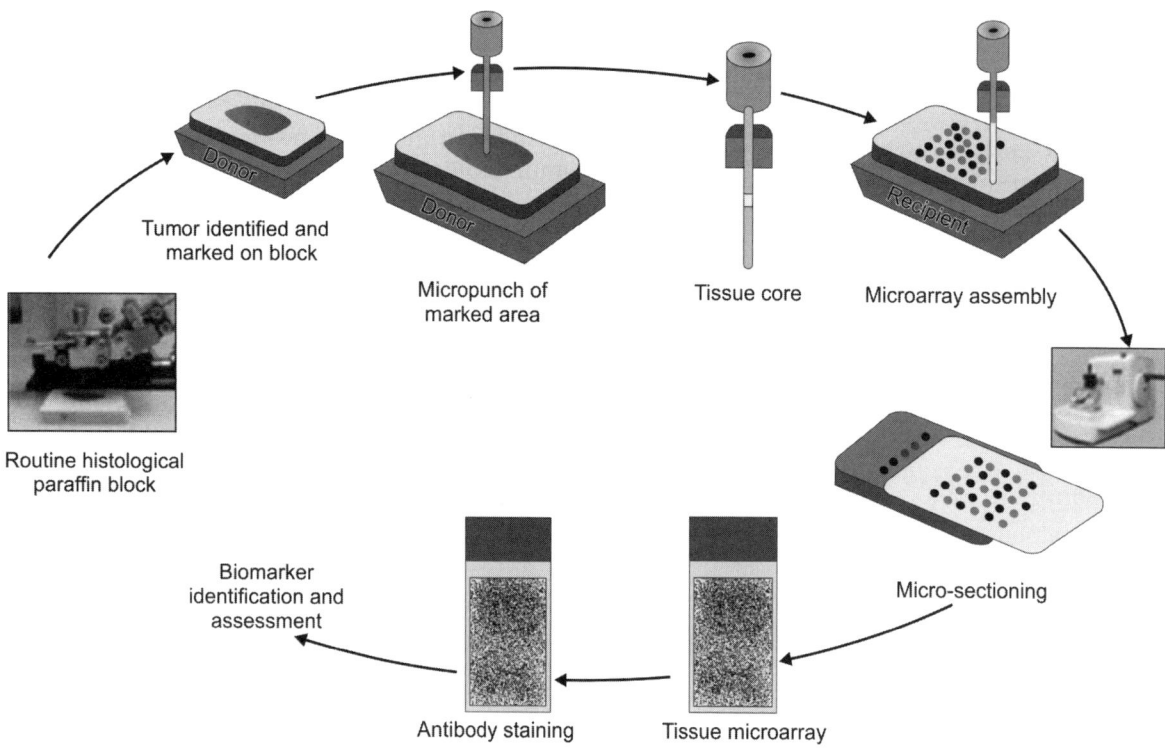

Fig. 14.9: Tissue microarray method

Applications of Tissue Microarrays

- Immunohistochemistry
- Staining of: H and E, HC, ISH,
- In situ hybridization
- Fluorescent in situ hybridization (FISH)
- In situ PCR
- RNA or DNA expression analysis
- TUNEL assay for apoptosis
- Morphological and clinical characterization of many patient tissues.

Advantages of Tissue Arrays or Tissue Chips

- Experimental uniformity.
- Allows amplification (and conservation) of scarce tissue samples.
- Saving the assay volume.
- Reduces the number of slides examined (conventional slides tissue paraffin).
- High-throughput.
- Analysis can be automated and data can be computerized.

Types of Tissue Microarrays

- **Cryo-tissue microarrays (cryo-TMAs):** Cryo-TMAs uses frozen tissues which are embedded in an optimal cutting temperature compound. These cryo-TMAs due to their freezing are superior to formalin fixed tissues for RNA and protein analysis. Also the antibodies work much better with frozen tissues.
- **Multi-tumors tissue microarrays:** Multi-tumor TMAs have many different types of tissues aligned on the slide. The technique was first used by Kononen et al. 1998. Kononen used this type of TMA to detect 6 gene amplifications. p53 expression was also examined in breast cancer tissue.
- **Progression tissue microarrays:** This type of tissue microarray examines different stages of tumor (or disease) progression within a given organ. For example, examination of tumors in the breast. These slides can then be assayed for markers of interest, or biochemical analysis of the samples can be done.
- **Prognosis tissue microarrays:** Disease samples such as tumor biopsies can be taken from patients and examined. These samples can be used in clinical follow-ups to monitor the patient's progression. Data is then analyzed and compared with other clinical data.

EXCERCISE

1. Describe microwave (MW) irradiation of primary tissue fixation with respect of principle and advantages.
2. What is ultrasonic decalcifier? Write its advantages
3. Describe procedures for decalcification of bone marrow biopsy by ultrasonic decalcifier.
4. Write a short note microwave stimulated tissue processing. Write advantages of it.
5. What is ultrasonic stimulated tissue processing? Give schedule for it.
6. Describe an automatic knife sharpner.
7. Describe ultramicrotome in short.
8. Describe automatic staining machine. Give a schedule of staining by automatic stainer.
9. What is endoscopy? Give its importance in cytopathology.
10. What is the purpose of endoscopy? Write types of endoscopy.
11. What is colposcopy? What is the purpose of colposcopy? How is it performed?
12. Define autoradiography. Describe the methodology of autoradiography in short.
13. What do you mean by immunohistochemistry? Write applications of it.
14. Give the immunohistochemical protocol for formalin fixed, paraffin embedded tissues.
15. Write a descriptive note on TMA.
16. What is tissue microarray? Write its types, applications and advantages.

OBJECTIVE QUESTIONS

1. Domestic microwave ovens operate at _____ GHz and at 100 watt output.
   a. 4.86
   b. 2.45
   c. 8.98
   d. 1.25

2. Ultrasonic decalcification promotes rapid destruction of _____ structures.
   a. Crystalline
   b. Nuclear
   c. Cytoplasmic
   d. None

3. In ultrasonic decalcification the tissue is maintained at _____ during the process.
   a. 0°C
   b. 35°C
   c. 17°C
   d. 25°C

4. With ultrasonic decalcification, the decalcification time can be reduced by _____ compared with conventional procedures.
   a. 40–50%
   b. 60–65%
   c. 80–90%
   d. 10–20%

5. The ultrasound gives best effect at frequency of _____.
   a. 100kHz–1Mhz
   b. 10kHz–100Mhz
   c. 1kHz–10Mhz
   d. 1kHz–1Mhz

6. In ultramicrotomy the microtome is combined with a _____.
   a. Fluorescent microscope
   b. Student microscope
   c. Simple microscope
   d. Binocular microscope

7. The tissue thickness in ultramicrotomy is in _____.
   a. Nanometer
   b. Micrometer
   c. Centimeter
   d. Millimeter

8. _____ and diamond knives are used in ultramicrotomy.
   a. Steel
   b. Glass
   c. Plastic
   d. All

9. In ultramicrotomy _____ advance mechanism is used instead of mechanical advance mechanism.
   a. Electrical bar
   b. Magnetic bar
   c. Thermal bar
   d. None

10. _____ is a device used to provide lighting and visualization of the interior of a joint.
    a. Microscopy
    b. Endoscopy
    c. Colposcopy
    d. Microtomy

11. _____ is the diagnostic procedure used in the prevention of cervical cancer and involves the use of a magnifying device.
    a. Colposcopy
    b. Microscopy
    c. Endoscopy
    d. Microtomy

ANSWERS

1-b, 2-a, 3-c, 4-b, 5-a, 6-d, 7-a, 8-b, 9-c, 10-b, 11-a.

CHAPTER 15

Solution and Reagents

IMPORTANT DEFINITIONS

■ Solution

When a solute is dissolved in a solvent, then the mixture formed is called a solution. The solute is the substance which is dissolved and present in small quantity while solvent is the bulk substance in which solute is dissolved and present in large quantity.

■ Reagents

Reagents are chemical compounds or mixture of compounds usually solutions employed in chemical analysis or for detection of biological constituents.

■ Stock and Working solution

A stock solution is a concentrated solution from which different types of working solutions can be prepared by simple dilution.

■ Normal Solution

One normal solution is defined as 1 g equivalent of a substance in 1 liter of distilled water. These are solutions which are used as a reference standard solution for the preparation of fresh normal solution. For example 2/3 N H_2SO_4 or 0.3 N barium hydroxide are used for the preparation of protein-free filtrate.

■ Molar Solution

One molar solution is defined as 1 g molecular weight of a substance in one liter of solution. 1 M solution is prepared by dissolving amount of chemical equal to the molecular weight in 900 mL distilled water and make up the volume to 1 liter and store in clean and dry container.

PREPARATION OF STANDARD SOLUTIONS

■ Preparation of 1N HCl

It is prepared by using commercially available concentrated hydrochloric acid. Concentrated HCl is available in a liquid form. Add 87 mL of conc. HCl in about 900 mL of distilled water and make the final volume 1 liter by using volumetric flask. Standardize the normality of HCl by titrating with 1 N sodium carbonate.

■ Preparation of Standard Sodium Carbonate

1 N sodium carbonate is prepared by dissolving 53 g sodium carbonate in distilled water in a volumetric flask and making the final volume to 1 liter with distilled water. Standard sodium carbonate should be stored in a polyethylene container at room temperature. Table 15.1 gives values useful in preparation of normal and moral solutions.

■ Preparation of Percent Solution

Weight by Volume (W/V)

Dissolve for example 10 g of sodium tungstate in 90 mL distilled water and make up the volume to 100 mL by measuring cylinder to make 10% sodium tungstate and store is clean dry container.

Volume by Volume (V/V)

About 2% acetic acid is prepared by mixing 2 mL of acetic acid in 98 mL water and store in a clean and dry container.

Table 15.2 gives molecular weights and equivalent weights of important chemicals.

Buffer Solutions

A buffer solution is the one that resists change in pH on adding a small quantity of acid or alkali. Buffer solution are required to carry out a biochemical reaction at a particular pH. Buffer solutions are prepared by combination of:
- A weak acid and its salt with strong base.
- A weak base and its salt with strong acid.
- A acidic salt and a basic salt. Tables 15.3 and 15.4 shows some important buffers used.

Dilution of Stock Solution

If a series of working solutions are needed with varying strengths, then they should be prepared by dilution of the stock solution. For example: varying strengths of alcohols are needed in the processing of specimen for histological examination. Commercially available alcohol is 95%.

Preparation of 70% alcohol from 95% alcohol:
Rule: Dilute the stock with the solvent in the ratio of:
- Volume of stock solution equivalent to the strength of the diluted solution (70 mL) and
- Difference between the strengths of stock solution and dilute solution (95–70 = 25 mL).

Table 15.1: Values useful in the preparation of normal and molar solutions

Substance	Specific gravity	% by weight	App. normality	mL required for 1 N solution/Liter
Sulfuric acid	1.84	98	36.8	27.2
Nitric acid	1.42	70	15.8	63.3
Hydrochloric acid	1.18	36	11.65	85.8
Glacial acetic acid	1.05	99.5	17.4	57.5
Phosphoric acid	1.7	85	45.6	21.9
Ammonium hydroxide	0.90	58.6	15.1	66.5

Table 15.2: Molecular weight and equivalent weight of some chemicals

Substance	Formula	Molecular weight	Equivalent weight
Hydrochloric acid	HCl	36.50	36.500
Oxalic acid	$H_2C_2O_4$	90.00	45.00
Oxalic acid	$H_2C_2O_4.2H_2O$	126.05	63.025
Sulfuric acid	H_2SO_4	98.00	49.000
Sodium hydroxide	$NaOH$	40.00	40.000
Ammonium hydroxide	NH_4OH	35.04	35.040
Potassium hydroxide	KOH	56.00	56.00
Sodium carbonate	Na_2CO_3	106.00	53.00
Sodium bicarbonate	$NaHCO_3$	84.00	84.00
Sodium thiosulfate (anhydrous) hypo	$Na_2S_2O_3$	158.00	158.00
Sodium thiosulfate (hydrous) hypo	$Na_2S_2O_3.5H_2O$	248.20	248.20
Potassium dichromate	$K_2Cr_2O_7$	294.210	49.035
Copper sulfate (anhydrous)	$CuSO_4$	149.71	149.71
Copper sulfate (anhydrous)	$CuSO_4.5H_2O$	249.71	249.71
Silver nitrate	$AgNO_3$	169.87	169.87
Sodium chloride	$NaCl$	58.45	58.45
Disodium salt of EDTA	$Na_2H_2C_{10}H_{12}O_8N_2.2H_2O$	372.24	

Thus, by mixing 70 mL of 95% alcohol and 25 mL of water will yield a solution of 70% strength. This will give total volume of 95 mL of 70% alcohol. For getting 1000 mL 70% alcohol mix

25/95 × 1000 = 263.3 mL of distilled water with

75/95 × 1000 = 736.7 mL of 95% alcohol to give a total 1000 mL of 70% alcohol.

Table 15.3: Some important buffers

Sl. No.	Constituents of buffer	PH of buffer
1.	0.05 M HCl + 0.09 M KCl	2.07
2.	0.1 M Potassium tetraoxalate	1.48
3.	0.1 M Potassium dihydrogen citrate	3.72
4.	0.1 M Acetic acid + 0.1 M Sodium acetate	4.64
5.	0.01 M Acetic acid + 0.01 M Sodium acetate	4.7
6.	0.01 M KH_2PO_4 + 0.01 M Na_2HPO_4	6.85
7.	0.05 M Borax	9.18
8.	0.025 M $NaHCO_3$ + Na_2CO_3	10.0

Table 15.4: Buffer solutions covering a range of pH value

Sl. No.	Name of buffer	Range of pH
1.	Hydrochloric acid—Sodium citrate buffer	1.0–5.0
2.	Citric acid—Sodium citrate buffer	2.5–5.6
3.	Acetic acid—Sodium acetate buffer	3.7–5.6
4.	Disodium hydrogen orthophosphate Sodium dihydrogen orthophosphate	6.0–9.0
5.	Aqueous ammonia—Hydrochloric acid	8.2–10.2
6.	Sodium tetraborate—Sodium hydroxide	9.2–11.0

EXERCISE

1. Define the following terms: Solution, reagent, normal solution, molar solution, standard solution and buffer solution.
2. Describe the procedure for preparation of 70% alcohol from 95% alcohol.
3. What is buffer? Enlist important buffer solution.
4. How will you prepare 10% sodium tungstate and 2% acetic acid solution?

Bibliography

1. Baker FJ, Silverton RE. Introduction of medical laboratory technology. 5th edition. Butterworths, London; 1976.
2. Baker JR. Cytological techniques; John Wiley & Sons, Inc, New York; 1950.
3. Baker JR. Principle of biological technique Methuen. John Wiley London;1958.
4. Bancroff JD, Stevens A. Theory and practice of histological technique. Churchill, Livingston; 1982.
5. Bancroft JD, Stevens A. Theory and practice of histological techniques. 3rd edition. London: Churchill Livingstone; 1990.
6. Bansal S. New Illustrated Medical Dictionary; AITBS Publishers, Delhi.
7. Bharuch C, et. al. Handbook of medical laboratory technology. Christian Medical College, Vellore; 1970.
8. Bourne LD. Exfoliative cytology in: theory and practice of histological techniques.Churchill, Livingston; 1982.
9. Carleton HM, Leach EH. Histological techniques. Oxford University Press; 1947.
10. Chayen J, Bitensky L, Butcher RG, Paulter LW. A guideline to practical histochemistry. Philadelphia: JB Lippincott Co; 1969.
11. Clayden EC. Practical section cutting and staining. Edinburgh: Churchill Livingstone; 1967.
12. Conn HJ, Darrow MA, Emmel VM. Staining procedures. 2nd edition. Baltimore: Williams and Wilikins Co; 1960.
13. Conn HJ. Biological stains 2nd edition. Baltimore: Williams and Wilikins Co; 1969.
14. Cowdry EW. Laboratory techniques in biology and medicine. 3rd edition. Baltimore: Williams and Wilkins Co;1952.
15. Culling CEA. Handbook of histopathological and histochemical techniques. 3rd edition. London: Butter Worth; 1974.
16. David SK. Handbook of histological and histochemical techniques. CBS Publication and Distributors; 1991.
17. Disbrey BD, Rack JH. Histological laboratory methods. London: E & S Livingstone; 1970.
18. Drury RA, Wallington EA. Carleton's histological technique. 4th edition. London: Oxford University Press; 1967.
19. Glick D. Techniques of histo and cytochemistry. New York and London, J Nat Cancer Inst, 10, 321. Interscience, Publishers; 1949.
20. Godkar PB, Godkar DP. Textbook of medical laboratory technology. 2nd edition. Bhalani Publication House: Mumbai; 2004.
21. Gray PY. Handbook of basic microtechnique. 2nd edition. McGraw-Hill; 1958.
22. Gridley M F. Manual of histologic and special staining techniques. 2nd edition. The Blakiston Division, Mc Graw-Hill Book Co, New York; 1960.
23. Henry JB. Clinical diagnosis and management by laboratory medhods. Philadelphia: WB. Saunders Co; 1984.
24. Brown HS. Recent advanves in microwave decalcification protocols.
25. Lillie RD, Fullmer HM. Histopathologic technique and practical histochemistry. 4th edition. McGraw-Hill: New York; 1976.
26. Lillie RD. HJ Conn's Biological Stains. 8th edition. Baltimore, Williams and Wilkins Co; 1969.
27. Line JJ, Ringsrud KM. Basic technniques for the medical laboratory. 2nd edition. Mc Graw-Hill, New York;1979.
28. Linne JJ, Ringsrud KM. Basic techniques in clinical laboratory science. 3rd edition. Mosby Year Book: USA; 1992.

29. Luna LG. Manual of histological staining methods. 3rd edition. Mc Graw-Hill: New York; 1968.
30. Lynch MJ, Raphael SS, Spare PD. Medical laboratory technology & clinical pathology. 2nd edition. In Wood MJ 14 , Philadelphia: W B Saunders; 1969.
31. Lyon H. Theory and strategy in histochemistry. Birlin: Springer-Verlag; 1991.
32. Manual for cytology. National Cancer Control Programme; 2006.
33. Manual of basic techniques for a health laboratory.World Health Organization; 1980.
34. Manual of histologic and special staining techniques. 2nd edition. The Blakiston Division, McGraw-Hill, Book Co: New York; 1960.
35. Mayers CP. Histochemical fixation by microwave heating. J Clinical Pathology. 1970; 23:273-5.
36. Moore RJ. Histochemical localization of oesteoclasts in EDTA decalcification. J Histochemical Technology; 1990.
37. Mosby CV. Mosh's Medical, Nursing and Allied Health Dictionary. 6th edition. 2001.
38. Mudherjee KL. Medical laboratory technology: a procedure manual for routine Diagnostic test. Tata Mc Graw-Hill; 2000, Vol III.
39. Neiburgs HE. Cytological techniques for office and clinic; New York: Grybe abd Stratton Inc; 1956.
40. Ochei J, Kolhatkar A. Medical laboratory science: theory and practice. Tata McGraw-Hill.
41. Pantin CFA. Notes on microscopical technique for zoologists.Cambridge University Press; 1946.
42. Papanicolaou GN. Atlas of exfoliative cytology science. Cambridge Mass, Common Wealth Fund. 1960;95:732.
43. Pearse AGE. Histochemistry: theory and applied. 3rd edition. Churchill Livingstone. 1972; Vol II.
44. Pearse AGE. Histochemistry: theory and applied. 4th edition. London;Churchill Livingstone; 1980, Vol I.
45. Pulvertaft RJV. Museum technique: a review. J Clinical Pathology. 1950.
46. Ramzy. Clinical cytopathology and aspiration biopsy. 2nd edition. McGraw-Hill, Book Co: New York;1990.
47. Rogers A. Techniques of autoradiography. Elsevier, North Holland. 1979: pp. 429.
48. Sharma A. Abhinav's Medical Dictionary; R Lall Book Depot, Meerut.
49. Taber's cyclopedic medical dictionary; 18th edition: Jaypee Brothers Medical Publishers(P) Ltd.
50. Thompson SW. Selected histochemical and histopathological methods. CC Thomas:Spring Field; 1966.
51. Verdenius HHW, Alma L. A quantitative study of decalcification in histology. Clinical Pathology. 1958.
52. William H. Cell biology laboratory manual; Heidcamp, Biology Department, Gustavus Adolphus College, St.Peter, MN 56082.

Glossary

Abrasive	Which produces abrasion, i.e. wearing away of the material.
Absorption	Uptake of substances into or across tissues.
Acid-fast	Not readily decolorized by acid after staining.
Acute	Having severe symptoms and a short course.
Adipose	To fat.
Adjuvants	They are substances which are added to hasten or increase the action of the principal ingredient.
Adsorb	To attract and retain other material on the surface.
Aerosol	A colloidal system in which solid or liquid particles are suspended in gas.
Affinity	Force causing a substance to elect one substance rather than another with which to unit.
Aggregation	Clustering or coming together of the substances as clustering of the blood cells especially the platelets or RBCs
Amphoteric	Being able to react as both an acid and a base.
Anesthesia	Insensible condition.
Anaplasia	A change in the usual nature of a substance as by the adding of acetone. A change in the structure of cells and in their orientation to each other (malignancy).
Anatomical	Related to the structure of the organism.
Anoxia	Absence of oxygen.
Antibody	An immunoglobulin molecule that reacts with specific antigen that induces its synthesis.
Antigen	Any substance that is capable of inducing a specific immune response.
Argentaffin	Are cells that react with silver salt taking a brown or black stain.
Artefact	Any structure or feature produced by the technique used and not occuring naturally.
Autolysis	Self-dissolution or self-digestion that occurs in tissues or cells by enzymes in the cells themselves.
Auxochrome	Are ionizing group which increases the intensity of the color.
Axillary	Pertaining to the axilla
Bevel	Instrument for measuring angles.
Bilirubin	A yellow colored pigment derived from the substances present in hemoglobin, liberated from break down of RBCs.
Biopsy	Removal and examination of tissues from the living body.
Birefringent	Substance which split a ray of light and throw in different directions unequally.

Bone marrow	A soft organic substance filling the bone cavities.
Buffer	A substance of which the acidity or alkalinity is not changed upon addition of a small amount of acid or alkali.
Cancer	Any malignant or cellular tumor.
Carcinogen	Any substance which cause cancer.
Catalogue	Alphabetical list.
Celloidin	A concentrated preparation of pyroxylin.
Chromophore	A chemical present in a compound which gives a definite color to the compound.
Chylous	Pertaining to or of the nature of chyle.
Cilia	Minute hairlike processes that extend from the cell surface.
Clearing agent	Any substance which causes elimination.
Coagulant	Which causes coagulation of fluid.
Coagulation	The process of clotting of fluid.
Collagenous	Pertaining to collagen.
Colloidal	A homogenous solution in which the fine particles of a substance are dispersed in a solvent uniformly.
Conductivity	Capacity for conduction.
Contrast	Difference in radiography the difference between the densities of the part of the body radio graphed and of the radiographic film.
Cornified	Converted into horny tissue.
Corrosion	Wearing away slowly of a thing by a destructive agent.
Corrosive	Which causes corrosion.
Cortex	Outer layer.
Cristae	A crest of ridge.
Cryogen	Substance which produces low temperature.
Cryoprotectant	Substance capable of protecting from the effect of cold.
Curetting	Material removed from a cavity or a diseased surface with the help of a spoon shaped scraping instrument.
Cutaneous	Pertaining to the skin.
Cytology	Study of the formation, structure, function and pathology of cells.
Cytopathology	Study of cellular changes in disease.
Dealcoholization	Removal of alcohol from a substance.
Degenerate	A change from higher to lower form.
Dehydration	Removal of water from a substance.
Denaturation	A change in the usual nature of a substance by the addition of acetone or alcohol to make it unfit.
Deparaffinization	Removal of paraffin from the tissue.
Diagnosis	Determination of the nature of a cause of a disease.
Differentiation	Distinguishing of one thing from another.
Diffusion	The tendency of molecules of a substance to move from the region of high concentration to one of lower concentration.
Digenesis	Reproduction in which alternate generations are sexual.
Diploid	Having two sets of chromosomes.
Disease	Any deviation from or interruption of the normal structure or function of any body part, organ or system.

Glossary

Disinfectant	The chemical substance which prevents infections by killing bacteria.
Emanation	The act of coming out of anything from the body or emission or radiation.
Embedding	To place a tissue in a firm medium such as paraffin in order to keep it intact during section cutting.
Endoscopy	Inspection of the inside of the hollow organs or cavities of the body by using an endoscope.
Enzymes	These are biocatalyst produced by living cells, which increases the rate of chemical reaction without undergoing utilization and required in very small amount.
Equator	An imaginary line encircling a globular body, midway between its poles.
Excision	Removal by cutting.
Exfoliation	A falling off in scales or layers.
Exudate	Thin fluid escaped from the blood vessels and deposited in the tissues as a result of inflammation, containing protein, cellular debris and other solid materials.
Fibrillary	Pertaining or consisting of fibrils, small fibers or filaments.
Fibrocyte	A fibroblast, any cell producing fibers of the connective tissue.
Fibrosis	Formation of fibrous tissues.
Fission	Act of splitting.
Fluorescent	Emitting light or shining when exposed to other light rays.
Fungus	Vegetable cellular organisms living on organic matter marked by the absence of chlorophyll and the presence of the rigid cell wall, e.g. moulds, yeast, etc.
Gauze	A light, open meshed fabric of muslin or similar material.
Genotype	A group of individuals who resemble each other in genetic constitution.
Granulation	Division of a hard substance into small particles or small, rounded masses of tissue formed during healing of the wound.
Haploid	Having half the normal number of chromosomes found in the somatic (diploid) or body cells such as in the germ cells, ova, or spermatozoa.
Hereditary	Transmitted from one generation to another.
Histochemistry	Chemistry of cells and tissues.
Histology	Microscopic study of the minute structures of the tissues.
Hydrophilic	Water loving.
Hydrophobic	Water hating.
Hygroscopic	Absorbing moisture readily.
Hyperplasia	Abnormal increase in the number of normal cells.
Hypersensitivity	Excessive susceptibility or sensitivity.
Hypertonic solution	A solution having a greater osmotic pressure than that of the cells or body fluids, so it draws water out of the cells shrinking their cytoplasm.
Hysterectomy	Surgical removal of uterus.
Hypotonic solution	A solution having a less osmotic pressure than that of the cells or body fluids, so it causes water to enter the cells and thus inducing swelling and rupture of the cells.
Illumination	The lighting up of a part or an organ of the body or an object for inspection.
Image	An idea representing a real object or the picture of an object such as that produced by a lens or mirror.
Immersion	Dipping, to place a body under water or other fluid.
Impluse	The act of driving onward with sudden force or a sudden uncontrollable determination to act.
Impregnation	Saturation.
Incision	A cut or a wound made by cutting with a sharp instrument or with a knife.

Infiltration	The diffusion or accumulation in a tissue or cells of substances not normal to it.
Irritability	Abnormal sensitiveness to stimuli or capability or reacting to a stimulus.
Isotonic solution	A solution having same osmotic pressure as that of the cells or body fluids.
Kinetochore	Centromere.
Lesion	Any pathological or traumatic discontinuity of tissue.
Ligament	A band of strong fibrous connective tissue which connects the articular ends of the bones and forms the joint and serves to facilitate or limit the movement of the joint.
Lithotomy position	The position in which the patient lies on the back with the thighs flexed on the abdomen and the legs on the thighs and the thighs are abducted. It is employed usually in women in operation on genital organs.
Lobulation	Formation of vacuoles, the condition of being vacuolated.
Lubricant	Substance which makes surface smooth.
Lymph	A colorless, transparent, clear, alkaline fluid within the lymphatic vessels.
Magnification	The process of increasing an object in size, especially while seeing by the microscope.
Malignant	Becoming worse and ending in death.
Mammography	X-ray examination of the breast.
Mastectomy	Excision of the breast.
Matrix	The intracellular substance of a tissue as bone matrix.
Meiosis	A type of cell division of the germ cells wherein, over two successive cell divisions, each daughter nucleus receives half of the number of chromosomes present in somatic cells.
Melanin	A dark pigment giving color to the hairs, skins, choroid of eyes, etc. It is present in some tumors like melanoma.
Membrane	A thin, soft layer of the tissue that covers an organ or structure, lines, a tube or cavity, divides a space or organ or structure, or separates one part from another.
Metabolism	The sum of all the physical and chemical processes taking place within an organism. The process by which the food materials are transformed into the body tissues and energy for growth, repair and general functions of the body.
Metallic	Composed of metal or pertaining to the metal.
Microscopy	Examination with the microscope.
Microtome	An instrument for cutting thin sections of the tissues for microscopic study.
Microtomy	The cutting of thin sections.
Microwave	A wave between a wavelength of 1 mm and 30 cm.
Mitosis	It is multiplicative division or replica division as the two daughter cells produced resembles the parent cells.
Mordant	A substance that fixes a stain or dye like phenol.
Morphology	The science of the form and structure of organisms.
Mounting	Process of preparing slides of the specimens for the microscopic examination.
Mucin	A glycoprotein which is the chief constituent of mucus.
Museum	Building used for storing curiosities of art or science or nature.
Mycellium	The mass of thread-like processes (hyphae) constituting the thallus of the fungus such as that of the molds.
Necrosis	Reversible depression of the central nervous system produced by drugs.
Necropsy	Examination of body after death.
Neoplasia	The formation of a neoplasm.
Nomenclature	System of the technical or scientific names.

Organelle	A specialized structure of a cell which perform a definite function as mitochondria, etc.
Organization	The process of organizing or of becoming organized.
Orientation	Adjustment of oneself in an environment with regard to time and space.
Osmotic pressure	The pressure that develops when two solutions of different concentration are separated by a semipermeable membrane.
Osteoblast	A cell arising from mesoderm that is concerned with the bone formation.
Parasite	A plant or animal that lives upon or within another living organism called host from where it obtains some advantage.
Parfocal	Characteristic of a microscope which allows the rotation from one objective to another and only requiring a small, fine focus adjustment to be in focus.
Pathogenic	Producing a disease.
Phagocytosis	Ingestion and digestion of bacteria and foreign particles by phagocytic cells.
Pigments	Any coloring matter in the body.
Polarized light	The light rays in which its vibrations are parallel to each other in only one plane.
Polyclonal	Derived from different cells.
Polymerization	The process of forming a polymer.
Porosity	Condition of being porous.
Preservation	The act of preserving.
Proliferation	Reproduction and multiplication of similar forms, especially the cells.
Propel	To drive forward.
Protist	Any member of Protista kingdom
Putrefaction	Enzymatic decomposition of, especially of proteins, with the production of foul smelling compound.
Pyknosis	A thickness, especially degeneration of cell in which the nucleus shrinks in size and the chromatin condenses to a solid mass.
Radiation	Process by which energy is propagated through a space or matter or emission of rays or energy in all directions from a common center.
Radiolucent	Semi-transparency to radiant energy.
Reagent	A substance used to produce a chemical reaction to detect the presence of another substance.
Refract	The turn back or to cause to deviate.
Refractive power	The degree to which a transparent object deviates the rays of light from a straight path.
Reproduction	Process by which animals and plants produce offspring or creation of a similar structure or situation.
Resect	To cut out a part of an organ or a structure.
Resolution	The ability to distinguish two very small and closely-spaced objects as separate entities.
Restoration	To return to a previous state, as a return to health or replacement of a part to its normal position.
Sarcoidosis	A disease of unknown cause characterized by granulomatous lesions that may affect any organ or tissue of the body.
Secretory	Pertaining to or promoting secretion.
Sectioning	The cutting of very thin sections of tissues for examination under the microscope.
Septicemia	Blood poisoning or systemic disease associated with the presence and persistence of pathogenic microorganisms or their toxins in the blood.
Serrations	Process of formation of dents or teeth on a sharp margin.
Sexual reproduction	Reproduction by means of sexual or germ cells in which a male germ cell (spermatozoon) fuses with a female germ cell (ovum/egg).

Shrinkage	Contraction.
Solute	The substance dissolved in a solvent to form a solution.
Solution	A homogenous mixture of solid (solute) and liquid (solvent).
Solvent	Dissolving or forming a solution.
Spatial	Pertaining to space.
Spicule	A small, sharp needle-shaped structure.
Spillage	An overflow.
Spindle	A fusion—shaped or tapering at both ends.
Spirochetes	Microorganisms of the order *Spirochaetales*.
Sputum	Matter expelled from the mouth by coughing which comes from the lungs.
Stain	A dye or a pigment used in coloring tissues or cells to be identified or studied under the microscope.
Tampon	A pad or plug made of cotton, sponge or other material used to arrest hemorrhage or for the absorption of secretions.
Tendon	A cord of fibrous connective tissue continuous with the muscle and attaching it to a bone or other parts.
Tilt	Sloping position.
Tomography	Obtaining of X-ray picture by a special X-ray apparatus, of a tissue section or of particular depth of a tissue or of an organ.
Topography	Description of a part of the body.
Translucent	Semi-transparent.
Transmission	The transfer, as of a disease, from one person to another.
Transparent	Transmitting light rays so that things at the back of the substance are visible.
Traumatic	Caused by or pertaining to an injury.
Truncate	To amputate or to deprive of limbs or having the end cut off squarely.
Tuberculosis	The disease caused by *Mycobacterium tuberculosis*, which most commonly affects the lungs, but other body parts such as gastrointestinal tract, bones, joints, nervous system, skin, lymph nodes, etc. are also involved.
Tumor	Swelling or one of the cordinal signs of inflammation.
Ultrasonic	The science dealing with the study of inaudible sounds with frequencies of more than 20,000 cycles per second.
Ultrasound	Inaudible sound with the frequency of 20,000 to 100,000,000,00 cycles per second.
Utricaria	Hives, needle rash or a vascular reaction of the skin characterized by transient appearance of wheals attended by itching, caused by certain food, drugs, infection or emotional stress.
Vapor	Steam, gas or medical substance for inhalation.
Virtual image	The image produced by the imaginary focus of the rays.
Vital	Pertaining life or essential for life.
Wavelength	The distance from the top of one wave to the top of the next one.

Index

Page numbers followed by *f* refer to figure and *t* refer to table.

A

Abrasive
  powder 81
  stones 81
Absolute alcohol 106, 108, 147
Absolute ethyl alcohol 147
Acetic acid 45, 178
Acetone 58, 59
Acid
  alcohol 20
  concentration of 55
  fast bacteria 120, 126
  fast staining 120
  fuchsin 105
  phosphatase 126
    staining for 117
  thionin method 152
Acidic stains 102
Acidified ethanol solution 122
Acidified toluidine blue method 119
Acridine orange 105
  fluorescence method 153
Acrolein 46
Acrylic resins 74
Adhesive, types of 83
Adipocytes 8
Adipose 181
  connective tissue 9*f*
  tissue 8
Aerosol sprays 95
Affinity 101
Agar 68
Agar-ester wax double infiltration 74
Agar-paraffin wax double embedding 74
Agent
  chelating 54
  clearing 60, 182
  decalcifying 51, 53
  dehydrating 58

Agitation 55
Agranulocytes 12
Albumen 83, 84
Alcian blue 36, 105
Alcohol 58
  descending grades of 107
Alcoholic pinacyanide 124
Aldehydes 42
Alizarin red 105
Alkaline phosphatase 116, 125
Alpha-naphthol 117
Alternative embedding media 68
Alum hematoxylins 108
Alumina 81
Aluminium
  hematoxylin 108
  oxide 81
Ammonium hydroxide 177
Amphoteric 181
  stains 102
Amyl acetate 61
Amyloid 104, 124
Anabolism 5
Anaphase 3, 5
Anaphylactic 119
Anaplasia 181
Anesthesia 181
Anhydrous 177
Aniline blue 105
Anoxia 181
Antibody 172, 181
  primary 173
  secondary 173
Antigen 181
  retrieval 173
Apathy's medium 131
Aperture iris diaphragm 18
Aqueous ammonia 178
Aqueous media 68

Araldite embedding solution 74
Areolar connective tissue 8, 8*f*
Argentaffin 181
Artefact 47, 114, 181
Arthroscopy 170
Artificial exfoliation 135
  applications 135
Artists' grade pigments 36
Aspiration procedure 143
Auramine O 105
Autopsy 33, 34, 38
  clinical 34
Autoradiography 171
  method 171
  steps of 172*f*
Auxochrome 102, 181
Axolemma 14
Axon 14
Axoplasm 14
Ayre's spatula 139*f*
Azo Dye 102
  coupling method 116, 117
Azocarmine G 105

B

Bacteria 119, 126
Bacterial decomposition 40
Barr bodies 151
Basal cells 136
Basophils 12
Belgian stones
  blue 82
  yellow 82
Benzene 60
Benzidine method 117
Benzoquinone 46
Bevel 181
Biebrich scarlet 105
Bile pigments 115, 125

Bilirubin 181
Biogenic amines 47
Biopsy 32, 33, 48, 181
    core 33
    curettings 51
    excisional 34
    incisional 34
    open 34
    small 51
    stereotactic needle 33
    testicular 48
Birefringence 29
Bismarck brown 105
Block holders 85f
Block to block holder, mounting of 85
Blood 11
    analyze 38
    cells, types of 11f
    films 153
    vessels 119
Body tube 19
Bone 10, 51
    compact 11
    cross-section of 11f
    forming cells 11
    marrow 48, 96, 182
    spongy 11, 11f
Borrelia recurrentis 121
Bouin's solution 45
Brain 96
    fixation of 157
Breast 96
    cyst aspiration 142
    secretions 142
Bronchial brushings 142
Bronchial washings 142
Bronchoscopy 170
Broom like device 139
Buccal smear 152
Buffer solutions 177
    covering range 178t
Buffered neutral formalin 44

C

Calcite crystals 30
Calliphoridae 33
Cambridge rocking microtome 78f
Canada balsam 130
Canaliculi 11
Cancer 182
Candida 126
Carbohydrate 112, 125
    catabolism 6
Carbol fuchsin 120
Carbon dioxide gas 95
Carborandum 81
Carbowax 68, 147
Carcinogen 182
Carcinoma 136f
Cardiac muscle 13, 14f
Carnoy's fixative 147
Carnoy's fluid 45
    composition of 45

Cartilage 10
Catabolism 6
Catalogue 182
Cedar wood oil 61
Cell 1
    division 2
    during malignancy 135
    intermediate 137
    membrane 1
    metabolism 5
    of normal genital track 136f
    structure of 1, 1f
Celloidin 69, 72, 182
Cellosolve 59
Cells, superficial 137
Cellular abnormalities 136f
Cellular pathology 32
Cellulose 83, 84
    nitrate 68, 69
Centrosomes 2
Cerebrospinal fluid 38, 141
Cervex brush 139f
    device 139
Cervical material 140f
Cervical/vaginalsmear, collection of 139
Cervix 96
    visualization of 138
Champy's fluid 45
Chemical classification of dye 103t
Chemical hazards 161
Chemical oxidation 107
Chemical pathology 32
Chemical production 103
Chemical storage 161
Chemical waste disposal 161
Chiasma, singular 5
Chloroform 61, 63
Chrome deposits 114
Chromium
    oxide 81
    trioxide 57
Chromogen 102, 173
Chromophore 182
Chromyl chloride 46
Chylous 182
Cilia 182
Ciliated columnar cells 137
Ciliated epithelium 7, 7f
Citrate-citric acid buffer 54
Citric acid 178
Clove oil 61
Coagulant 182
Coating fixatives 147
Cold microtome 79
Cole's hematoxylin 108
    composition of 109
Collagenous 182
Colloidal 182
Colonoscopy 170
Colposcopy 170, 170f
    purpose of 170
Columnar cells 137
Columnar endometrial cells 137

Columnar epithelium 7, 7f
Common sense 160
Compound fixatives 42, 44
Condenser 18
    focus knob 19
Confocal microscope 29f
Confocal scanning optical microscopy 28
Connective tissue 8, 96, 104, 110, 125
Coplin jar 107f, 144
Coulombic attractions 100
Counter stains 109, 109t, 173
Covalent bonds 101
Coverslipping 173
Coverslips 133
Cresyl fast violet method 152
Crohn's disease 119
Cryoelectron microscopy, development of 27
Cryofixation 27
Cryogen selection 94
Cryoprotectants 94
Cryostat 79, 93, 97, 98f
    sections
        advantages of 98
        disadvantages of 98
        fixation of 98
        procedure 98
Cryo-tissue microarrays 174
Crystal violet 105
    stain 120
Cuboidal epithelium 6, 6f
Cutaneous lesions, multiple 119
Cystoscopy 170
Cytobrush 139, 139f
Cytochrome oxidase catalyses 117
Cytogenetic study 48
Cytokinesis 3, 5
Cytological changes 135
Cytological fixatives 42, 45
Cytological specimens 144
Cytological staining techniques 148
Cytology 136, 162
Cytopathology 135
    advances in 165
Cytoplasm 2
Cytoplasmic changes in cancer 136
Cytoplasmic fixatives 42, 45
Cytoplasmic inclusions 2
Cytoplasmic reticulum 2
Cytoplasmic stains 109

D

Dark field illumination, reflected 23
Decalcification 51, 163
    technique of 51
    treatment after 54
Decolorizer 120
Deconvolution microscopy 29
Dehydrating fluids 58
Dehydration 27, 58, 107, 110, 182
    completion of 59, 60f
    precaution during 59
Dehydrogenase 126
    demonstration of 118

Denaturation 182
Denatured alcohol 58, 146
Dendrites 14
Deparaffinization 110, 172, 182
Diacetyl 46
Diamond 81
    knives 80
Dichromate, fixatives containing 57
Diethyl pyrocarbonate 46
Diethylene dioxide 59
Dimethyl sulfoxide 69
Dimethyl-para-phenylenediamine 117
Dimmock embedding mould 70f
Dioxane 58, 59
Disinfectants 161
Disodium salt 177
Disposable blades 80
Disposable plastic pipette 140f
Distilled water 108, 147
Distrene 130
Draw tube 19
Dunn Thompson method 114
Dyes, types of 101

E

Ebner's fluid 53
Efferent neurons 14
Ehrlich's hematoxylins 108
    composition of 108
Elastic cartilage 10
    connective tissue 10f
Elastic connective tissue 9, 10f
Elastic fibers 125
Electric cryobath–isopentane 95
Electrolytic decalcifications 54
Electron microscope
    reflection 27
    types of 26
Electron microscopy 25
Elftmann's fluid, composition of 46
Embedding 67
    media 68, 69
    moulds 70f
Endocervical brush 139, 139f
Endocervix 137
Endogenous peroxide quenching 173
Endogenous pigments 114
Endometrial aspiration 140
Endometrial cells 137
    stromal 137
Endoplasmic reticulum 2
Endoscope 169f
Endoscopic biopsy 170
Endoscopy 169
    purpose of 170
    specimens 142
    types of 170
Enzymes 5, 47
    staining of 116
Eosin 37, 109
    azure 148
    procedure 123
    staining 123
        method 110
Eosinophils 12
Epithelial
    mucins 104
    tissues 6
Epithelium
    keratinized stratified 7
    simple 6
Epoxy resins 74
Equipment hazards 162
    electrical 162
    mechanical 162
Equipment required for section cutting 83
Erythrocytes 11
Erythrosin 37
Esophagus 142
Ester wax 68, 69
Ethanol 46, 58
Ether alcohol mixture 146
Ethoxyethanol 59
Ethyl alcohol 43, 58, 146, 147
Ethylene glycol monoethyl ether 59
Euparal 130
Evaporation rate 41
Exfoliate 135
Exfoliation, types of 135
Exfoliative cytology 135
Exogenous pigments 114
Eyepiece 19
    adjust 22
    tube 19

F

Farrant's medium 131
Fat catabolism 6
Femur 10
Ferric chloride solution 111
Fetal maturity 141
Fibro cartilage 10
Fibroblasts 8
Fibrocartilage connective tissue 10f
Fibrocyte 183
Fibrosis 183
Fibrous, white 9
Fick's law 57
Filter holder 18
Fine focus knob 19
Fine-needle aspiration 34
    cytology 142
        technique of 143f
Fire hazards 161
First aid action 163
Fission 183
Fixation before processing, completion of 57
Fixation, duration of 41, 48
Fixative
    concentration of 41
    functions of 40
    properties of 40
    simple 42
    special purpose 147
    types of 41
    volume of 48
Fleming's fluid 45
    composition of 45
Floating water bath 83
Flow cytometry study 48
Fluid
    abdominal 135
    amniotic 141
    transfer processor 65, 65f, 65t
Fluorescence microscope, components of 25f
Fluorescence microscopy 24
Fluorescent 183
    antibody technique 25, 26f
    protein, green 25
    staining 104
Fluorochrome 25
Fluorochroming 25f
Forensic autopsy 34
Formaldehyde 42, 46
Formalin pigment 114
    removal of 44
Formic acid 53
    solution 53
Freeze-etch 27
Freeze-fracture 27
Freezing, theory of 93
Frozen section 37, 48, 93
    advantages 93
    applications 93
    disadvantages 93
    mounting of 96
    staining of 123
    storage of 97
    technique 163
Frozen tissue, storage of 97
Fructose 20
Fungi 121, 183

G

Gastric washings 135
Gastroscopy 170
Gelatin 68, 83, 84
    embedding 72
Gendre's fluid 46
    composition of 46
Genital tract, normal 136
Germinal cells 136
Giemsa 105
Giemsa's stains 121, 144, 153
Glacial acetic acid 108, 147, 177
Glass knives 80
Glass slide 35
Glutaraldehyde 43, 46
Glycerin jelly 131
Glycerol 130, 131
Glycogen 2, 46
Glycol ethers 59
Gmelin's method 115
Golgi apparatus 2
Gram's iodine 120
Gram's stain 119
Gram-negative bacteria 120
Gram-positive bacteria 119, 120

Granules, secretion 2
Granulocytes 12
Grocott's silver methanamine method 123
Gut 96
Gynecological sample collection 138

H
Haemoglobin, staining of 114
Hage-Fontana silver 121
    method 121
Hand microtome 79
Hardening effect of fixative 48
Harri's hematoxylin 108, 126, 148
    composition of 108
Haversian canal 11
Haversian systems 11
Heart 96
    fixation of 157
Heidenhain susa fixative 44
Heidenhain's hematoxylin 109
Helly's fluid 44
Hematoxylin 105, 123, 108
    procedure 123
    solution 109, 110
    stains 107
    standard 110
Hemoglobin 125
Hemosiderin 115
    pigments 125
Histopathology 32
    advances in 165
    laboratory, safety in 160
Histotechnicians 38
Hollow viscera, fixation of 157
Honing 82
    technique of 82, 82f
Hormonal assessment, stains for 150
Hormone receptor assays 48
Hot plate 83
    method 89f
Humerus 10
Hyaline cartilage 10, 10f
Hydration 110
Hydrocarbon slurry 95
Hydrochloric acid 177, 178
Hydrogen bonding 101
Hydrophilic media 129
Hydrophilic mountants 130
    disadvantages of 129
Hydrophobic
    bonding 100
    media 69
    mountants 130
Hydrous 177
Hyperplasia 183
Hypersensitivity 183
Hypertonic solution 183
Hypotonic solution 183
Hysterectomy 183

I
Ice crystal artefact 98
Immersion oil 19
Immunofluorescence 25

Immunohistochemistry 172
    applications of 172
Impregnation oven 62, 62f
Impression smear preparations 37
Indigo-carmine 105
Infectious hazards 160
Infiltrating media 96
Inhibisol 61
Interstitial lamellae 11
Ion beam milling 27
Ion exchange resins 54
Iris diaphragm 18f
Iron hematoxylins 108
Isopentane 94
Isopropanol 146
Isopropyl alcohol 58, 59
Istochemical fixatives 42

J
Jars, staining 107f
Joint fluid 141

K
Kaiser's glycerin jelly 131
Kaiserling's fixative 157
Kaiserling's method 157
Kaiserling's solution 157
Karo corn syrup 131
Karyopyknotic index 151
Ketones 59
Kidney 96
Knife 80f
    adjustments 86
    back 80f
    edge 82
    handle 80, 80f
    sapphire 80
    sharpening 81, 82
    sharpner, automatic 168, 168f
    steel 80

L
Lactic acid orcein technique 152
Lacunae 11
Laparoscopy 170
Laryngoscopy 170
Larynx 142
Lead hematoxylins 108
Leishman stain 144
Leishmania 123
Lens 22
    systems 19
Lesion, immobilization of 143
Leuckhard embedding boxes 70
Leuko dyes, colorless 102
Leukocytes 11
Levulose syrup 131
Limb 20
    fixation of 157
Lip 96
Lipid 2, 46, 112, 125
    stains for 152
Liquid
    based preparations 35

    connective tissue 11
    nitrogen 94
Liver 96
    biopsies 48
Lubricants, types of 81
Lung 96
Lymph 12, 12f
Lymph node 48, 96
Lymphocytes 12
Lysochromes 103
Lysosome 2

M
Macrophages 8
Magnesium oxide 81
Masson-fontana ammonical silver
    reaction 115
Mast cell 8, 119
    demonstration of 119
    granules 104
Maturation index 151
Mayer's glycerol albumen 84
Mayer's hemalum 116, 126
Mayer's hematoxylin 108, 126
    composition of 108
Meiosis 3, 5, 184
    stages of 4f
Melanin 115, 184
    pigments 125
Membrane 30, 184
    filters 146
Mercuric chloride 43, 147
Mercuric oxide 108
Mercuric pigments 114
    removal of 45
Metabolism 184
Metachromatic staining 104
Metal boat mould 70f
Metallic impregnation 104
Metaphase 3, 5
Methacrylates 74
Methanol 58, 146
Methenamine silver nitrate method 121
Methyl
    alcohol 43
    benzoate 61
    green 106
    salicylate 61
    violet 124
Methylated spirit 58
Methylene blue 106, 126
    wet film technique 150
Microanatomical fixatives 42, 44
Microorganisms, staining of 119
Microphages 12
Microscope
    slides, cleaning of 20
    care of 20
    compound 21
    parts of 18, 20f
    bright field 21, 21f, 22
Microscopy 17
    advantages of dark field 23
    applications of phase contrast 24

basic terminology in 17
dark field 22, 23, 23f
types of 21
Microtome 77, 79, 86
base sledge 78, 78f
freezing 78, 95, 95f
knife 79
care of 81
profiles 79, 79f
types of 80
parts of rotary 77f
rocking 78
setting 84
sliding 78, 78f
vibrating 79
Microtomy 77, 163
Microwave
fixation 165
irradiation 165
tissue processing 166f, 167
Microwave-stimulated
processing 167t
tissue processing 166
Mineral acids, dilute 53
Mitochondria 2
Mitochondrion, structure of 2f
Mitosis 3
stages of 3f
Molar solution 176, 177t
Molybdenum hematoxylins 108
Monocytes 12
Mononuclear leukocytes 12
Mordant staining 104
Motor neurons 14
Moulds for embedding 70
Mount specimen 21
Mountant, types of 129
Mounting of block 85f
Mounting sections, methods of 131
Mounting, techniques of 132f
Mucin 2
Mucocele fluid 144
Muco-substances 46
Mucus
content 144
low 144
Multi-tumors tissue microarrays 174
Muscle 96
biopsies 48
Muscular tissues 12
Museum
safety in 159
techniques 156
basic 156
Mycobacterium 120
leprae 120
tuberculosis 120
Myelin 14
Myelinated fibers 14
Myofibrils 12

N

Nadi' reaction 117
Nasopharynx 142

Natural dyes 101
Natural exfoliation 135
Natural oxidation 107
Necropsy 34
Needle 143
biopsy 33
Nerve 119
biopsies 48
cell 14, 14f
Nervous tissues 13
Neurilemma 14
Neuroglia 13
Neuron 13, 14
afferent 14
types of 14
Neutral EDTA solution 54
Neutral stains 102
Neutrophils 12
Nipple discharge 142
Nitric acid 53, 177
solution 53
Nitro dyes 102
Nocardia 120
asteroids 120
brasiliensis 120
Non-ciliated endometrial cells 137
Non-corrosive knives for cryostats 80
Non-gynecological sample collection 140
Non-keratinized stratified epithelium 7
Non-myelinated fibers 14
Nuclear
changes in cancer 136
fixatives 42, 45
stains 109
Nucleic acid 5, 47
stains for 153
Nucleoplasm 2
Nucleoproteins 47
Nucleus 2
Numerical aperture 17
Numerous dehydrating agents 58

O

Oil red method 152
Omentum 96
Optical microscope 17
Oral lesions 142
Orange cells 141
Osmium tetroxide 43, 46
Osmolarity 41
Osseous tissue 10
Osteoblasts 11
Osteocytes 11
Oven, drying 83
Oxalic acid 177
Oxidases 126
staining for 117
Oxidizing agents 42
Oxitol 59

P

Pancreas 96
Papanicolaou method 148
Paper boat 70f

Parabasal cells 137
Paraffin blocks, storage of 71
Paraffin embedded tissues 172
Paraffin embedding 62
wax 69
Paraffin sections 106, 110
Paraffin wax 63t, 68
embedding 70
processing 163
removal of 106
Paraplast 68, 69
Parasites 122, 126, 153
Pathology museum, functions of 156
Penetrating lesion 143
Perani's fluid 53
Periodic acid
Schiff reaction 112
solution 112
Perl's prussian blue method 115
Peroxidase 117, 126, 173
pH value 178t
Phagocytosis 2
Phase contrast microscopy 24, 24f
Phosphate, fixatives containing 57
Phosphoric acid 177
Photosensitive resins 130
Picric acid 43, 126
fixatives containing 58
Pigments 2
particulate 36
staining of 114
Plasma cells 1, 8
Plastic embedding 73
cassettes 70
moulds 70
Plastic ice trays 70
Plastic spatulas 138
Plasticizer 130
Pneumocystis 123
carinii 123, 140
Polarization light microscopy 29
Polychrome methylene blue 123
Polyester wax 69
Polyethylene glycol 59, 147
Polyfin 70
Polymorphonuclear leukocytes 12
Polyvinyl alcohol 68, 131
Post-fixation procedures 57
Potassium
aluminium 108
dichromate 43, 177
hydroxide 177
Proctoscopy 170
Prometaphase 3
Propanol 146
Prophase 3, 5
Propylene glycol staining 112
Prostate 96
Prostatic secretion 135
Protein 46
catabolism 6
content 144
denaturing agents 42
Protozoa 122

Q

Quick papanicolaou staining technique 149
Quinonoid dyes 102

R

Radiations hazard 161
Reaction
    rate of 101
    temperature 55
Reagent 176
    accidents 163
    loss, rate of 101
Refract 18
Refraction, index of 19
Refrigerated contact 95
Rehydration 172
Resin 83, 84
    embedding 73
Resin-embedded tissue 130
Restaining 133
Reticular connective tissue 8, 9f
Reticulin 113, 125
Ribonucleic acids 6
Ribosomes 6
Ringing media 133
Romanowsky stains 150
Rose Bengal 37
Rossman's fluid 46
    composition of 46
Rotary microtome 77
Routine fixatives 146
Ruge's fluid 121, 122

S

Safranine 126
Sample collection, technique of 139
Sarcoidosis 119, 185
Sarcophagidae 33
Sarcoplasm 12
Scanning electron microscope 26, 27f
Schauddin's fixative 122, 147
Schwann cells 14
Secretory cells 137
Section adhesives 83
Section cutting, technique of 84
Seminal fluid 142
Sensory neuron 14
Septicemia 185
Serous effusions 141
Serrations 185
Sex chromatin, stains for 151
Sexual reproduction 185
Shorr staining technique 149
Silicon carbide 81
Silver nitrate 36, 177
    staining 113
Skin 96
    biopsy 34, 48
    with fat 96
Slide 83, 143
    labeling of 133f
Smear 147f, 151
    of cell samples, mounting of 154
    preparation of 37, 144, 145

Smooth muscle 12, 13f
Sodium
    acetate buffer 178
    bicarbonate 177
    carbonate 177
        preparation of 176
    carboxy methyl cellulose 68
    chloride 177
    citrate 141
        buffer 178
    hydroxide 177, 178
    salicylate 83
    silicate 84
    tetraborate 178
Solid organs, fixation of 157
Spatula 139
Specimen 144
    analyze 38
    collection 33
    containers 35
    fixation of 156
    fresh 37
    labeling of 35
    logging of 34
    mounting of 158f
    organization of 158
    preparation of 156, 157
    preservation of 157
    reception of 156
    restoration of 157
    thick 145
    with low pH 144
Spillage of reagents 161
Spirochetes 126
Spleen 96
Spray fixatives 147, 147f
Spreading, method of 145f
Sputum 135, 140
Squamocolumnar junction 136f
Squamous cells of ectocervix 136
Squamous epithelium 6, 6f
    functions 6
Squash preparations 37
Staff training 160
Stainer, automatic 169f
Staining 100, 110, 151
    automatic 149
    direct 104
    dish 106, 107f
    equipments 106
    method
        automatic 169
        special 110
    procedures 106, 163
    processes, types of 103
    racks 106
Stains 102
    basic 102
    precipitates 114
    special 150
    types of 101
Starch 83, 84
Stock methenamine silver nitrate
    solution 121

Stock solution 153
    dilution of 177
Stomach 142
Stratified epithelium 7
Stratified squamous epithelium 7, 7f
Streaking 145
    method of 145f
Streptavidin 173
Striated muscle fibers 12, 13f
Stropping 82, 83f
    technique of 83
Substances, colored 103
Substrate 173
Suitable impregnation medium 62
Sulfuric acid 177
Sulfurous acid solution 112
Sweet's stain 113
Synapse 14
Synthetic
    dyes 101
    resins 68
Syringe 143
    holder 143

T

Teased preparation 37
Teeth 52
Telophase 3, 5
Temporary mountant 131
Thermoelectric cooling 95
Thionine 123
Thoracoscopy 170
Thrombocytes 12
Thyroid 96
Tissue 1, 6, 32
    agitate 67
    areolar 8
    arrays, advantages of 174
    blocks, size of 63
    calcified 52
    chips 174
    components
        nature of 103t
        stain 100
    containers 66
    dense
        connective 9
        regular connective 9, 9f
    density 62
    embedding center 70, 70f
    examination of 37
    fixation of 40, 48, 96
    fixation, primary 165
    fixed 37
    fresh 162
    identification 35
    in block 71, 71f
    labeling of 57
    loose connective 8
    manually, clearing 67f
    marking 36
        substances 36
    microarray 173
        applications of 174

method 174f
prognosis 174
progression 174
synthesis 173
types of 174
mounting 96
orientation 36
processing 57
    automatic 64, 66
    manual 66
    schedules for 64t
    steps of 57
    ultrasonic-stimulated 167, 167t
proteins 129
sample 35
    special 48
selection of 51, 57
size of 48
storage of 48
supporting connective 10
transfer processor 64, 64f
with alcohol 59
Toluene 61
Toluidine blue 123
Toxoplasma 123
Transfer processor 64t
Transitional epithelium 7
    stretched 8f
    unstretched 8f
Transmission electron microscope 26, 26f
Transmitted dark field illumination 23
Trichloroacetic acid 53
Trichrome stain 122
Troubleshooting cryostat freezing procedure 97t
Tuberculosis 119
Tungsten
    carbide 80
    hematoxylins 108
Typanosoma 123

U

Ulcerative colitis 119
Ultramicrotome 79, 168, 168f
Ultrasonic decalcification 165, 165f
Urea, fixatives containing 58
Uric acid 48
Urine 38, 135, 140
Uterine
    cervix 136f
    curettings 96
Uterus 96
Utricaria pigmentosa 119

V

Vacuum impregnation 63
    oven 64f
Vacuum, creation of 143
Vaginal pool smear, collection of 140
Vaginal secretion 135
van der Waal's forces 100
van Gieson's stain 111
Vapor fixatives 46
Verhoeff's elastic fiber stain 111
Verhoeff's stain 111
Veronal acetate solution 117
Viscosity 41
    nitrocellulose, low 72
Vital staining 103

W

Water 107, 130
    bath method 89, 89f
    soluble
        media 68
        waxes 68
    tolerant media 69
Watery specimen 145
Wax dispenser 62
Weigert's hematoxylin 109
Weigert's iron
    hematoxylin 109
        composition of 109
Weigert-Van Gieson staining 110
Wooden Ayre's spatulas 138
Working solution 153, 176

X

Xylene 60, 130
    removal of 106

Z

Zamboni's fixative 98
Zenker's solution 44
Ziehl-Neelsen's stain 120